Learning from the Wounded

CIVIL WAR AMERICA

Gary W. Gallagher, Peter S. Carmichael,
Caroline E. Janney, and Aaron Sheehan-Dean, *editors*

Learning *from the* Wounded

The Civil War and the Rise of American Medical Science

SHAUNA DEVINE

The University of North Carolina Press *Chapel Hill*

© 2014 THE UNIVERSITY OF NORTH CAROLINA PRESS

All rights reserved. Designed by Sally Scruggs and set in Calluna by codeMantra. Manufactured in the United States of America. The paper in this book meets the guidelines for permanence and durability of the Committee on Production Guidelines for Book Longevity of the Council on Library Resources. The University of North Carolina Press has been a member of the Green Press Initiative since 2003.

Library of Congress Cataloging-in-Publication Data
Devine, Shauna, author.
Learning from the wounded : the Civil War and the rise of American medical science / Shauna Devine. — First edition.
p. ; cm. — (Civil War America)
Includes bibliographical references and index.
ISBN 978-1-4696-1155-6 (cloth : alk. paper) — ISBN 978-1-4696-1156-3 (ebook)
I. Title. II. Series: Civil War America (Series)
[DNLM: 1. History of Medicine—United States. 2. American Civil War—United States. 3. History, 19th Century—United States. WZ 70 AA1]
R151
610.973—dc23
2013035601

18 17 16 15 14   5 4 3 2 1

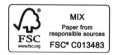

Contents

Tables and Illustrations

Acknowledgments

This study had its beginnings a few years ago while I was at McMaster University. This is where I was first introduced to the history of medicine, and I would like to thank David Wright, Ken Cruikshank, and Jim Alsop for their support of my early Civil War medical research. Jim has been a great mentor and friend and has served as an exemplary intellectual presence at every turn. His contribution to my development as a scholar extended well beyond my initial work on the health crisis in Andersonville Prison, and I am ever grateful for his support and friendship.

The research for this book had its origins while I was a graduate student at Western University, and I am grateful for the support I received while there. I would especially like to thank Margaret Kellow for her guidance and mentorship. To Neville Thompson, who served as an exemplary editor, replete with smart advice, I am greatly indebted. Throughout my years at Western, Neville has been a great friend, constant source of support, and wonderful lunch companion. I am truly thankful for his encouragement in the research and writing of this project.

I very gratefully acknowledge my mentor and friend Shelley McKellar. By providing expert guidance and incisive feedback throughout the development of this project, Shelley made this work much stronger. I will always be thankful for her insights, warm encouragement, and careful engagement with my work.

Very special thanks to Dale C. Smith. Dale read the book manuscript at various stages of production and offered invaluable feedback along the way. I am deeply indebted to him for his advice and constructive suggestions and thank him for giving me the benefit of his extensive knowledge of nineteenth-century medicine. I am also very happy we have become good friends along the way.

I am appreciative to the groups that have listened to my talks and indebted to the many people whose perceptive questions and comments I had not anticipated in my work. I particularly welcomed the opportunity to present parts of this work at Lakehead University, the University of Alabama at Birmingham as the Reynolds Lecturer, Georgia Health Sciences

University, North Carolina State University, Duke University, the University of Virginia, the London Historical Medical Association, the Army Medical Department and School, and the National Museum of Civil War Medicine. I have also presented parts of this work at the annual meetings of the Society for Civil War Historians, the Canadian Society for the History of Medicine, the Society for Military History, the Society for the Social History of Medicine, and the American Association for History of Medicine. Questions, discussions, and ideas from the members of these groups were extremely helpful in developing this book. In particular I would like to thank Mark Harrison, Geoff Hudson, Michael Flannery, Sanders Marble, Bill Rothstein, Todd Savitt, Michael Bliss, John Harley Warner, Eva Ahrén, Jeffrey Baker, Mindy Schwartz, and especially, Michael Sappol.

Research librarians and archivists played a key role in the making of this book. I would like to thank the staff at the National Archives and Records Administration in Washington, D.C., the Library of the College of Physicians in Philadelphia, the Library of Congress, the National Library of Medicine, the American Philosophical Society, and the National Museum of Health and Medicine. In particular, I would like to thank Brian Spatola, Kathleen Stocker, Gary Morgan, Tim Duskin, Charles Greifenstein, Sofie Sereda, Joan McKenzie, Stephen Greenberg, and most especially Michael Rhode, who spent many of his lunches in the archives so I could keep working.

I owe a special thank you to the entire team at University of North Carolina Press, especially Caitlin Bell-Butterfield, Ron Maner, Brian MacDonald, Mark Simpson-Vos, and David Perry. David's questions, advice, and feedback through the early revisions of this manuscript made the work much stronger. The press has offered advice and suggestions at various stages, and I am very appreciative for the many good insights and questions. I would also like to thank the two anonymous readers engaged by UNC Press for their careful reading of this work and their extraordinarily helpful suggestions. I am indebted to them for their time and professionalism.

Many thanks to my entire family for their support through this academic journey. I would especially like to thank L.B., Marilyn, and Stuart for the emotional support but also the diversions on *Union Jack*.

I most especially thank Gary, whom I can always count on. I truly appreciate his unwavering support of my work. I am lucky to have him in my corner and dedicate this book to him.

Learning from the Wounded

Medical Education and the American Civil War

*I had sawn all across the forehead and then swept the saw gradually towards the temple.
With the first full sweeps of the saw to and fro suddenly the patient loudly champed his
jaws at us several times: My assistant instantly dropped the head and leaped backwards
holding up both hands in horror and exclaimed "good god isn't he dead." My heart gave
one great convulsive leap then stood still then began to beat at race horse speed while I
was gasping for breath. . . . But a moment's reflection explained the matter. I had failed
completely to sever the fibers of the temporal muscles. . . . The body being absolutely
limp from the absence of any rigor mortus, the lower jaw at the middle of its movements
would drop only to snap vigorously against the upper jaw when the muscle was made
taught again. In a few moments we had sufficiently regained our self command to realize
that the man was surely already dead and to continue the post mortem, but it was with
unsteady hands and perturbed minds.[1]*

In popular conceptions of the American Civil War, such a story, told by
war physician W. W. Keen years after the conflict, seems to confirm
the impression of Civil War medicine. It has become commonplace to
associate this war with inexperienced physicians and surgeons hacking off
limbs with unsanitized medical equipment while patients clamped down
on bullets trying to suppress the pain. New estimates of the Civil War death
toll, and how those men died, seem to support this impression. As many as
750,000 soldiers died as a result of the war, a number that would be propor-
tional to 7.5 million people today.[2] More Americans, in fact, died during the
Civil War than in all other major wars combined,[3] and two-thirds of these
deaths were due to diseases like gangrene, pyemia, tetanus, diarrhea, and
dysentery, some of which followed from wounds suffered in the war and
others from unsanitary conditions.

The medical history of the war, captured in the letters, diaries, case histories, the medical and surgical specimens that were prepared, and the photographs of diseases and unique operations that were submitted to the new
Army Medical Museum confirms the impression of a medical profession

unprepared to deal with the demands of the war. Without being sentimental, it is fair to say that the doctors are the unsung heroes of the Civil War. The war was overwhelming in its scope, and physicians were forced to deal with diseases and injuries that differed both quantitatively and qualitatively from their usual practice patterns in civilian life. Civil War doctors practiced tirelessly in the new general hospitals or the temporary field hospitals; they treated the dying and wounded after horrific battles such as Antietam—where more than 23,000 men were either killed or wounded as a result of the one-day battle. From the beginning of the war, doctors managed the catastrophic wounds of battle, but an equally important objective of their practice was to arrive at new understandings of and ways of coping with the unfamiliar diseases that abounded in the camps and hospitals as the war raged well past the prophesied three months.

Many physicians realized early on that their limited knowledge of the body and disease was inadequate to care for the thousands of patients created by the war. But as the war went on and physicians gained experience performing surgeries or studying diseases, they also developed new ways to produce and record knowledge about the causes, treatment, management, and prevention of disease. These included dissection, microscopic analyses of organs and tissues to produce finer distinctions about disease, chemical investigation into disease processes, therapeutic trials, and medical experimentation. In the process, Civil War physicians, especially northern physicians, transformed American medical science. The Civil War created the context for the most significant medical experience of the nineteenth century in the United States and in the process set American medicine on a new course.

So who were the doctors who arrived to treat Union troops in 1861? A physician trained in America would have had some kind of formal education and have met at least a few basic standards. Though there were numerous medical schools and societies in the country, most schools offered generally weak curricula, and societies were unlicensed and unlike the professional organizations common today.[4] However, as Rosemary Stevens demonstrates, it was from this "apparently poor but potentially fertile ground that the future structure of medicine ... was to emerge."[5] When the Civil War erupted in 1861, there was an infrastructure in place that would support the improvements in American medical education and science that were just ahead.

Beginning in the early nineteenth century, proprietary medical schools emerged in the United States, supplementing the informal apprenticeship system that had previously dominated medical training. Individual physicians who wanted not only the distinction of being a medical school professor but also money from student tuition established these schools, which were not attached to a university or hospital but operated independently.

As more schools emerged, and competition among the proprietors intensified, it became common practice to reduce medical school requirements. Eventually, to gain entrance to a medical school, one only had to be able to pay the tuition fees. There were no standardized tests, and a college education, or even literacy, was not a requirement.[6] Most proprietary medical schools consisted of two four-month terms of lectures, with the second set of lectures identical to the first. The standard courses offered generally included anatomy, botany, chemistry, diseases of women and children, materia medica, obstetrics, physiology, principles and practices of medicine, and principles and practices of surgery. Faculties were small, usually five or six physicians who taught what they preferred rather than what was needed. Because very few of these schools were associated with or had access to hospitals, the chief method of teaching and learning was through the didactic lecture. In fact, as the historian Martin Kaufman has shown, it was possible to obtain a medical school degree in this period without ever having been in a hospital, delivered a baby, witnessed a surgery, or even examined a patient.[7]

Anatomy was the cornerstone of medical training in antebellum America, and as Michael Sappol has demonstrated, the best physicians in the country were proficient in anatomy. However, most American Protestants refused to see the dead body in medical terms. Thus, medical professionals and students always struggled with the lack of available bodies. Physicians and medical students were forced to snatch bodies from graves, a ghoulish undertaking that in the end did not produce enough bodies for the many American medical students. As early as 1831, some states began passing anatomy acts, which legally allowed medical schools to dissect unclaimed bodies. Most states, though, opposed the passage of these acts, leaving only two states with such legislation on the eve of the Civil War.[8] Thus, while most elite physicians had performed dissections or were familiar with the body, most of the rank and file were not.

By the 1830s and 1840s medical standards had been lowered further yet. In response to the attacks on elitism and the professions in Jacksonian America, most states had abandoned licensing laws and state recognition of medical societies, which meant that a medical degree was all that was required to practice medicine.[9] One historian has observed that "the United

States seemed to accept the market as the sole criterion of professional skill."[10] The absence of legal regulations for medicine not only lowered educational standards but also encouraged the proliferation of competing sects, including unorthodox practitioners such as homeopathists, eclectics, and Thompsonians.[11] Before the war, these sects were remarkably popular with the public and posed a serious professional and financial threat to the orthodox physician.

In the absence of a national framework to support better educational models, particularly for medical science, elite physicians increasingly looked abroad. It became a rite of passage for many elite physicians between 1830 and 1860 to study at the Paris Clinical School. What American students most wanted in Paris, as John Harley Warner has demonstrated, was access to bodies, patients, and hospital instruction from the leaders in French science and medicine. Students at the Paris Clinical School had the opportunity to actively examine thousands of patients in the large hospitals using stethoscopes and other medical equipment, and they learned to compare symptoms studied at the bedside with lesions observed postmortem. Thus while most American physicians still practiced "Hippocratic methods," which consisted of passive observation at the bedside, the Paris School took physicians further by making the autopsy essential for understanding diseases and symptoms. But because fewer than 1,000 American physicians made the trip overseas to learn the correlation of clinical symptoms with pathological anatomy, "the great majority of medical students in America had no systematic hospital teaching and little or no legal access to cadavers."[12]

Both the influence of the Paris Clinical School and the degraded educational standards at home led elite American physicians to begin pressuring for the reform and development of American medical education. Very slowly, the American Medical Association (AMA) coalesced into an organization that would help to develop and reform American medicine. At first, the AMA influenced the formation of local medical societies and medical journals, which did offer the possibility of professional affiliation for regular physicians.[13] There were also some improvements in the East Coast hospitals—particularly in Boston, New York, and Philadelphia—which facilitated ideas on the progress of medical science. This institutional support for medicine would become even more important during the Civil War for disseminating the new ideas, medical and surgical techniques, and results of experiments and investigations that came out of the Civil War hospitals.

During the war years, and in the great Civil War hospitals, Paris medicine became known or understood by the rank-and-file physicians and would provide a foundation for a social transformation in American medicine.[14] This story includes these physicians and their Civil War experience, but it is also a story of the elite and new elite in American medicine, who saw firsthand the limitations of the Paris Clinical School, prompting the development of new models of medical science that would characterize American medicine in the final third of the century. These new models, or rather the Civil War medical model, came to include the medical "experiment," specialization and more sophisticated concepts of infectious disease and disease management, and the national and international transmission of knowledge. The war, then, was more than a broad school of experience; it was also a conduit for the production, development, and dissemination of new medical ideas.

THE CIVIL WAR AND AMERICAN MEDICINE

The impact of war on medicine is widely debated, usually focusing on specific contributions of wartime research to medical science and practice (World War II and the development of penicillin is the most frequently cited example).[15] Although there is a historiographical and perhaps a philosophical debate concerning whether any "good" can come from war,[16] historians have less commonly considered the impact of war and medicine on physicians as members of a practicing community.[17] While American historians have been less comfortable dealing with the Civil War and American medicine, it has been long accepted that the Civil War had a profound impact on America's social, cultural, economic, and technological development. This book is a first step in reexamining the impact of the war on the American medical profession but also the increasing influence of science in the practice of medicine.

For almost 150 years, historians and physicians alike have wondered why American medical science did not "take off" in the 1840s and 1850s. Historians have looked at various educational opportunities, such as the Paris Clinical School,[18] the formation of the AMA, the expansion of medical schools,[19] and the response to epidemics.[20] Historians have cited specific examples of pioneering scientific developments in antebellum America, especially the clinical work of Austin Flint Sr.;[21] the similar contributions of Elisha Bartlett, William Pepper, and Alonzo Clark; the surgical work of Samuel Gross, Valentine Mott, Ephraim McDowell, and Daniel Brainerd;

William Gerhard's revolutionary distinction between typhus and typhoid fever;[22] and the increasing attempts to improve courses in physiology and microscopy in select American medical schools in the 1850s.[23] But while there were innovative or successful practitioners, they were too few in number to change the overall orientation of the medical community before the war. American medicine was still hampered by the lack of regulation on education and practice and the diversity of medical providers including the regulars or allopaths, homeopaths, botanics, hydropaths, naturalists, wise women, and even self-treaters.[24]

The efforts of the Parisian generation to instill an interest in pathological anatomy and the science of medicine as taught in Europe also largely failed to take root within the larger American medical community because most antebellum doctors were concerned with medical practice, not science. As one example, one of the most influential Parisian American disciples, W. W. Gerhard, had a telling experience with his 1836 lectures and book, *On the Diagnosis of Diseases of the Chest*. The first edition was a failure, but once he recast it as *Diagnosis, Pathology and Treatment of the Diseases of the Chest* in the 1850s, it was a success. The key change was in the 1852 introduction by Morrill Wyman of the techniques of thoracentesis (draining fluid from the chest). Wyman's account gave accurate diagnosis a therapeutic importance.[25] In other words, it was science with a direct benefit to medical practice to which most physicians could then relate. However, there were too few of these therapeutic examples, and thus the primary concern for most antebellum physicians was to develop and keep a practice. Thus, despite all the efforts of historians, there is no evidence of any major change in the nature of the profession on a national basis by 1860.[26] Most studies of the period overwhelmingly associate the rise of American medical science with the laboratories and universities in Germany,[27] to such a degree that the Civil War's larger impact on American medicine has yet to be fully explored.[28]

The most striking feature of the literature relating to nineteenth-century medicine is not how the war is framed but rather that the role of Civil War medicine in the larger development of American medicine lacks almost any analysis.[29] Until recently, it was assumed that the war was a medical disaster.[30] That the quality of American medical care was poor during the Civil War is actually a tradition that goes back to the late nineteenth century, when American doctors were busy convincing patients that conditions were now much better than they had been just a generation before. Also, because the study of the Civil War has developed as a specialty area within the history of medicine,[31] most studies on scientific development in the nineteenth century neglect to tackle the war directly despite the fact that most elite physicians at the time were connected in one way or another to Civil War medicine.

This volume builds on a rich literature, as numerous aspects of the war have been well documented, including the development of American hospitals,[32] the development of nursing and the role of women and gender during the war,[33] the health of the black soldier,[34] Civil War pharmacy,[35] the institutional history of the war,[36] the war's effect on public health,[37] perceptions of death as a result of the war,[38] and surgery and disability.[39] But few studies have examined science in the practice of medicine within the broader context of American medicine in the nineteenth century.[40]

During the last quarter of the nineteenth century, the social regulation of American medicine came back, and the modern medical profession emerged as a social force in the United States, which historians have been studying ever since. The regular profession emerged as the dominant force. Physicians had won the prewar sectarian competition to a degree that they could not have anticipated in 1860. There is no question that the practical value of antiseptic surgery and the role of bacteriology in public health and asepsis supported the last push to professional prestige in the 1890s and early twentieth century. But most of the postwar generation of American medical students and physicians who went to study in the German laboratories and universities did not reach professional maturity until the mid- to late 1880s. In fact, the crucial social changes in American medicine predated the influence of these physicians. Just after the war, there was a "reconstruction of medical school curricula . . . and a more vigorous defense of the value of physiology training for the future practitioner."[41] The emphasis on physiology in the early postbellum period represents the changing ideas about how to study disease processes and the body that developed with the Civil War. Through the 1860s there were also pressures to replace the didactic lecture with actual laboratory work.[42]

In 1867, beginning with Pennsylvania, state after state began passing anatomy acts, making unclaimed bodies available to medical schools for teaching and research. By 1881, fourteen more Union states had passed anatomy acts along with one former Confederate state (Arkansas). There were still reports of body snatching throughout the 1870s (medical knowledge moved faster than legislation), but with the increasing medical authority of practitioners and the new prominence of medical science, states continued to strengthen old anatomy acts or create new ones. The Civil

War demonstrated that with access to bodies, and thus a deeper understanding of the body, there were new possibilities for medicine. By 1890 most northern states had passed anatomy acts, and by 1913 every state in the United States except North Carolina, Alabama, and Louisiana had done so.[43] "Anatomical dissection, so fiercely contested for much of the eighteenth and nineteenth centuries, was made invisible, regularized. And so it remains today."[44]

What accounts for this apparent transformation in American medicine—and in such a comparatively short time? The United States (Union) Army Medical Department was the preserve of the regular profession, and despite the efforts of homeopathic professional organizations and individual providers to break into the community during the emergency, Civil War medicine was essentially regular medicine. Senator Henry Wilson of Massachusetts suggested early in the war that "if it were desirable to bring in medical men of the new school, as we have been asked to do this year by a number of petitioners . . . the difficulty would be in having these diverse systems of practice in the Army. It would lead to great confusion. I think it better to have it all one or all the other."[45]

Thus, while homeopathists and other sectarians fought to maintain the equal or even superior status they had achieved in relation to the orthodoxy before the war, they were effectively excluded from medical positions that were sanctioned by the government and the Army Medical Department.[46] As A. M. Woodman of New York pointed out, "there is so much animosity existing between the two schools in this city, physicians with homeopathic diplomas have been refused for examination from the board in this city."[47] Woodman went on to note that he would be willing to "practice the other school" or "work with a colored regiment if accepted into the service,"[48] but the regulars were adamant about maintaining the corps' exclusivity. The social and political power that resulted from this service in the postwar period by the regular profession should not be underestimated—"it was not so much that the physicians were obviously effective as it was that they were there and their competitors were not."[49] The public's conception of the orthodox physician was reshaped with the war.

The doctors in the units and the hospitals were removed from the stresses of practice in the competitive civilian environment (that is not without importance),[50] but the physicians functioned in a hierarchical system that exposed them to European-inspired science. In 1861 most people recognized that the military was not ready for war; not only did recruits get sick in camps, but surgeons saw wounds of such destructive nature that they had no frame of reference for the care and treatment of the patients. In response, Surgeon General William Hammond was appointed, and as part of his effort to improve the care of soldiers, he immediately began restructuring Union—and American—medicine.

This volume follows the medical experiences of American physicians who served in the Union Medical Department—volunteer and regular physicians, elite and rank and file—through the Civil War to investigate how the experience affected the way individuals practiced and studied medicine. As the story unfolds, the complex questions that led to the shift in emphasis from pathological anatomy, experimental physiology, chemistry, microscopy, and medical specialization will be revealed. Rather than a survey of Civil War medicine, this is the story of how medicine and understandings of disease were structured, investigated (both formally and informally), and taught and learned during the war, and how this medical knowledge was disseminated in the later nineteenth century.

Finally, the boundaries of this book should be mentioned. The Civil War as a stimulus to American scientific medicine is largely a northern story, and thus the South is not considered in the present volume. Confederate surgeon general Samuel Preston Moore, like William Hammond, saw the opportunity presented by the war for reforming medicine. After all, before the war many southern physicians had traveled abroad to study medicine or studied in the leading centers in the North including Boston, Philadelphia, and New York. During the war, a few southern physicians, including Joseph Jones, Francis Peyre Porcher, Samuel Stout, and Richard Bolton, were given both opportunity and encouragement from headquarters to conduct small research projects with the hopes that the findings would benefit not only the soldiers but also southern medicine.

The Confederate Medical Department, however, was shaped by its lack of resources and faced tremendous shortages in medicines and food, hospital beds, blankets, and personnel throughout the war. While the North expelled competing sects, the southern physicians served alongside slaves, eclectics, homeopathists, and wise women. Even if physicians wanted to research or perform medical experiments, there was little opportunity—physicians struggled most of the time trying to offer comfort and proper treatment. The central goal, then, was to provide immediate care to the troops in order to preserve manpower. The many (and continual) shortages in the South meant that no large-scale research projects were formed. There was no equivalent to Circular No. 2 or the Army Medical Museum to foster medical developments on a larger scale. Southern physician Joseph

Jones eagerly visited the Army Medical Museum in the postwar period and perhaps summed it up best when he commented on the "magnificent operations" performed by the Union surgeons, noting that they were "in striking contrast to our cramped and imperfect labors."[51]

Chapter 1 introduces the various effects of Surgeon General William Hammond's Circular No. 2, particularly the directive to collect and dissect bodies and specimens, which created a framework for a kind of research society among the physicians in the war. The development of clinicopathological investigation, networks of knowledge, and the production and transmission of this knowledge during the war are also described. Chapter 2 discusses the development of pathological anatomy and its parameters. As the limitations of localized pathology alone were realized, some physicians began to think differently about disease and searched for new ways to understand, study, and document wartime diseases and disease processes. In a medical culture that had been largely indifferent to research, some physicians now found in the war a supportive community in which to develop new methods; they were encouraged to learn and pursue investigative medicine and benefited from both institutional and organizational support.

Chapter 3 turns to the state of medical knowledge in the second half of the nineteenth century and the dynamism of the war years in relation to theories of disease and investigative medicine. Physicians learned from the Civil War body and, in the process, produced a new set of guidelines for medical knowledge. This chapter explores how the initiatives to develop investigative medicine through the study of gangrene and erysipelas created a model for the integration of laboratory results and clinical observation. Chapter 4 analyzes how the wartime medical model supported the development of specialty study and how unfamiliar diseases and medical challenges fostered an environment that encouraged, even demanded, specialization, as well as the role of the Civil War hospital and the Army Medical Museum in supporting the development of specialized knowledge, giving these new modes of practice legitimacy.

Chapter 5 takes a closer look at Civil War bodies and frames this examination of bodies within the evolving ideas about death during the war. A particular focus is the military's assumed ownership of Civil War bodies and the various ways in which knowledge was supported and contested. Chapter 6 demonstrates that the medical model developed during the war led to a pattern of recording events, experiences, challenges, research ideas, and problems, and to the transmission of this knowledge. The focus is on the military's response to the 1866, 1867, and 1873 cholera outbreaks, particularly how wartime practices, principles, and patterns were adapted in the postwar period. These new methodologies became institutionalized and found further support for their development.

Chapter 7 explores how some medical professionals formed a powerful identity through their wartime work and found themselves arbiters of scientific knowledge. War physicians were part of a shared experience that included the collection and study of specimens, mandatory case reports, publications based on their wartime experiments, and newfound knowledge, reflecting a deeper understanding of anatomy, physiology, biology, disease, and the human body.

Many physicians came into the war without the underpinnings of a proper education or practical experience in managing hospital diseases and wound trauma. There was no appreciation of a science-based practice, which naturally evolved in the Civil War hospitals. To manage septic infections in the Civil War hospitals, physicians were ordered to use disinfectants—locally on the wound but also in the environment. In the process, cases of hospital infections were drastically reduced, results that promoted numerous debates about whether agents such as bromine reacted with tissues or blood or rather worked by killing an external agent. Physicians developed new ideas as the war progressed, and the thinking of many American physicians coalesced around a new understanding of American medical science. They saw that if they got it right—diagnosing, treatment, prevention, or management—it could make a difference in medical care. In the process, American physicians caught up to their European counterparts. The Civil War prompted major developments in the life and work of northern physicians who doctored in the war and in the process transformed American medicine and medical research.

A NOTE ABOUT SOURCES

Before embarking on my first research trip to the National Museum of Health and Medicine (NMHM) and the National Archives, I read through the six-volume *Medical and Surgical History of the War of the Rebellion*. My first impression concerned the great scope of Civil War medicine. The editors included every imaginable subject in their account, including diseases, wounds, surgeries, autopsies, hospital construction, and therapeutics. I looked closer at some of the autopsy reports. They were generally very short, just a few descriptive lines of the procedure. At first, then, I was impressed with the high number of autopsies recorded in the war but not with the detail of the autopsies. When I got to the NMHM, I pulled a series of "specimen histories." These were case histories that accompanied medical and surgical specimens and the results of autopsies. I was at first surprised at how long, detailed, and analytical many of the case reports were. The physicians posed questions throughout, pondered what they did not understand, and hypothesized on the nature of diseases and wounds that they were managing. But the overarching message in these reports was the drive to understand disease processes; there were debates about germ theories, preventatives, and the best way to investigate disease. I realized I was looking at the long version (sometimes ten or more pages) of the few lines that had been synthesized and published in the *Medical and Surgical History*. It was almost like reading about a different war. The same pattern followed with the manuscript sources at the National Archives and Records Administration, the College of Physicians, the American Philosophical Society, and other institutions.

The editors of the *Medical and Surgical History* wanted to tell the story of the Civil War, and the result was a large encyclopedia of Civil War medicine; however, in the process they edited away the rigorous epistemological dynamism that distinguished Civil War medicine. Numerous case histories are included in the six-volume series, but they are short, heavily pared down, and largely a description of medical and surgical cases. This realization shaped my research, and while the published sources remain critical, this book has largely relied on the unpublished case histories, narratives of service, personal papers, memoirs, and correspondence, which reveal the doctors' attempts to better understand wartime medicine, but also the strides made in producing knowledge and managing medicine itself. Physicians were challenged every day by what they saw, and they questioned, agonized over, and shared this knowledge. They used and explored medical science and were desperate to learn from the medical challenges presented by the war and from each other. Throughout this work, specific case histories, physician experiences, and medical challenges are often quoted to bring to life the dynamism of the war and to provide the reader with a fuller understanding of both Civil War doctors and war medicine.

CHAPTER ONE

Circular No. 2 and the Army Medical Museum

The Union Medical Department was ill-prepared when the Confederate batteries fired on Fort Sumter, April 12, 1861. The department initially had a tremendously difficult time organizing both the volunteer and regular physicians and was inept at managing the new hospitals and training camps. Endemic and epidemic diseases were a part of life in antebellum America, and Americans were used to living with illness to some extent.[1] However, the war brought thousands of men together from all parts of the North, who were then housed in new training camps. Within these camps, overcrowding, exposure, unsanitary sewage disposal, and a lack of resistance to infectious diseases among the soldier population created ideal conditions for diseases to thrive—and they did. Diarrhea, dysentery, measles, typhoid fever, and pneumonia abounded, killing many new recruits before they even reached the battlefield.[2] The first major challenge, then, was finding a way to both understand and control the considerable amount of illness.

During the first year of the conflict, ranking medical officers routinely noted how difficult it was to organize and instill authority among many of the medical practitioners. Soldiers were dying, and it was argued that the laissez-faire medical culture among some physicians was contributing to the high rates of mortality and morbidity.[3] In his narrative of service, J. T. Calhoun noted that the records of the medical department of many of the regiments were "so imperfect as to be absolutely unworthy . . . it was rare for any of us to keep a proper set of books."[4] The medical department was pitifully small in 1860 and inadequate to deal with the medical challenges of the war.[5] The head of the Army Medical Department, Thomas Lawson, was over eighty years of age and was generally opposed to spending money on scientific advances. He died shortly after the outbreak of the war and was succeeded by the very conservative Dr. Clement Finley, the next in line in seniority of service, who was, according to one observer, "utterly ossified and useless."[6]

Finley was hugely unpopular and, like Lawson, opposed any type of scientific advance within the medical department.[7] More problematically, he refused to support the use of civilian organizations or women in the hospitals and was regularly accused of hindering the progress of the medical department.[8] Frederick Law Olmsted lamented: "I believe men are dying daily for the want of a tolerable Surgeon General."[9] These deaths were vividly reported in newspapers and magazines. Americans had only a few years earlier read about the similar disastrous medical care of British soldiers during the Crimean War in American newspapers, medical journals, and pamphlets and were well aware of the importance of effective medical care, sanitation, proper diet, and medical treatment. To help manage the medical problem, a group of civilians formed the United States Sanitary Commission.

The commission determined early on that its objective was to "prevent the evils that England and France could only investigate and deplore. This war ought to be waged in a spirit of the highest intelligence, humanity and tenderness, for the health and comfort, and safety of our brave troops."[10] The commission proposed several reforms, including comprehensive medical exams for recruits, the use of women as nurses in the army hospitals, and the hiring of medical cadets.[11] Perhaps most significantly, the Sanitary Commission pressured Secretary of War Edwin Stanton to remove Surgeon General Finley and replace him with someone who would energize the medical department.[12] The Thirty-Seventh Congress was debating Bill No. 188 (the Wilson Bill), which proposed to "increase the efficiency of the medical department of the Army," the objective being to get "the right men wherever they may be found, whether in the Army or the volunteer force to take these positions."[13] It was argued that "Army surgeons, having their places for life, had less inducement to improvement, and they have had fewer opportunities to improve, than surgeons in civil life . . . therefore if you want good officers enlarge your circle."[14] After some debate, Congress decided that all physicians would be appointed on merit rather than on the seniority system, which opened the door for the appointment of William Alexander Hammond.[15]

Hammond had spent the first few months of the war organizing military hospitals in the Northeast, where his organizational ability, openness to innovation, and scientific talents caught the attention of the Sanitary Commission. He was also one of the few military doctors who understood the important medical contribution that the Sanitary Commission could make. This was partly because he was sympathetic to both military and civilian medical needs. He had entered the Army Medical Service as an assistant surgeon in 1849 and served in various posts over the next ten years; he resigned from the army in 1860 to take the chair of anatomy and physiology at the University of Maryland, Baltimore. When the war broke out in April 1861, he helped treat members of the 6th Massachusetts after they were attacked by a mob of Confederate sympathizers while passing through Baltimore. He immediately resigned his professorship and rejoined the army.[16]

Hammond was considered a particularly good candidate because of his long-standing interest in medical and scientific investigation.[17] Before the war, he had regularly conducted laboratory experiments, written numerous essays and articles on physiology (one winning a prize), routinely collected specimens for his peers at the Philadelphia Academy of Science and the Smithsonian Institution, and observed European army hospitals in 1858.[18] As physician W. Welch noted in his letter of support, "Assistant surgeon Hammond is eminently qualified for the post. . . . I have no personal or other interest in him beyond the knowledge that he possesses such a rare assortment of good qualities as would enable him to relieve you of much care and do important service to the army if he is appointed."[19] Indeed, Hammond had a forceful personality and was known for getting things done. All this well fitted the objectives of the commission, whose express purpose was to "avoid delay and circumlocution for the purpose of accomplishing efficiency and directness of action."[20] With the support of the U.S. Sanitary Commission, Hammond was officially appointed surgeon general of the U.S. Army on April 28, 1862, and he became the central architect of reform for the Union Medical Department.[21] The appointment was eloquent testimony to the developing support for scientific medicine within the medical department.

WILLIAM HAMMOND AND THE DEVELOPMENT OF UNION MEDICINE

Hammond's energetic approach to wartime medicine included the formal restructuring of the medical department; the development of a national military hospital system; the creation of chemical laboratories; improved record keeping; the hiring of female nurses, storekeepers, washwomen, and medical cadets to meet the demands of war; and the introduction of specialty hospitals. As the physician Silas Weir Mitchell observed, "Whatever else may be thought or said of Hammond, nothing is more sure to me than that he duly saw and used a great opportunity; that he served his country as few could ever have done; that he created the Army Medical Museum; that he saw the need for and advised the foundation of the Army Medical School; that he pointed out the men who were to direct the Army Medical Museum and the medical library." Mitchell concluded, "Until the end of his army career, [Hammond] was the unfailing friend of scientific study," even creating "special hospitals for diseases of the heart, lungs and neural maladies."[22]

Before the war, American medical reformers were faced with a clear difficulty: the lack of government support for the medical profession. Each state had its own ideas about how to legislate, license, and train physicians— and many states, as described earlier, had abandoned licensing regulations altogether. By 1860 there was a decline in professional morale among the elite about both the state and direction of medicine. Elite physicians knew they had to lead the charge for reform—but how? What conditions would allow for a social transformation in American medicine? Hammond saw government support for wartime medicine as a unique way to initiate the reform of American medicine and to establish common standards for American physicians. He thus sought to foster an environment that would support the improvement of knowledge and practice. He did this first by formally organizing military medicine along more scientific guidelines. The development and enforcement of the wartime medical reforms enabled the Office of the Surgeon General to transcend many of the limitations in medicine that had plagued American physicians before the war.[23] Furthermore, institutions that could cultivate the development of American medicine were for the first time supported by the government.[24] And these new ideals and support excited some of the American physicians, who similarly viewed the diseases and bodies produced by the war as an unprecedented opportunity to learn valuable lessons that would benefit medicine as a whole.[25]

Hammond was incredibly ambitious, smart, and, above all, fearless in taking on the military establishment. After all, for a generation the Army Medical Department had refused to support any radical departure from the accepted and accustomed mode of operation. Hammond, by contrast, almost immediately saw the benefit of not only marshaling all of the medical talent in the Civil War North but also practically training American physicians. He decided, as part of his early reforms, that all physicians were to be scrutinized in a manner they had not been before. They were subject to strict medical examining boards, which were staffed by elite physicians who valued science as the foundation of the profession. In order to ensure that professional standards were enforced within the Army Medical Department, Hammond explicitly, and controversially, ordered examiners to exclude from practice those deemed unacceptable because of poor medical qualifications.

On July 2, 1862, Congress enacted "an act to provide for additional medical officers of the volunteer Service," authorizing medical boards to examine candidates before the appointment of surgeons and assistant surgeons.[26] Physicians looking for regular army commissions or seeking promotion were also required to sit for a multipart examination, which consisted of a written examination on the basic principles of anatomy, surgery, and the practice of medicine; an oral examination on anatomy, surgery, and the practice of medicine and pathology; another oral examination on chemistry, physiology, hygiene, toxicology, and materia medica; a clinical, medical, and surgical examination at a hospital; an examination on a cadaver; the performance of a surgical operation; and an essay.[27] The board was permitted to deviate from this general plan when appropriate (usually if a well-known physician applied) "in such manner as it is deemed best to secure the interests of the service."[28] Candidates failing one examination were permitted a second examination after two years, but never a third.[29]

If candidates were successful, they were appointed by the secretary of war as surgeons or assistant surgeons (as determined by the examining board). Hammond's insistence that candidates "who passed the best examinations" should be given precedence according to their examination results as reported by the examining boards proved to be a point of contention between the volunteers and the regulars.[30] As John Brown recalled when Hammond was finally ejected from the service, "Hammond has been the Lucifer who had endeavored to promote discord."[31] Brown was referring to what he perceived as the "interference of the volunteers" in assuming prestigious hospital posts, but Hammond did not mind making enemies. He wanted scientifically minded physicians who would best support his efforts, regardless of seniority of service.[32]

As revealed by the letters they wrote to the Surgeon General's Office, numerous physicians agonized over the results of their exams.[33] Those physicians who failed often provided excuses and asked to be retested; others who had not received their results wrote repeatedly to inquire why; and still others asked for a second chance on their exams.[34] Joseph Woodward, a prominent physician, had his examination delayed and wrote to his wife saying how anxious he was to have his exam completed as he nervously waited in his hotel room.[35] The physician R. Weir too recalled that "as soon as I appreciated that the military contest would last longer than the three months prophesied at the beginning . . . I went up for the required examination. . . . I was lucky enough to pass and came out fifth in the long list, thinking perhaps I might have done better had I had time . . . to read up for the trial."[36] John Shaw Billings similarly remembered, "I came before the Board, and at about noon by the second day I began to feel rather comfortable and thought I was getting on very well; but by noon on the third day there was a consultation between examiners, and they began all over again, going back to anatomy and to the beginning of things. That went on for three days more and made me very uneasy."[37] Billings worried needlessly, as he later secured a position with the president of his board of examiners, Dr. McClaren.

His examination was in fact so impressive that in the spring of 1862 two men came into the hospital where he was then working and asked to see his cases. Billings remembered that they had "an air of importance," so he obliged them with a tour. After a few minutes the men asked Billings if he knew the results of his entrance examination, to which he replied that he did not. The two proceeded to enlighten Billings, "At the end of the first day [of the exam] they [the examiners] concluded that probably you would pass, but hoped it would not be necessary to change the order of precedence in the roll, and that you could come in at the bottom. The second day they thought they would have to put your name higher up, and on the third day they concluded that you would be at the head of the class." Billings soon learned that the two callers were Hammond and Dr. Jonathan Letterman, medical director of the Army of the Potomac, and Billings was informed by Hammond that he was to be promoted. "You will be sent some contract doctors, and you are to go to the Cavalry barracks at Cliffburne . . . and turn them into a hospital."[38] Thus, not only were the boards important for structuring Civil War medicine; a good exam result could also make (or break) a doctor's career.

In addition to the regular exam, physicians also wrote an essay. Lavington Quick was asked to discuss the symptoms, diagnosis, pathology, and treatment of erysipelas, a relatively unfamiliar disease for many Americans, and his essay was surprisingly detailed.[39] Similarly, Roberts Bartholow was questioned on the varieties, symptoms, causes, diagnosis, pathology, and treatment of phrenitis.[40] Joseph Woodward was asked to write an essay on the diagnosis, causes, pathology, and treatment of gangrene.[41] Not having had the benefit of access that the war would provide, Woodward commented on the difficulty: "In conclusion the writer must express his regret that the subject which has fallen to his but related to a disease of which he has never seen a well marked case, which has compelled him to rely for his account upon the recollections of his reading, a very imperfect substitute he well knows for those personal recollections which he thinks he retains of almost every other surgical affection of importance."[42]

Those who obtained posts and were found to be unqualified were often reported to the surgeon general (though there were, of course, those who slipped through the cracks), but the evidence is overwhelming that the examining boards' stringent requirements were important in the development of American medicine because they put proficiency in scientific medicine at the forefront of the requirements, while simultaneously setting the standards upon which Civil War medicine would develop. Moreover, those who were found to be unqualified had a difficult time moving forward professionally during the war. Physicians, Hammond argued, were crucial for the development of American medicine—ideally they would understand Paris medicine: "The Surgeon-General presumes that every surgeon who has passed the medical examining board is capable of judging the intrinsic value of any pathological specimen."[43] Further, and perhaps most importantly, the boards helped to ensure that the orthodoxy had almost exclusive ownership of medicine through the war years.

One of the most important new avenues to support this professional development was in the wartime hospitals. In America, urbanization and permanent hospitals had not developed at the same rate as in Europe, and physicians did not have significant hospital opportunities before the war. Until the Civil War, hospitals in America were small, private institutions, and hospital training was not considered essential or even important for most American physicians.[44] Thus, the basic features of early nineteenth-century hospital medicine, including anatomical pathology and specific diagnostic techniques such as percussion, auscultation, and palpitation, while well known among elite medical practitioners, were slow to take root, and medicine overall remained much as it had been in the first decades of the century.[45] Charles Rosenberg, however, has suggested that "at mid-century every aspect of the relationship between medical knowledge and the hospital was uncertain and subject to future negotiation."[46]

Thus, the time was ripe for a rigorous epistemological intervention, and the war created a new medical context to which all Americans had to adapt. Medicine was no longer community medicine; soldiers were scattered throughout the United States. Laymen were not able to perform the necessary surgery that was often required after battle. And households were not able or equipped to manage the war convalescents, making the hospital necessary for a new class of patients and physicians.[47] Whether physicians had desired hospital experience before the war was irrelevant; during the war they had no choice. There was a huge demand for physicians and thus ample opportunities to develop a program of clinical inquiry. Indeed, even those physicians who had studied in Paris clamored for hospital posts, having found upon their return from France that it was difficult to continue their training owing to lack of hospital opportunity. The methods of the Paris Clinical School, then, for many, found their first application in the hospitals of the Civil War, a medical system that was highly compatible with military medicine.

Most Civil War patients arrived at the hospitals in critical condition or were long-term convalescents, which meant that doctors were required to provide extended treatment, keep detailed records, and closely monitor and study symptoms, diseases, and patients. Physicians in charge of hospitals were directed to make a report of all operations and treatment and keep a register of the sick and wounded; in addition, they had to give a full record of the cases, including condition of the patients at the time of any operation (description of wound, mental state, and constitutional state), followed by the progress, treatment, and result of the cases.[48] Physicians were also given diagnostic and technical equipment. Later in the war, John Shaw Billings commented that all "medical officers of the U.S. Army are to be furnished by the government with clinical thermometers. . . . I wish the instruments to be of first class workmanship, accurate and corresponding with each other."[49] Indeed, physicians worked daily and tirelessly within the new hospitals, but it was here that they could build their careers.

Walt Whitman served as a nurse, visitor, and confidant to hospital patients in Washington for more than three years during the war and observed that "any one of these hospitals is a little city in itself. Take for instance Carver Hospital. . . . It has more inmates than an ordinary country town. The same with the Lincoln hospital or the Finley hospital or Armory square hospital under Dr. Bliss (one of the best anywhere). It must have nearly a hundred tents, wards, sheds, and structures of one kind and another."[50] Whitman observed that some physicians rose to the challenge of war quite well: "I meet with first class surgeons in charge of many of the hospitals, and often ward surgeons, medical cadets, and head nurses are fully faithful and competent. Dr. Bliss, head of Armory Square, and Dr. Baxter, head of Campbell, seem to me to try to do their best, and to be excellent in their posts. Dr. Bowen, one of the ward surgeons of Armory, I have known to fight as hard for many a poor fellow's life under his charge as a lioness would fight for her young. I mention such cases because I think they deserve it, on public grounds."[51]

Whitman also noted that the government was "full of anxiety and liberality toward the sick and wounded. The system in operation in the permanent hospitals is good and the money flows without stint. . . . I find no expense spared, and great anxiety manifested in the highest quarters to do well by the national sick."[52] He observed that while incompetence sometimes prevailed in the operation of some of these institutions, he believed that they were "generally well conducted."[53] As one observer similarly recalled, "If the National Government had done nothing else during the last four years, through its Medical Department, but organize and maintain this superb hospital service, it alone would, wherever there are intelligence and experience to appreciate the difficulties to overcome, have secured for the country a high place among the nations, for successful achievement in this path of military effort."[54] Most hospitals in America were for the first time controlled by a bureaucracy, but not the credentialed administrators who govern the institutions today; rather, the military provided the necessary structure that allowed the institutions to develop and be dominated by medical professionals, who in turn used the hospital to fulfill their professional needs.

CHANGING THE PRODUCTION OF WARTIME MEDICAL KNOWLEDGE

"Very soon after his appointment, Surgeon General William Hammond saw the great scientific advantage that would accrue to the cause of scientific medicine and surgery by rendering the enormous experience of the war available for future study. Hardly ever in the history of the world has such an opportunity been offered for obtaining specimens illustrative of pathological anatomy."[55] So remarked the army assistant surgeon Harvey E. Brown in regard to Circular No. 2, which was issued May 21, 1862, by Surgeon General Hammond. Circular No. 2, which provided for the establishment of the Army Medical Museum, grew out of the necessities of wartime.[56] The museum was constructed for the purpose of "illustrating the injuries and diseases that produce death or disability during war, and thus affording materials for precise methods of study or problems regarding the diminution of mortality and alleviation of suffering in armies."[57] Military medicine was complex, and most surgeons had little to no experience treating bullet wounds or camp and hospital diseases. The museum was created to teach physicians the basic principles of military medicine.[58] However, once the project got under way, American physicians saw the museum as a new source of medical vitality, a center of learning that could institutionalize pathology and lay the national foundation to both reform and develop American medicine along more scientific guidelines.[59]

Circular No. 2 directed medical officers to "diligently collect and forward to the office of the Surgeon General all specimens of morbid anatomy, surgical or medical, which may be regarded as valuable; together with projectiles and foreign bodies removed; and such other matter as may prove of interest in the study of military medicine and surgery."[60] The circular gave physicians unprecedented access to specimens and bodies on a scale never before experienced in American medicine and created new opportunities in which to develop ideas about medicine and disease. The Union Medical Department's programmatic attempt to develop medical science brought an unprecedented number of American physicians intentionally into the domain of medical science—and began the process of setting American medicine on a new course.

There was palpable enthusiasm for the project almost immediately. The noted physician Elisha Harris recalled in 1864 that "the plan of the Museum originated with Surgeon General Hammond, and may be regarded as one of the fruits of that effort which placed at the head of the Medical Department a thoroughly scientific man as well as accomplished medical officer."[61] It was noted in 1878 by an investigative committee on military affairs that the medical museum was regarded as an "institution universally admitted to be one of the proudest scientific monuments in any age or country."[62] As one observer similarly recalled, "the museum is a great, systematically arranged object-lesson, in which the physical history of man in health and disease, and at all stages of development, is given and illustrated, [and] it becomes no longer a place in which to gratify a morbid curiosity, but one [in] which to pursue, under the most favorable circumstances, one of the most fascinating of studies."[63]

INDEX OF CONTRIBUTORS

Physicians took their antebellum medical education seriously, but there were few opportunities to develop varied forms of medical knowledge. When Circular No. 2 was issued in 1862, the educational opportunities had not developed significantly in the United States, which highlights both the importance of Hammond's directive and the unprecedented opportunity to regulate the further education of American physicians. Importantly, with the exception of a few career medical officers, all the wartime practitioners were civilian allopathic physicians before and after the war, in 1860 and 1866. It is well known that some of the more familiar and more renowned physicians sought posts during the war, but these years also supported the development of the next generation of elite physicians who helped shape not only Civil War medicine but American medicine.[64]

The prominent physician Jacob Da Costa, for example, wrote Hammond: "I beg to offer my services as attending physician by contract for one of the military hospitals in Philadelphia."[65] Benjamin Woodward (who later did fascinating work in his experiments with gangrene) also wrote Hammond: "I am anxious to be in some department of the army while the war lasts."[66] Woodward left a "good practice to come into the service," but welcomed the opportunity to use the war to develop his interests and skills.[67] Similarly, Samuel Gross, chair of Surgery at the Jefferson Medical College and the founder of the Pathological Society of Philadelphia, the Philadelphia Academy of Surgery, and the later American Surgical Association, wrote Surgeon General Finley in 1861, "It will afford me great pleasure to be made chief of one of the military hospitals located in this city. My time will not permit me to visit Washington to apply in person, nor do I deem it necessary to procure credentials, as my character I suppose is well known to that department. The salary is no special object; I want the situation on account of the opportunities it could afford me to study the nature and character of camp diseases in reference to the cooperation of a work on scholarly medicine and surgery."[68] He wrote Finley once again a few months later to remind him "of the kind promise you made me four or five weeks ago to appoint me to one of the government hospitals in this city. I find these institutions are now being opened and it will afford me much pleasure to be placed in charge of one."[69]

Gross, an eminent surgeon, worked in a number of capacities during the war, including training military surgeons to perform amputations and treat gunshot wounds. He also studied the results of surgical operations, camp diseases, and hospital administration and published his observations. Though it was a great demand on his time, he, like many others, wanted both the experience and the opportunity to contribute, and his enthusiasm was evident when he received one of his appointments, "I accept with much pleasure your kind offer to act as a member of the medical board of Philadelphia. Although the position may as you observe involve some sacrifice of time, I shall care nothing for it if I can be instrumental in rendering the government some service by providing it with efficient and competent medical officers."[70]

Although there were more than 12,000 physicians who doctored on the Union side during the war, four groups can be retrospectively contrasted for the purpose of analysis (though these groups were by no means static). The top of the pyramid was the elite, those men who had been to Europe, edited journals, wrote textbooks, founded and developed medical societies, taught private courses, and occupied posts at medical schools and hospitals. For these men, the war provided the opportunity to develop or showcase the medical skills and expertise that they had acquired either at home or abroad. They included Samuel Gross, Austin Flint Sr., Valentine Mott, Joseph Leidy, and Silas Weir Mitchell. Before the war these men guarded their seniority and were often reluctant to share hospital positions or the limited access to bodies that they had. During the war they assumed a new role as teachers, responsible for educating the more-junior physicians who were now charged with treating Union soldiers. This meant they instructed physicians; wrote textbooks, articles, and instructive essays; consulted on autopsies; and held posts at the newly created specialty hospitals (as discussed in chapter 4).

Another identifiable group comprised those physicians who aspired to be elite and become practically acquainted or more accomplished with the medical sciences—John Brinton, W. W. Keen, Joseph Woodward, Middleton Goldsmith, Benjamin Woodward, Roberts Bartholow, and George McGill among them. The war was critically important for these two groups because it provided an opportunity to distinguish themselves among the many American physicians, advance their own careers, learn the intricacies of the medical sciences, and in the process develop American medicine. Most of these men held a medical degree, studied with a faculty preceptor, had taken private courses, or studied in Europe. This group closely followed scientific developments abroad and had for some years wanted to move medicine and the profession forward by reforming American medicine. The next two groups comprised the "rank and file," the bulk of the medical practitioners in the country. Both the skill level and interest in the basic sciences varied widely in these groups. Many of these men studied with a "community preceptor" (usually serving an apprenticeship with a more senior physician). Some of these men may have also sought out some kind of private instruction in hospitals or anatomy rooms. Some of them held a medical school degree, while others had attended medical school but not graduated, and others still had never set foot in medical school. As William Rothstein has demonstrated, many of the practitioners before 1860 who lived in rural areas or small towns "were less likely to have degrees."[71] Moreover, before the war less than half of the students attending medical school actually received a medical degree.[72]

Some of these practitioners, however, did want to become familiar with scientific medicine, to contribute and be part of the profession in a more significant way, and perhaps to become better known through the process. Physicians lamented about the state of antebellum medical education that there was little benefit to be obtained at a medical school so why bother going. There was a drive for improved clinical education, and some men had argued for better practical teaching and more resources, including faculty, equipment, and patients. Though there had been minor improvements in the American medical schools between the years 1820 and 1860, they were slow to take shape. Raising the standards in this group of physicians was crucially important for the development of American medicine, and the Civil War hospitals created a social transformation and the promise of new possibilities for many of the rank and file.

Finally, there were those practitioners who volunteered for war service out of a sense of duty or because they wanted to receive steady income for their medical work. These men may or may not have attended a course of medical lectures but did not possess a real knowledge or desire to understand scientific medicine.[73] Most of the members of this group were trained with some kind of preceptor, and what mattered most for these men was skill, or the appearance of skill, in bedside or community medicine. They had no hospital experience, could not afford or lacked the desire to engage in extensive private instruction or travel abroad to study medicine, and thus possessed a minimal knowledge of medicine, disease, and the body.

All of the physicians in these four groups, under the terms of the new Wilson Bill, were placed under the direct authority of the medical department and the surgeon general and were officially organized into seven categories:

1. Surgeons (ranking of major) and assistant surgeons of the regular army (ranking as first lieutenant)
2. Surgeons and assistant surgeons of volunteers
3. Regimental surgeons and assistant surgeons commissioned by state governors

4. Acting assistant surgeons (civilian physicians employed by the Union army as part-time or full-time surgeons under contract)
5. Medical officers of the veterans corps
6. Acting staff surgeons
7. Surgeons and assistant surgeons of colored troops

In order to meet the demands of field and hospital service, Hammond also created the function of brigade surgeon, a senior role in the Union medical corps. Because the role was medical supervision, candidates were required to take an exam before a board of medical officers and, if successful, were placed in an upper-level position, such as managing a hospital, training junior officers, or serving as a medical director of an army. They also made sanitary inspections, organized field and general hospitals, and supervised junior physicians. Some of these men earned the rank of surgeon (ranking as major), but the role was not rank dependent.

By far the largest category of physicians included the volunteer or acting assistant surgeons and assistant surgeons of the regular army (ranking as first lieutenant). These groups worked in both general and field hospitals and were in charge of treating wounded patients after battle or sick patients in hospital wards; they also prescribed medicine and performed operations, but only the surgeons had administrative duties in the hospitals. The acting assistant surgeons were those physicians who did not have a military commission and were under contract on a temporary basis—and, as noted earlier, they were not particularly popular among the regulars. As W. W. Keen recalled, "I did not want to make an Army career and declined commission in the regular army and was appointed Acting Assistant Surgeon or as we were usually called by the regulars 'damned contract doctors.'"[74] The skill level varied widely in this group. Some men were very proficient in medical matters, whereas others were forced to learn the intricacies of medicine and disease on the job and sometimes at the expense of the patient. The important point, however, is that, within the context and structure of wartime medicine, the range of contributors crossed all experience levels from the elite to the very inexperienced.

Moreover, not just regular and volunteer physicians benefited from experience and education during the war; it was also common practice to contract medical students, who had minimal education and practical experience, to act as hospital stewards or medical cadets.[75] After the formation of the corps of medical cadets was approved by Congress in August 1861, American medical students clamored for posts. Medical cadets were either noncommissioned officers or civilians contracted with the medical department for at least three months of medical service (called acting medical cadets). Regular and acting medical cadets generally assisted physicians, acted as wound dressers and ambulance attendants, and helped in postmortem exams by preparing specimens and issuing medicines. Thus, for these men, too, it was an unparalleled educational and practical intervention. One young cadet, for example, waited anxiously for wounded soldiers from the Battle at Brandy Station in June 1863: "If we get the Rebel wounded, so much the better, for a great many of them were stuck by Rush's Lancers in the first charge they made, and lance wounds are rather a great luxury in military surgery."[76]

Some young students were even recruited to work in specialized areas of medicine. Joseph Woodward wrote to Professor Leidy at the University of Pennsylvania and Silas Weir Mitchell at the Jefferson Medical College in the hope of filling a position at the newly formed medical museum to assist with microscopial preparations. He asked for someone with "neatness and mechanical tact" and "some knowledge of microscopial work," though given the limitations in this area of study before the war, he did concede that "this is not an indispensable."[77] The successful applicant was to be paid $90 per month, receive the title of hospital steward, and be granted time to "prosecute his studies" for admission to "civilian medicine" or the "medical corps."[78] There was also the opportunity to partake in "field work"; for example, in January 1863 John Brinton wrote C. M. McDougall inquiring as to whether he knew of any "young men in New York, of pathological instincts, who would collect for the museum with interest."[79]

Some of the war physicians, then, contributed to the project initiated by Circular No. 2 because they were merely obeying orders; however, numerous others got caught up in the general desire for improvement and advancement that characterized the project. During the war, all physicians were faced with new responsibilities, challenges, and opportunities; however, to maintain a position in the Union Medical Department, they were all required to follow the orders of the surgeon general. This in many ways bridged the social gap between American physicians by bringing the wartime educational requirements under one common standard. One way to measure the sheer impact of the project stimulated by Circular No. 2 is through the examination of the voluminous materials that were submitted to the Army Medical Museum by both volunteer and regular army physicians.

It is an impossible task to describe each case report, narrative of service, autopsy report, or essay that was submitted as per the orders of Circular No. 2. The index of contributors found in the Army Medical Museum catalog[80] or the *Medical and Surgical History of the War of the Rebellion* is long and speaks to the enormity of the project.[81] As one example, volume 2 of the *Medical and Surgical History of the War of the Rebellion* lists 2,754 reporters and operators, most of whom submitted multiple specimens and case histories.[82] As George Otis noted in 1865, "The extent of these materials is simply enormous. The returns are of as huge proportions as the armies that have been engaged in active operations for the last four years. The great body of the medical officers have made the reports required of them with commendable diligence and promptitude, and their zeal is the more deserving of praise when the engrossing nature of their field duties is considered. The result has been the accumulation of a mass of facts and observations in military surgery of unprecedented magnitude."[83]

To support this professional drive among the profession, Hammond placed clinical instruments, medical texts, and current medical journals such as the *American Journal of the Medical Sciences* and the *Medical News and Library* on the army medical supply table; he also supported the publication of numerous educational treatises during the war to train and educate physicians. Among numerous others these included: Roberts Bartholow, *A Manual of Instructions for Enlisting and Discharging Soldiers* (1863); John Brinton, *Consolidated Statement of Gunshot Wounds* (1863); Henry Clark, *Inspection of Military Hospitals* (1863); Jacob M. Da Costa, *Medical Diagnosis* (1864); Charles R. Greenleaf, *A Manual for the Medical Officers of the United States Army* (1864); William A. Hammond, *A Treatise on Hygiene* (1863); DeWitt Peters, "Interesting Cases of Gunshot Wounds" (1864); Joseph Janvier Woodward, *The Hospital Steward's Manual* (1862) and *Outlines of the Chief Camp Diseases of the United States Armies as Observed during the Present War* (1863).[84] Hammond also distributed essays and pamphlets about quinine for the treatment and prevention of malaria, epidemic diseases, pneumonia, and amputation and the treatment of surgical wounds. These were written by the elite, most of whom had studied in Europe, for the benefit of the rank and file who were doctoring during the war.[85] Hammond continually encouraged individual physicians to institute projects that might develop medical knowledge.[86]

The project, then, brought numerous American physicians together as they attempted to master the problems and challenges presented by the war, creating an unprecedented continuing educational experience for

American physicians but also a new type of cohesion among them.[87] The project of building the medical museum had deep roots and thus broad implications for American medicine.

CONTEXTS OF KNOWLEDGE PRODUCTION:
The "Circular" and the Civil War Case Report

The diseases that attacked the troops and the institutional support provided by the Army Medical Museum and the new hospitals created a dynamic medical environment, which led to innovative intellectual and conceptual responses to the challenges. Knowledge was produced in a variety of ways, and the form in which it was organized, developed, and transmitted was one of the most important facets of Civil War medicine. This knowledge was at the core of the interaction between physicians within the wartime environment and was crucial in supporting a new foundation for American medicine.[88] Circular No. 2's directive to collect and dissect bodies and specimens supported a research community among physicians in the war. Research during the war differed from research that had been conducted by traditional urban research societies in antebellum America, which were generally very small (and tended to exclude the rank and file).[89] By contrast, wartime research projects often took the form of large, structured collective investigations of material and knowledge. The war doctors were at the forefront of this type of collective investigation.[90]

The medical department issued hundreds of circulars requesting that physicians study various subjects for the purpose of constructing knowledge relating to diseases, treatments, diagnoses, hospital construction, bodies, and specimens, as well as circulars requesting investigations into specific areas proved extremely effective in amassing knowledge.[91] The individual physician's experiences and findings could then be evaluated in relation to the larger body of developing knowledge. Physicians submitted their reports, and the staff at the Army Medical Museum, Surgeon General's Office, or those charged with the study of specific diseases and treatments would compare the incoming data in analyzing various diseases, wounds, and treatments. There were numerous case histories that provided an empirical account of soldiers and patients, allowing for a synthesis of the wartime medical environment. Each patient's case history represented a branch of knowledge that could be developed.

Throughout the war, then, American physicians eagerly sought to share and learn from the larger wartime medical program. The transmission of this knowledge was a central aspect of this project and was, in fact, crucial for a number of political and professional reasons: it was an attempt to reorganize American medicine so that it was more unified, to orient it to scientific guidelines, and to create a network of knowledge that linked American physicians with each other and international physicians. In conjunction with Circular No. 2, Circular No. 5 was issued and directed that the research at the museum be published in the *Medical and Surgical History of the War of the Rebellion*.[92]

The most effective vehicle of transmission was the Civil War case report. Circular No. 5 required that *all* physicians write and submit a case history or essay along with each specimen that was submitted to the museum. The circular stated, "All medical officers cooperate in this undertaking by forwarding to this office such sanitary, topographical, medical and surgical reports, details of cases, essays and the results of investigations and inquiries as may be of value for this work, which full credit will be given in forthcoming volumes." Indeed, the generation of this medical knowledge had to move through the profession somehow, as Hammond concluded, "It is scarcely necessary to remind the medical officers of the regular and volunteer services that through the means in question much may be done to advance the science which we all have so much at heart, and to establish landmarks which will serve to guide us in the future."[93]

The case report was important in constructing a profile of expertise while creating a picture of the prevailing wartime diseases and interesting cases. The broad range of cases and even the practice of case writing created a community of physicians dedicated to the mastery of tissues, organs, and disease processes, both the stable and unstable, the commonly encountered and the unexpected outcomes.[94] In the nineteenth century, case reporting was fairly common among elite physicians;[95] however, as already discussed, many physicians drawn into this project were well below this level, and by engaging in this work they developed a strong identification with medicine and science particularly relating to practical instruction, diagnosis, treatment, and the dissemination of knowledge.

Especially early on, then, Hammond used the authority of the medical department to ensure that compliance with these instructions was enforced. For example, he issued Circular No. 10 as a follow up to Circular No. 2 on August 10, 1862, in which he noted that "many medical officers, both regular and volunteers have partially disregarded previous circulars from this office. These circulars are explanatory orders and in future, officers neglecting to comply with their directions will be proceeded against for disobedience of orders."[96] It is important to remember that this was wartime. The structure of the military was new and intimidating for many volunteers and helped to ensure compliance: "Not long after taking charge, one Saturday afternoon about 4 o'clock I received an order to report at the office of Dr. Letterman, the Medical Director of the Army of the Potomac, in Washington. I had had so little experience in army orders that I almost trembled at the formal and peremptory character of the order. I feared that without knowing it I had done something to displease Mr. Stanton, the Secretary of War, who was a good deal of a bogy to most people at that time, for he has a way of putting them sometimes into Fort Delaware or other similar close quarters, without giving any reasons too, which was very disagreeable."[97]

But Hammond was clever. Circular No. 5 promised that all contributing medical officers would have their case studies published in the *Museum Catalogue* and the *Medical and Surgical History of the War of the Rebellion* and perhaps national and international medical journals. As Hammond stated, "It is therefore confidently expected that no one will neglect this opportunity of advancing the honor of service, the cause of humanity, and his own reputation."[98] John Shaw Billings suggested, "Every medical man in this country should help a little and provide for the perpetuation of his name as that of a physician interested in the progress of the profession by sending at least one specimen to [the museum]."[99] Woodward noted that once the case reports and specimens were submitted to the museum, the "officers entrusted with the labor of digesting these observations, and preparing them for the press, have constantly endeavored, in all their publications, to give full credit to their brother officers at the various military posts, whose original labors are the foundation of all the scientific work that has been done, and all that can be done at the Surgeon General's Office."[100]

As Hammond anticipated, physicians sought and savored this potential recognition: it was a chance to be known, make contacts, and distinguish themselves in a medical world that was rapidly transforming. The process of collecting, analyzing, and diagnosing conferred and demonstrated a new commitment, experience, and knowledge of anatomy, physiology, and pathology, giving physicians' authority and mastery of the body grounded in science—the epistemological foundation upon which wartime medicine was developed.

There is an enormous amount of material contained in the case histories. All were handwritten; some were short and descriptive, whereas others were pages long, very detailed, and analytical.[101] Case reports generally

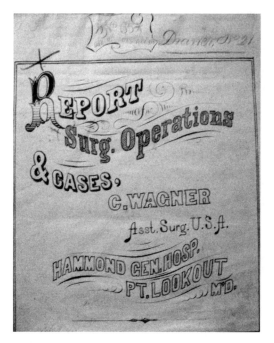

Report of surgical operations and cases, case notes of Charles Wagner (Courtesy of the National Archives, Washington, D.C.)

included the name of the patient, date of admission, name or description of the wound or disease, progress of the case, course of treatment and remedies, type of operation performed, the immediate outcome, and an autopsy report if appropriate. Finally, the case report included the name of the practitioner. Much of the material studied and collected consisted of medical reports and illustrations of these reports generally in the "shape of pathological specimens, drawings and models."[102] The data consisted of numerical returns illustrating the different types of wounds, diseases, accidents, and injuries; quarterly reports detailing the various wounds, diseases, and surgical operations; sanitary reports; and numerical lists of the wounded. Physicians also submitted case histories extracted from their own case books and miscellaneous reports, usually the result of independent observation or research, which included "reports and dissertations on new methods and modes of treatment; modifications of surgical apparatus and appliances; [and] pathological researches on morbid processes" pertaining to surgery or unfamiliar diseases, such as gangrene, osteomyelitis, and pyemia.[103]

The case studies and the eventual publication of the *Museum Catalogue* and the *Medical and Surgical History* structured the collection of specimens, which by war's end was a routine activity. And physicians were accountable for their decisions.[104] In the performance of an operation or amputation or the administration of therapeutics, if they deemed a patient "cured" and he rejoined his regiment at the front, the doctor was then accountable to himself and the patient.[105] The case report also made the doctor accountable to the government, the surgeon general, and the public; however, perhaps most importantly, the doctor was accountable to his profession, which sought to elevate medicine onto a more scientific stage.

Perhaps for the first time on a significant scale, American physicians were making important strides toward earning the respect of the public: they were doctoring, even risking their own lives, to save the soldiers still alive and fighting for the preservation of the Union. Pathologists working in the hospital or museum laboratory promised detection of the cause of disease and perhaps improved treatment, and this is how scientific medicine was framed during the war. It was a concept that was important for the development and the efficacy of both the orthodox physician and the medical sciences.

CIRCULAR NO. 2 IN PRACTICE

It is perhaps not surprising that, as physicians responded to the mandates of Circular No. 2, the weakness in the training of American physicians was quickly exposed; however, because the circular demanded that physicians deal with the basic principles of disease such as causation and development, this focused study of diseased structures provided a unique opportunity to teach physicians the basic principles of medicine: understanding, diagnosing, treating, and managing some of the effects of the pervasive microorganisms encountered on American soil.[106] Training physicians properly to diagnose disease and understand the dynamics of disease and wounds thus became *the* central component of the project.

The medical portion of the museum was assigned to Joseph Woodward of the Army of the Potomac, the surgical section to John H. Brinton of the volunteers on duty with the Army of the Mississippi.[107] Brinton and Woodward were granted full authority to develop the project, and medical officers were "directed to comply with the requests made of them."[108] Before the war, Woodward was a professor of the theory and practice of medicine at the University of Pennsylvania, where he received his medical degree in 1853. His research interests included pathological histology and microscopy, and he formed classes for instruction in the use of the microscope and the study of pathology. He was also demonstrator in operative surgery, in charge of

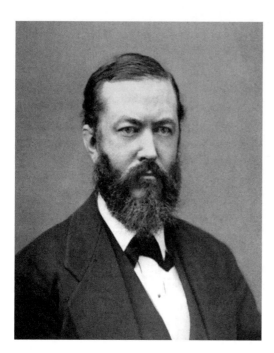

Joseph Woodward (Courtesy of the National Museum of Health and Medicine, Washington, D.C.)

the surgical clinic of the university, and a member of the Pathological Society. He had published extensively on the microscopic aspects of cancerous growths and the anatomical diagnoses of cancers and further developed his expertise within the museum.[109] At the outbreak of the war, he entered the army as an assistant surgeon and, after serving in several battles, on May 19, 1862, received his appointment as curator from Hammond, opening up new realms of possibilities for Woodward.

The surgical section was assigned to John H. Brinton, the museum's first curator. Brinton received his medical degree in 1852 from Jefferson College in Philadelphia and obtained postgraduate training in Paris and Vienna. He was a professor of the principles and practices of surgery at Jefferson Medical College before volunteering for services in the Brigade of Volunteer Surgeons in August 1861.[110] On August 1, 1862, Hammond sent Brinton official orders in which he was directed to "collect and properly arrange in the military museum all specimens of morbid anatomy, both medical and surgical, which have accumulated since the commencement of the rebellion in the various hospitals, or which may have been retained by any of the medical officers of the Army."[111] Hammond also dispatched a number of medical officers[112] to various hospitals to obtain from the surgeon in charge "all specimens that had accumulated since the establishment of that

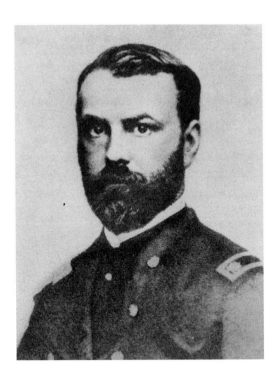

John H. Brinton (Courtesy of the National Museum of Health and Medicine, Washington, D.C.)

hospital."[113] They were also charged with going to the battlefield, usually following a large conflict, where they would both elucidate the overall importance of the project and engage in a series of demonstrations on how to prepare specimens, even digging out trenches where corpses had been buried. As one observer recounted, initially, "Woodward failing to get material from the army camps, gathered up a company of darkies, hired some mule teams, drove to the battlefield nearby, exhumed buried limbs and bodies, and brought the pathological specimens to Washington himself";[114] however, because evacuation was often slow, such action was rare, and bodies were in any event usually quite accessible.

In his memoirs, Brinton recalled the method under which specimens were collected and prepared: "First of all the man had to be shot, or injured, to be taken to the hospital for examination, and in a case for operation, to be operated upon. If all this were taking place in a city hospital, or a permanent general hospital, the bones of a part would be removed would be partially cleaned and then with a wooden tag and carved number attached, would be packed away in a keg, containing [clear] alcohol, whiskey, or sometimes salt and water."[115] Once procured, specimens were turned over to the depot quartermaster for transport to Washington under the provisions of

General Order No. 27. A representative of Adams Express Company was then contacted to deliver the specimens to the museum.[116] General Order No. 116, issued May 22, 1863, set up the museum and working laboratory, where the specimens would be prepared, verified, recorded, dissected, and studied when the corresponding case history arrived days later.[117]

Hammond requested medical specimens of disease illustrating morbid processes of every kind including diseased organs; a series of specimens illustrating disease of the brain, nervous system, heart, tubercles of the lungs, cancers and tumors of internal organs; and specimens illustrating enteric fever and chronic diarrhea, parasites, concretions and calculi, including microscopial preparations, which were to be mounted on slips of glass. Healthy specimens taken after autopsy for comparative purposes were also requested.[118] For the surgical section, specimens illustrative of surgical injuries and affections including fractures, excised portion of bone, diseased bones and joints, the structure of stumps, wounds and vessels from nerves, and any extraordinary injuries were requested.[119]

Recognizing the importance of this undertaking, Joseph K. Barnes, who succeeded Hammond as surgeon general in late 1863 (he was officially appointed August 18, 1864) expanded the project as one of his first official orders.[120] Under his jurisdiction, the work of collecting material for the Army Medical Museum was pushed vigorously. He issued General Order No. 306, which confirmed both that medical officers had command of general hospitals and that they were ordered to procure and submit all specimens.[121] Circular No. 26, issued November 26, 1863, similarly reminded all medical officers in charge of general hospitals of the importance of preserving medical and surgical specimens for the museum. In 1864 Barnes broadened the directives of the collection to include human anatomy, physiology, pathology, somatological anthropology, instruments and apparatus, and illustrations of methods of teaching connected with special departments of practical medicine.[122]

The project, though, began slowly, as Brinton remarked, with "just three dried varnished specimens placed on the little shelf—it was a bit of a joke at first—no idea that it would become the magnificent military museum, which I believe influences and will influence to no slight degree the future of American military surgery."[123] Initially, many physicians did not see the point of collecting and dissecting bodies and specimens.[124] After all, most of the rank and file were unfamiliar with pathological anatomy, and thus its relevance as a medical system was unknown. Importantly, however, Brinton suggested that, once the project got going, there was a shift in thinking among American physicians; the museum's immediate purpose was to furnish information that would benefit Union soldiers, but there was also profound recognition of the advantages in this undertaking.[125] Indeed, Otis noted in 1865 that "the several circulars requesting medical officers to forward preparations to the Army Medical Museum met with very general and liberal responses."[126]

This directive provided a model for change. And it was a specific medical model that physicians understood: they were required to diagnose, monitor, and treat conditions, record patient progress, and perform autopsies when necessary, culminating in the delivery of the specimen to the museum along with a case report.[127] The new museum evolved to support medical research and investigative medicine. Woodward noted that "it would meet a want long felt by every medical man in America who has ventured in the domain of original research."[128] Billings too recognized the vigor of medical science and the potential for the medical profession generated by the new museum: "The necessities of modern progress in anatomy, physiology and pathology, have led to the creation of medical museums in all parts of the civilized world . . . it is certain that the securing and forwarding of [specimens] is a very useful thing to the physician who does it. It tends to keep him in touch with current living thought and work of the profession, to direct his attention to the connection between symptoms and the mechanism of their production, which is often so important in deciding on the remedy to be used, and, above all it gives him an interest in other men's work, and thus broadens his views and increases his pleasure."[129]

The war physicians pushed to make this a national, scientific project that would have far-reaching implications for American medical education. As Woodward concluded, "A cabinet of comparable anatomy furnishes the means for useful collateral studies, subordinate to the general purposes of a pathological museum; hence such cabinets are found in connection with most of the great pathological collections of Europe, and one has been commenced at the Army Medical Museum."[130] Importantly, there were two simultaneous levels of support or development unfolding during the war. First, the project allowed for the development of "mass" pathological anatomy—thousands of bodies filled the shelves, creating a large center for the study of pathological anatomy. But second, and of equal importance, these bodies and specimens were being prepared by individual physicians, who were closely studying individual diseases and individual patients as they attempted to master the wartime wounds and diseases. Physiological and bacteriological medicine was more individual than the pathological museums of Paris, and the wartime program began preparing physicians for this transition as well.

The process of collecting and the collection itself allowed for the creation of new forms of analysis, a new way to think about disease, and this promise for medicine had a profound effect on the individual physician. Brinton noted that "professional zeal had been excited" simply because collecting specimens placed physicians in the domain of scientific medicine; they were forced to identify with the gross pathological specimen, to see the object of disease. He noted that never before in American medicine had there been "so great an activity and development and so earnest an effort to master the unsolved problems of the past."[131] The physician Edward H. Smith also reasoned that "if there is any benefit from the sad struggle of the age, it is that medical officers can fully justify looking for information and present the information for the world's future use. . . . The use of limbs and organs, and operations once deemed experimental will in future use be instilled to our confidence because of the keen, careful, and honoring eye of experience."[132]

To understand why so many physicians searched for wartime opportunities, we must explore what the experience meant to the physicians themselves. One of the clear objectives was to enable American physicians to become, for the first time in a significant way, producers of medical knowledge. Physicians formed a powerful medical identity in the process. Billings observed that "the objects of a medical museum are to preserve, to diffuse and to increase knowledge."[133] As Hammond similarly noted, "A large number of memoirs and reports of great interest to medical science, and military surgery especially, have been collected and are now being systematically arranged. . . . The greatest interest is felt in this labor by the medical officers of the army and physicians at large."[134] The "mysterious" scientific educational opportunities abroad were now available in America to the "many" American physicians doctoring in the war. There was no longer a singular medical capital such as Edinburgh, London, Paris, Vienna, or Berlin but rather new domestic sources and opportunities to expand and produce knowledge.

The project, then, was as much about education as it was about identity and professional authority, which transformed the profession in these years. The physician C. Wagner wrote to Brinton that he was "desirous to be part of the surgical history of the war," reported that he was "keeping all specimens of interest, case notes written out carefully," and asked Brinton "for any suggestions" on how to contribute effectively so that his preparations would be of value.[135] Soon after, Wagner sent Brinton a detailed list of specimens: "Please find enclosed a list of the pathological specimens that I have at present on hand. I will have more after a while. The specimens, with a brief history of each case, will be forwarded in due time. I have had several interesting cases of gunshot wounds of the lungs, but cannot procure specimens because the cases will recover." He went on to note, however: "Today I performed an interesting operation: resection of the ulna; removed two-thirds of the bone, disarticulating it at the elbow. I have more operations in prospect. I will send you one very pretty specimen, a portion of the cranium from a case of resection of the cranium."[136] By 1865 Wagner had become one of the chief contributors to the museum: "I have the honor to transmit by express one half barrel containing anatomical specimens. Reports of both cases of amputation at the hip joint were forwarded several days ago with the quarter's report of surgical operations, in which, cases from whom the specimens were obtained are represented by hospital numbers 6654 & 1995."[137]

There were also the very interesting cases:

I take this opportunity to send you the bones of the leg which Brig. General T. W. Sherman U. S. V. lost in consequence of a gunshot wound received May 27, 1863 at the first assault of General Banks upon Port Hudson. I regard the specimen of interest both from the distinguished reputation of the patient and from the extraordinary character of the treatment which he received. The wound in his leg which was extensive and greatly lacerated (having apparently been produced by a conoidal ball) was very tightly sewed up with a continuous suture, the cutting out of which gave exit to a large discharge of decomposing coagula pus and bone splinters. . . . He remained in a most discouraging condition for nearly two weeks when amputation through the middle of the thigh was performed by Dr. W. Stone, a civil surgeon, and resulted favorably.[138]

But most reports simply reflect the interest in being able to contribute to the project, to be part of the larger collaboration, and to produce knowledge that would benefit American medicine. A letter sent November 8, 1865, by James Armsby, a surgeon in the Ira General Hospital in Albany, New York, stated: "I have the honor to state that I have this day forwarded to your address, for the army medical museum, a box containing an album of photographs of morbid specimens and necrosed bones removed from patients treated in this hospital. Attached to each specimen is a case study."[139]

Physicians were, in fact, making tremendous progress in their ability, as identified in the case of William Williams Keen. Keen began at Jefferson Medical College in the fall of 1860, and as he pointed out, he was fortunate enough to have made friends with faculty members John Brinton (his preceptor), Jacob Da Costa, and Silas Weir Mitchell. Keen credited his mentors with instructing him in the basic principles of scientific medicine: "If I had not entered the office of Brinton and Da Costa I would have graduated without ever having looked through a microscope, ever having personally examined a patient or written a prescription."[140] Indeed, "two or three days later I was sitting at one of the windows with Gray's Anatomy [a new book then] on my lap and a skull in my hands beginning the study of bones. Minutes later Silas Weir Mitchell came in the room and asked if I wanted to help him with some experiments on snakes. This is the beginning of a friendship that has endured for over 52 years."[141] Keen became part of an alliance that was very interested in the pursuit of scientific medicine. They were able to transcend the limitations of the antebellum medical world by volunteering for medical service in the war.

Keen, like the bulk of American physicians, was very inexperienced when he sought, and received, a commission during the war. As he noted, "How vividly I recall my first operation on a living patient—a simple amputation of the forearm in an army hospital in 1862. I was greatly alarmed after the very first incision lest the patient might bleed to death before I could secure the arteries. . . . I shrunk from doing it because I was afraid of hemorrhage. I ended [the war] by being as little afraid of even the most furious hemorrhage as anyone could possibly be."[142]

As early as 1863 Keen was quite at ease with surgery and many other aspects of scientific medicine; during most of his service in the army, he was an agent of the Army Medical Museum and collected specimens from all the hospitals in Frederick, Maryland, and later Philadelphia and forwarded them to Washington.[143] He remarked after the war: "My own notes and specimens fill many a page and furnish many an illustration in the six splendid volumes of the *Medical and Surgical History of the War*."[144] Keen's developing proficiency and familiarity with the body progressed rapidly during the war. His reports to Brinton reveal his enthusiasm for the project: "I have received the catalogue of the museum and looked it over. I am glad to see such a valuable collection. Can you send me *another* copy for me to send to Dr. R. Davies, who was my temporary successor at Frederick? He has returned to England and I know he would like to have one [particularly because Davies published in *Hays American Journal* on specimen 881 of the catalogue]."[145]

Indeed, being associated with this work was important to Keen: "I sent a photograph of case 557 by mail. It is not noted I see, and if it was not received, Dr. Weir at Frederick can supply you with another and Dr. Gurdon Buck of New York can give you further information as to the case for he was to go there to have a plastic operation performed."[146] On another occasion, physician R. Weir wrote Hammond on behalf of Keen: "Dr. Keen forwarded today the barrel containing specimens from the General Hospital in Frederick and would like Brinton to forward all the numbers that these specimens will be catalogued as in order to ensure that the hospital gets due credit for the specimens, particularly because they are of value."[147] Keen, like many physicians, was able to use the war experience to develop a scientific identity. For others, it could be a source of professional embarrassment to be reprimanded for not participating. As one physician noted when asking for a copy of the circular, "I am constantly embarrassed in the performance of my duties for the want of them [circulars]."[148]

Physicians worked tirelessly developing the medical museum and building the collection, and the process altered conceptions of how to understand the body and how to produce knowledge. In 1865 Joseph Woodward wrote to Alfred Stillé, with whom he had enjoyed "agreeable intercourse" during their time at the Philadelphia Pathological Society, to discuss his ongoing work in the museum's laboratory related to pathological anatomy and histology: "I am desirous of inviting your attention to the studies at present in progress here under my supervision as to the diseases of our soldiers. The studies are assuming the more importance because of the bearing of the facts observed on general pathological doctrines."

Woodward, for example, wondered, "If for instance my preparations prove in the thickened peyers glands of our camp fevers and the swollen hardaceous connective tissue of the colon of our camp diarrhea, a cell multiplication of preexisting elements instead of the free cell development in a plastic exudation which appeared probable to those who teased fragments instead of cutting sections: this fact *once established* must lend its aid to the general reception of the modern doctrines of new formations, as versus, the older conception which is still so generally received in this country."[149] Woodward invited Stillé to Washington to examine the medical and microscopial collections that had been acquired in "ample proportions." He concluded, "I should much like to show you what we are doing and to converse with you on some of the views to which my observations are compelling me."[150]

While Woodward consulted with his peers, the rank and file consulted and learned from Woodward. American physicians had long sought private instruction from more elite physicians, and this type of education was facilitated for the large body of the war physicians through the medical museum. Woodward increasingly taught and questioned physicians on the basic principles of pathological anatomy. He wrote to Surgeon M. K. Taylor, for example, in regard to their differing diagnoses of chronic diarrhea based on independent pathological investigation: "The doctor is under the impression that you have found ulcerations of the intestine *very rare* in these cases. As a fellow-student of the same subject this statement has interested me very much and the more so because at the museum I have found ulceration the rule in cases fatal from the diarrhea, and this in specimens from the west and south as well as from the east. I have some hundreds of preparations in illustration of these views. . . . I shall be most pleased to receive the specimens at the museum whenever you are ready to forward them and their histories."[151]

The emergence of "expert authority" among the museum curators provided an opportunity to develop ideas about both pedagogy and wartime diseases while simultaneously pushing young physicians further. Woodward responded to Surgeon W. L. Faxon regarding a spleen he had sent to the museum. Woodward responded shortly after: "In reply to your note of March 6 which I have delayed to answer until I could study the spleen, I have this to say: The disease of the spleen on careful examination proved to be a metastic focus similar to the pyemic abscess. This condition of the spleen is not uncommon in an ulceration of the intestine and pneumonia both of which are present in this case."[152]

Similarly, on June 14, 1864, Woodward wrote to a young doctor in the field to correct him on his recently submitted case study: "I have to thank you for the interesting specimen in the case of Mason. You are however quite wrong in supposing the disease to be tubercular." Woodward went on to instruct the young physician: "Its characteristics the size, shape, of the tumor and the microscopial appearance all show the disease to be undoubtedly *medullary cancer*. You will I know pardon criticism on your diagnosis for the sake of truth. In a general way tubercules contain such size as these tumors. And, microscopically, the tubercule never contains such ulcerated cells as are presented in this specimen. I have had the specimen prepared for mounting and it will make by far the finest cancerous preparation in the museum, which is by the way enriched by numerous contributions from you."[153]

Woodward seemed to work endlessly answering and commenting on case reports and, as curator of the new national museum, reinforced a specific set of criteria by which to investigate disease processes. He liked especially to study cases from the field to both learn and confirm or correct diagnoses. In another interesting case, Woodward observed in a letter to Surgeon L. S. Todd, 4th Calvary Volunteers, San Francisco, on August 15, 1864: "Your specimen from Private Leo Monier Co. 'B' 4th cavalry voluntary infantry has come to duly to hand. You will be interested to learn that a profound and exhaustive microscopial examination of this specimen by assistant Surgeon E. Curtis of this office and myself has satisfied me that this specimen does not consist of detached mucous membrane, but of complete fibrinous cast of the bowels similar to what occurs from bronchial tubes in diphtheria. *Such casts are far from uncommon in dysentery, but this is the first which has been deposited in the army medical museum.* Thanking you for the specimen and history."[154] Indeed, Woodward offered clinical guidance throughout and long after the war: "Sections of morbid growths, and other specimens sent to the Surgeon General's Office by the medical officers of the Army for an opinion as to their nature, have been added, with a certain number of other specimens, especially in the direction of normal and pathological histology. The collection now contains about 7,000 permanently mounted microscopial slides."[155]

These examples could go on and on, but it is the general pattern as revealed by these case histories that is important. Physicians unambiguously embraced this new medical expertise and, while more subtly, so did the government and the larger public. Physicians adopted a powerful discourse about wartime medical care: perhaps through this program of research and investigative medicine the men in blue still alive and fighting the war might be saved. As one observer noted, "The necessity of prompt measures to secure the health and thus promote the efficiency of the vast army of volunteers who, in defense of the nation's life, clustered around the old army as a nucleus, not only invoked the best efforts of the authorities in Washington and the zealous cooperation of the State governments, but stirred the masses everywhere. The purpose to provide for the soldiers comfort had no rival in popular consideration."[156] Army surgeon Jonathan Letterman (who would later revolutionize the ambulance system) wrote Hammond, "It always affords me pleasure to cooperate with you in any way possible to advance the interests of the museum, which does so much."[157] Like many physicians, Letterman felt the opportunity of the war should not be lost: "I shall be glad to cooperate with you in any way in my power to amass something out of the dying in this war."[158]

The campaign to train and teach young, inexperienced physicians was an important ideal in the wartime program of medicine and medical research. But this institutional support for medicine, this drive for new knowledge, also benefited the elite physicians, as illustrated in the case of physician Henry Hartshorne.[159] Hartshorne was a prominent Philadelphia physician who received his A.B. from Haverford College in the early 1840s and his M.D. from the University of Pennsylvania in 1845. His thesis entitled "Water and Hydropathy" was well received by his peers.[160] His many medical experiences and career choices demonstrate the many different opportunities that physicians looked for in these years, and his Civil War medical service was an integral part of his development as a physician.

Hartshorne served as resident physician at Pennsylvania Hospital from 1846 to 1848, while simultaneously operating a medical practice. In 1853 and 1854, he became a professor of the Institutes of Medicine at the Philadelphia College of Medicine, and the following year he worked in Columbia, Pennsylvania, during a cholera outbreak there. In 1855 he became a consulting physician and lecturer on clinical medicine at the Philadelphia Hospital, and from 1857 to 1858 he lectured on natural history at the Franklin Institute. In 1859 he became professor of the theory and practice of medicine at Pennsylvania College in Gettysburg, a post he held until the war broke out in 1861.[161] During the Civil War, he worked at two government hospitals in Philadelphia and volunteered his services after the Battle of Gettysburg (July 1–3, 1863). Like all attending physicians, he was required to submit all of his case histories: "According to the instructions, I submit the following remarks upon cases occurring in the ward to which I have been attached as medical officer since July 10, 1862."[162]

By doing so, he was forced to really think about the dynamics of disease: "Difficulty must exist sometimes insurmountably in making out an accurate diagnosis of cases brought to a hospital from a distance often with a sickness of several weeks duration, of the character of the early symptoms of which little or no account can be obtained. I confess therefore to a considerable delay in making up my mind as to the true character of these cases which have afforded us the most painfully interesting study."[163] He then prepared a long and detailed report regarding "scorbutic marasmus" including symptoms, diagnosis, treatment, and postmortem appearance, which he subsequently compared with a report prepared by Dr. Samuel Gross. The two found a series of coincidences "too striking not to indicate a pathogenic association." These related to a combination of follicular colitis with double pneumonia of the posterior portions of the lungs—but the usual symptoms associated with this affection (cough, pain in the chest, expectoration, or delirium) were not well marked. Instead, and interestingly, they commented on the "hepatization found in the lungs," with "commencing suppuration" after death, a finding Gross and Hartshorne found both unique and puzzling, and one that demanded further study.[164]

Physicians could distinguish themselves among the profession through this project, and those who aspired to eminence in the profession benefited tremendously from the directives of Circular No. 2. John Shaw Billings, for example, had just graduated from the Medical College of Ohio in 1860. Shortly after the disastrous First Battle of Bull Run, he applied for an army commission in September 1861 and, after his successful exam, was appointed a contract surgeon. In April 1862 he was commissioned first lieutenant and assigned with the task of converting the cavalry barracks at Cliffburne into a hospital, after which he was ordered to Philadelphia, where he remained for almost a year.[165]

Billings worked at the West Philadelphia Hospital with Joseph Leidy, who taught Billings the basic principles of microscopy, a research tool that in 1862 was very new to Billings.[166] He made a number of valuable contacts while in Philadelphia. Silas Weir Mitchell, with whom he would form a lifelong friendship, noted, "My first acquaintance with John Billings was in the early days of the war—the exact date I cannot give you—but he was for a time attached to Philadelphia Hospitals and either then or previously was the excellent and warm friend of my brother, a medical cadet, Edward Kearsely Mitchell. He had charge of him during a part of his fatal illness and I remember with gratitude his tenderness and his close relation to this brilliant young life. This was the beginning of a life-long friendship and opportunities of helping each other in a great variety of ways."[167]

By 1874 Billings was "regarded as the foremost authority in public hygiene in America" and had an international reputation for hospital construction.[168] Also highly regarded for his surgical work, he was the first American surgeon successfully to perform an excision of an ankle joint (on January 6, 1862).[169] His high standing in public health and surgery was an exceptional attainment for someone so young, and an examination of his wartime work provides an interesting insight into his development.

In May 1862 Billings reported to the Cliffburne hospital and submitted a report of his work there to the surgeon general, dated July 1862. In his report he focused on "histories of cases of special interest," including operations, treatment, specimen analyses, and postmortem results.[170] Billings was meticulous in his reporting and recommendations. He took charge of

159 cases of gunshot wounds of "varying position, character and gravity," most of these belonging to Rebel soldiers who had been captured at the Battle of Williamsburg (May 5, 1862). All the wounds, Billings noted, were "suppurating and all the operations performed were necessarily secondary and performed on men too exhausted by a long journey and the pain arising from broken and splintered bones and despondent at being prisoners, all factors to be taken into account in estimating the percentage of mortality."[171] Eighteen cases developed erysipelas, which "responded to local circumscription with pure creosote and nitric acid" and an internal treatment of "quinine with full diet."

Billings was pleased with the results of the case of J. H. Miles of Virginia, who at the Battle of Williamsburg had been struck by a minié ball, which had "entered the left arm on its outer aspect about 4 inches below the outer third of the clavicle on the same side."[172] Billings noted in the case file that the "humerus was found so extensively split and shattered that amputation of the shoulder was clearly indicated—which operation I immediately performed by the oval method. Not more than two ounces of blood were lost. Five ligatures were used and the flaps closed by suture."[173] Billings prescribed "proper diet" and "simple cold water dressings," and the patient "improved steadily" and within 10 days was "walking perfectly convalescent." This case was later published in the *Medical and Surgical History of the War*.[174]

He also performed, for the first time in his career, a cranial procedure known as trephining.[175] William Rogers, a private from Company G of the 7th Ohio Volunteers, was wounded at the Battle of Fort Republic by a minié ball, which struck the "frontal bone one inch above the edge of the right orbit."[176] It is recorded in his case file that the patient was "rendered insensible for a few moments after being struck but soon recovered sufficiently to walk off the field"; on admission to the hospital June 15, the patient complained of "but little pain, pupils were normal, pulse regular"; however, "pulsation of the brain was evident, loose splinters of bone to be felt."[177] Billings thus decided to perform a cranial operation in which the "wound was enlarged and the fragments of bone were removed with the forceps." However, the ball which had "entered the substance of the brain" was not found. The patient developed an infection, continued his decline, and almost three weeks after being admitted to the hospital, died. During the postmortem, Billings examined the course of the wound and found the ball "much twisted upon itself lying in a sack of false membrane about one inch beneath the surface of the dura mater—the lateral ventricle of the right side having been opened." He studied the brain quite extensively, and even though he had barely touched a microscope before his service in the war, he studied the cyst containing the ball microscopically and noted that it consisted of "interlacing fibres, containing large cells."[178]

In March 1863 Billings received orders from Hammond to report to Jonathan Letterman for duty assignment with the United States Infantry, Second Brigade, Second Division, Fifth Corps.[179] He served in this capacity for nearly two years and was almost always in the field. He noted in his *Narrative of Service* that upon his arrival he immediately began scouting locations for hospitals and engaged in several surgeries, including "several amputations among these: two at the shoulder joint also one exsection of the same joint and one of the elbow."[180] During the Battle of Chancellorsville (May 1–3, 1863), shortly after Billings assumed his new post, he established a field hospital at the headquarters occupied by General Hooker (after Hooker had inexplicably retreated from the battle)[181] and found a brick house for the purpose. He noted that "at this place the most extensive shell wounds that I have ever seen came under notice. . . . In two instances the abdominal wall was entirely carried away and from a third I removed the entire head of a three inch shell which had passed into the abdominal cavity and was slightly impacted in the bodies of the lumbar vertebrae."[182]

Billings was clearly overwhelmed. He continued, "In a fourth case the fragment of a shell had passed through the pelvis from one trochanter to the other; while in another the arm had been torn entirely off and the brachial artery was hanging out three inches in length and pulsating to within one inch from the end. In two of them it proved difficult to return the protruded mass which in each case was as large as one's fist as the muscles of the abdominal wall were strongly and spasmodically contracted."[183] Conditions were difficult; however, Billings was able successfully to "lift the abdominal walls away from and over the tumor and close the wounds hermetically by means of sutures and collodion."[184]

He worked continuously after the Battle of Chancellorsville and was placed in charge of the corps hospital before being assigned to the 7th Infantry as a medical officer for the U.S. Army during the march toward Gettysburg (July 1–3).[185] Once in Gettysburg, Billings and his colleague Charles Wagner selected "what we supposed would be the most eligible position for a hospital."[186] When the battle began Billings "performed a large number of operations of various kinds and worked all night without cessation."[187] When his division moved on July 4, Billings stayed behind in charge of the hospital, which contained about 800 sick and wounded soldiers. He ordered seventeen hospital tents to be pitched, and in them he tended to the "most severe cases; about 17 in number." He noted that Medical Inspector John Brinton arrived with the much-needed medical supplies and that he was able to also procure clean, fresh straw, beef, and commissary stores from the town. He praised surgeons Ramsey, Whittingham, Bacon, and Prenneman, whose "energy and zeal made the labor of organizing the hospital quickly completed."[188]

It was here that Billings developed his most intensive experience as a surgeon. He lamented that there were too many operations to give details of them all, but he did comment on a few remarkable cases, including exsections of the shoulder joint.[189] He also commented on three cases of hemorrhage, in which he opened the flaps and secured the bleeding vessel. He saw six cases of gunshot wound of the thorax, which were handled by his colleague Assistant Surgeon Howard, who treated these men by hermetically sealing the orifice with collodion, a liquid adhesive. Billings was interested in these cases and thus made a postmortem of one to study further the effect of the wound, remarking on the unusual "abscess of the lung communicating with the pleural cavity which was filled with a sanio purulent fluid." He also commented on five cases of gunshot fracture of the cranium which involved the occipital bone, all proving fatal. He noted that in these cases the onset of death was preceded by a "low muttering form of delirium with occasional paroxysms of furious mania."[190]

Billings's adeptness as a surgeon and skill in hospital organization again did not go unnoticed. The medical director of the Army of the Potomac, Thomas McParlin (who had relieved Letterman), commented that Billings had "rendered me the most valuable, varied and constant aid in the discharge of general duties assigned and special ones that emergencies required."[191] After serving for a short time as medical inspector of the Army of the Potomac (where he was asked to collect specimens for the Army Medical Museum), he was officially transferred to the museum in the fall of 1864; there he assisted Woodward in the preparation of specimens, in particular in the microscopial section, which was rapidly developing.[192] It was here that Billings began his long service as one of the leading advocates of scientific medicine in the United States.[193]

When Billings helped design the new hospital and laboratory at Johns Hopkins a few years later, he was instrumental in designing the new curriculum, which focused on areas in which he had become skilled during the war, including record keeping and the development of physiological, microscopial, and pathological laboratories. Much of the efficacy of the

Johns Hopkins program "was its emphasis on learning rather than spoon fed teaching," and on the "laboratory, dissecting rooms and ward rather than the lecture room."[194] Stressing the ideal to "learn by doing" was a methodology not unfamiliar to Billings; indeed, medical practice during the war required industriousness, and the very essence of both wartime medicine and Circular No. 2 demanded that physicians "learn by doing." While Billings was later more successful than others, he was by no means atypical during the war.

THE DIFFUSION OF WARTIME MEDICINE

The broad picture of wartime medicine that emerges from these experiences was that in the sprawling wards of the Civil War hospitals and in the new medical museum, American physicians, for the first time, directed and facilitated a wide field of scientific investigation.[195] Civil War physicians were able to transcend what many physicians thought was the major limitation of the Paris Clinical School—weak medical museums.[196] By contrast, the elite and rank and file, teachers and students, together were able to augment their wartime clinical work with a medical museum of unparalleled scope.

The museum was in fact a unique educational center in the third quarter of the nineteenth century—not just in America but in the world. As one observer suggested, "Special work is being done in the several separate departments of the museum. One of the most important now in progress is the preparation of a series of sections through the human body, made in every possible direction." He further noted that the object of these preparations, which were completely unique, "is to show the organs of the human body from every possible point of view, thus in the complete series, exhibiting, as has never been done before, all the minute relations of adjacent organs. . . . This series of sections is being beautifully mounted, and when completed will be of great practical value to physicians and surgeons."[197] Those working at the medical museum strove to make sure the wartime specimens would be presented in a way that American physicians could learn about specific disease states. Of the medical series Woodward noted that "each preparation after careful dissection, in order that the lesion to be exhibited may be as clearly displayed as possible, is suspended in alcohol from a glass hook in the stopper of a fine glass jar." The case would then be numbered and displayed along with the case history.[198]

Of all the messages that American physicians relayed about this project, this grand undertaking, the one that resonated most was the drive for medical education and reform. The project in many ways organized the profession by providing the stability that medical societies were missing owing to their lack of licensing powers. Billings later suggested, "What should be the relation of this central national collection to those formed in different parts of the country, either in connection with medical schools, or with museums of broader scope? Certainly they should help one another, and this can be done in many ways." He continued, "I would say to the anatomist of a school, when you have made a copy for the national collection, . . . it will be seen by the anatomists of all schools and of all countries. To the pathologist of a medical school . . . after you have secured type specimens for your own collection put aside other good specimens for the National Medical Museum. On the other hand, the collections of the National Museum are available for study by any proper person, and its duplicates should be used to aid other museums which may be in special need of them."[199]

Physicians and aspiring medical scientists alike found support for scientific inquiry, and they were no longer professionally isolated: the prepared specimens and publications were vital in creating a network that linked physicians in America to the wider world of Paris, London, Vienna, and Berlin in a community of knowledge.[200] As an example, Dr. J. Murmich of Berlin, a surgeon in the Prussian army, traveled to America to observe medical practice in the United States as well as some of the recent work performed during the war. He was impressed with the wartime research and requested an exchange of German publications for copies of the *American Journal of the Medical Sciences.* As Joseph Henry noted, "I have informed him that the transmission of the two works, to and from this country can be counted on through the Smithsonian agency."[201] Woodward too commented that "this [anatomical collection] is not a museum of curiosities, it is a collection that teaches."[202] The collection received high praise from many visitors, including Dr. Meusal of Gotha, who stated:

> The art and manner with which the material was collected gives
> us a high opinion of our colleagues, who in the midst of the bustle
> of war have brought it together scientifically. . . . They lost no time
> in preparing specimens of interest and instruction to the observer.
> The abstracts of case histories are brief and clear, and the numerous
> illustrations excellent, and the aim to give complete information
> concerning the course of the disease and the result of an operation,
> deserves the greatest recognition. . . . Through the fact that

everybody is able to provide himself with a printed catalogue and that he may orient himself at home as to what he wishes to study, the museum becomes a common possession to all physicians.[203]

The idea that the museum could be a "common possession" for physicians was truly remarkable, and physicians strove to be part of the larger project. George Alexander Otis, who replaced Brinton as curator of the surgical and photographic sections of the museum in October 1864, noted: "The museum received contributions relating to collateral subjects . . . many pathological specimens not specially pertaining to military medicine or surgery and many preparations of human and comparative anatomy had been received, a cabinet of microscopial preparations had been accumulated, models and drawings of hospitals and medical and surgical instruments had been contributed."[204] In a report from Brinton to Surgeon General Barnes, he noted that a central part of the museum's value is that it is "used weekly and almost daily" by the civil profession throughout the country.[205] In his annual report to Congress, Joseph Barnes observed that between April and September 1867, 4,245 persons visited the museum, "many of them medical officers of the army and former officers of volunteers, eminent professional men from various portions of the United States and Europe."[206]

As news of the project proliferated, a system of exchanges was also made with numerous pathological societies, universities, hospitals, and museums in America, Britain, and Germany. Publications based on museum work were also sent around the globe, along with requests for scientific work of interest to be donated to the museum.[207] Those connected with this work made claim to having specialized knowledge and important information to share—a reflection of the confidence that this project generated among physicians. The publications were American and reflect America's identity as a producer of medical knowledge. This is not meant to be a triumphalist narrative, but one cannot help but get caught up in the general excitement generated by this project. In 1870 the *Medical and Surgical Reporter* noted of the medical literature, "In these publications it has been our aim to supply the wants of the greatest number of the profession . . . our course has been independent and American, and so it will continue to be."[208] The works produced during the war were referenced so frequently afterward that the publishers of the *Medical Gazette* felt compelled to address the issue, "We make no apology to calling so frequently the attention of our readers to the publications of the Surgeon General's Office, because they constitute such important accessions to our original medical literature."[209]

There was unparalleled loss caused by the Civil War. Throughout the war and after, Americans began the uneasy process of defining a new relationship with death, and the "living had to find meaning in the dead."[210] The museum was one way to make sense of the death, to find larger meaning in it, or to imbue the war dead with a sense of national importance. As one observer recalled, "We have visited the museum in its new and permanent location, and can cordially endorse the assertion of the Surgeon General that, 'by its array of indisputable facts, supported and enriched by full reports, it supplies instruction otherwise unattainable, and preserves, for future application, the dearly bought experience of four years of war,' and that, 'apart from its great usefulness, it is also an honorable record of those medical officers whose contributions constitute its value, and whose incentive to their self-imposed labors has been the desire to elevate their profession.'"[211]

The museum and Circular No. 2 were important in reorienting American medicine along more scientific guidelines. It was not long before this new scientific ethos among American physicians led to scientific advance. Collecting specimens and writing case reports encouraged American physicians to become more independent but also supported the development of new forms of specialized knowledge. As physicians studied various diseases in their hospital wards and prodded patients, trying to properly diagnose them, medical ideas started to become more sophisticated. For the rank and file in the thousands, this meant becoming familiar with hospital medicine and dissection, a domestic acquaintance that far transcended any foreign influence. For the elite practitioner, though, Parisian medicine was starting to seem limited in how far it could move the medical sciences forward, and some physicians worked to develop new tools to manage, understand, and investigate disease.

CHAPTER TWO

The Limits of Morbid Anatomy and the Development of New Medical Techniques

The war provided an abundance of bodies, and physicians eagerly dissected them. Before the war, dissection was largely "conducted on the margins of legality."[1] The practice was sometimes a contentious and volatile issue, as discussed in chapter 5. However, the context of anatomical study changed within the army during the war. It was no longer unsavory or associated with grave robbing under the cover of darkness; rather the Union's program of dissection was about advancing medical knowledge and learning and developing techniques that might translate into better care for the living. Rank-and-file physicians learned firsthand the methods of the Paris Clinical School, learned comparative anatomy, and saw diseased bodies and studied lesions in the hopes that the process might reveal the causes of the pervasive camp and hospital diseases that ravaged Union soldiers.

This opportunity to master the body was compelling for many physicians, but then there had always been a fascination with the postmortem both for its utility and for the sense of professional achievement this mastery provided. As Michael Sappol has demonstrated, knowledge of anatomy was the hallmark of the well-trained physician in 1860.[2] However, in the absence of adequate provisions for providing bodies, physicians increasingly traveled abroad for such access, which, as John Harley Warner has argued, transformed "American medical ideas, practices and, above all, epistemology."[3] Yet just under a thousand physicians studied in Paris, and while this influence was significant particularly among elite practitioners, Paris did not readily transform American medicine before the Civil War. There were thousands of individual physicians who knew Paris only at second hand, and in 1860 the bulk of American physicians still did not have equal access to hospital experience and bodies. Moreover, even the most elite physicians were often frustrated with the "meager opportunities for human dissection in America."[4] The eminent physician William Gerhard often complained, for example, of the difficulties of studying pathological anatomy with the "subjects so scarce in Philadelphia."[5] Thus while the orthodoxy did indeed seek to develop the "Paris Program" in America, particularly to be on the same footing with European medical science, the limitations already discussed made the development of dissection in American education and among American medical practitioners uneven at best. It was thus not until the war years that the options for anatomy changed for the "many" physicians.

During the war American medicine went through a rapid period of growth. Hundreds of hospitals were erected to manage the thousands of troops that needed treatment, but there were also thousands of bodies created by the war, as already discussed, leading to new educational opportunities. As Joseph Woodward observed, autopsies and the study of specimens allowed some doctors to see the pathological alterations of disease for the very first time.[6] When physicians brought pathology into medical practice on a large scale, it promised intellectual vitality, professional legitimacy, and perhaps superior medical care. The brilliant French physician Xavier Bichat once observed that "several autopsies will give you more light than twenty years of observation and symptoms."[7]

THE UNION'S PROGRAM OF DISSECTION

Knowledge of anatomy was necessary for understanding the structure and the function of the body in health and disease and was also the cornerstone of medical education at the time. Indeed, Hammond saw dissection as an essential part of both teaching and learning medicine and demanded that autopsies should be done in all "interesting" or "important" cases as a matter of professional interest.[8] Circular No. 2 proved significant in the development of this research tool and encouraged regular and volunteer, elite and rank-and-file physicians to become acquainted with and even proficient in anatomy. Since Circulars No. 2 and 5 required that physicians leave behind a record of their work, which was displayed in the museum and captured in the case notes, this work became visible not only to members of the profession but also to the larger public.[9] As homeopathists, among other sects, feared early in the war, this work or master narrative made the collection of specimens and autopsies routine and supported the emergence of a national medical identity rooted in scientific medicine.[10]

The Surgeon General's Office initially informed physicians that the body was not to be mutilated unnecessarily; examinations were to be made of "those parts that will furnish information regarding the nature and history of the case" and the context of wound or disease, the effect of disease, and rigor mortis; the expression on the face at the time of death (in the attempt to determine level of pain) and the external aspect of death were areas to be addressed in the case report.[11] There were two very different ways that physicians recorded their autopsies. The experienced physician, working in a general hospital, usually had many pages of observations relating to each autopsy, which were kept in a casebook or folder. They were detailed, thoughtful, and a mark of the physician's experiential separation from the "masses." These case reports were thorough analyses of the body; although the organ affected by disease received the most study, attention was given to the entire body both in general and in an attempt to understand either the path of the missile or the effect of disease. There was still reliance on clinical information, but because that was not always available, many reports were conducted in isolation from clinical facts and were primarily analytical.

The second set of sources consists of the standardized forms issued during the war as a tool to enable the less experienced physician to participate and to learn from this area of medicine.[12] In other words, there were very specific categories designed to guide physicians on how to dissect the body—much like "blueprints," the forms were basic but effective anatomy guides. They were often used at field hospitals, where there was less time for in-depth study and reflection. The focus was commonly on the immediate cause of death rather than on the entire function of the body. As such, tracing the missile through the body in the attempt to anticipate the damage caused by weapons was the primary objective, and the practice provides an interesting lens into postmortems in the field. Physicians, however, still used the body as a resource in which to develop military medicine for the benefit of treatment in future wars.

The physician John Woodworth, medical inspector of the Army of the Tennessee during the Atlanta campaign, performed and supervised postmortems at Field Hospital 15. Field hospitals, temporary and often very rough work sites—institutions, homes, or tents, usually located in close proximity to battlefields or camps—were especially chaotic and horrific after large battles. One woman, for example, commented on the trains carrying "bloody freight."[13] By 1862 Letterman had successfully reorganized the medical operations of the Army of the Potomac. Among his many reforms, medical operations were organized by division not regiment, field hospitals were set up before battle, and supplies were stockpiled (including blankets

Standard postmortem form (Courtesy of the National Archives, Washington, D.C.)

and tents). Captains were appointed to command ambulances in each corps, and sergeants managed divisions, brigades, and regiments.

Each regiment was supplied with a four-horse and two-horse ambulance and given instructions on how to proceed once the battle was under way. Ambulances were equipped with canned meat, milk, bread, and medical supplies. The members within the new ambulance corps, including a surgeon to supervise, were identified by a green band around the cap and half chevrons on each arm. They had the task of removing wounded men from the field and transporting them to the temporary hospitals.[14] The chaos after battle placed a premium on correct diagnoses—when performing triage, surgeons had to first evaluate the scope and severity of the wounds. They had to decide which men could be treated in the field hospitals and which cases needed to be transported to division hospitals located near the camps or to the large general hospitals located in cities. Within this improved organizational structure, physicians were able to perform autopsies in the field hospitals.

John Woodworth conducted or supervised postmortems in almost half of the cases that came under his attention.[15] The case reports are short and illustrate the wound, treatment, cause of death or complications, and postmortem. John Thompson, a private of Company B of the 83rd Indiana Volunteer Infantry, for example, was admitted to the hospital after being injured at Kennesaw Mountain on June 28, 1864. His case file noted that the wound "badly lacerated the muscles of the thigh," the femur was "fractured very high up," and the leg was "very painful and much swollen."[16] He was treated with cold-water dressings to the leg and morphine for the pain. The patient suffered with a fever and nausea until he died eight days after his admission to the hospital. During the postmortem, the femur was found to be badly shattered "from two inches below the greater trochanter (upper bony section) downwards, about four inches several fragments were entirely separated from their attachments." The muscles were "badly disorganized and a fragment of shell weighing nearly ½ lb. was found buried beneath the facia of the thigh." The report concluded: "I have the piece of shell, also the fragments of bones preserved which are at your disposal."[17]

Even within the chaos and confusion of battle and the inevitable difficulties of managing the dead and dying after battle, the desire of the physicians to learn and gain knowledge from these bodies was a pervasive theme. Sergeant J. K. Hillard, Company A of the 121st Pennsylvania Volunteers, had been wounded at the Battle of Gettysburg by a minié ball, which had entered on the right side of the chest, and which came out through the inner border of the scapula about two inches above its apex.[18] His case report noted that upon admission to the hospital the patient was "broken down in health; feeble, anemic, tongue furred and having a dusky hue of countenance"; while the "wound of entrance looked well the exit was sloughing and discharging ichorous pus and the soft tissue around the scapula were boggy."[19] He was treated with milk punch, beef essence, and tonics, and the wounds were dressed with a fermented poultice. The wound was cauterized to stop the spread of erysipelas and sloughing, which was followed by "profuse diarrhea and vomiting."

Despite continued treatment, the patient died three days later, and a postmortem was made eight hours after death. The report commented on the scattered tubercules found on each lung, along with some hypostatic congestion. All the other organs were healthy. On examining the course of the wound, it was found that the "ball had run round on the upper border of the third rib and out behind." The report also commented on a large abscess found "under surface of the scapula—that bone in fact denuded of its periosteum." Thus it was concluded that "death had evidently occurred from extreme exhaustion dependent on his condition."[20]

While some of the postmortems performed in the field lacked extensive analysis, that was not always the case; peculiar or unfamiliar cases provoked still more thorough examination. The case of Henry Johnson, a private from the Illinois Volunteer Infantry, was of particular interest. Henry Johnson entered the field hospital with a gunshot wound of the right arm fracturing the humerus bone that connects the shoulder to the elbow. A resection of the middle third of the humerus had been performed before his arrival at the hospital. Upon admission, his case file noted, the patient was "very pale emaciated, anemic, very restless and fitful complaining of pains in the legs and suffering from slight diarrhea."[21] He was treated with a usual course of quinine, milk punch, opium, ale tinc, and ferri chloride for a week, at which time it was noted that "the diarrhea is a little better, the pulse which had been very frequent and feeble all the time became a little less frequent and feebler." He was then given tapioca, wine, milk punch, and morphia. Twelve days after admission, his case report noted that "the wound which had looked well up to this time, now discharged a little chocolate colored fetid matter," which signaled a serious infection.

Henry Johnson died the next day. The doctors were concerned and puzzled by the case. It was observed that "his mind seemed somewhat deranged," and it was "learned that he acted strangely while with his regiment." The physician, curious about these symptoms, looked for clues as to why. He began with an examination of the lungs, heart, liver, stomach, intestines, and bodily fluids. He then moved on to the brain. He studied the dura matter, blood vessels, the cerebra, and the side ventricles and found that "the soft part of the cerebra opposite the crista galli contained between its layers a thin piece of bone, about one inch long, a quarter of an inch wide and as thick as a playing card, with smooth irregular edges" and that overall the "brain if anything was a little softer than usual."[22]

But for the most part the postmortems performed in the field hospital were largely empirical and provided thousands of observations on the effect of missiles, in the hope that the experts at the Army Medical Museum would profit from this information. These case notes give an excellent record of medical practice during the war, but they were equally important in the development of science: postmortems as a tool of inquiry became routine, allowing physicians the opportunity to become familiar with the body in new and unprecedented ways and conversant in pathological anatomy even in the most difficult circumstances. But equally important was the role of the postmortem in American medical education. So many of the war physicians came from diverse educational backgrounds and were shaped by the individualism of Jacksonian America that there were wide variations in treating, managing, and understanding disease. The directive to perform postmortems created a common experience for the rank-and-file American physicians and a chance to develop knowledge of gross human anatomy. The message was that this common set of experiences, rooted in a deeper understanding of the body, would create a new foundation for medical practice and education.

The general hospital records reveal that the order to perform postmortems led to a new medical model that supported both investigative medicine and pathological specialism. For elite physicians, this hospital experience was the apex of wartime medical science. General hospitals usually occupied large buildings and were constructed in large cities or near water or rail transport.[23] These new, large institutions furnished clinical material for analysis, and physicians were encouraged to study and learn from the bodies under their care. Thousands of autopsy reports were submitted to the Army Medical Museum, and in most cases postmortems were performed not longer than twenty-four hours after death but usually within twelve hours or less.

Medical inspector John LeConte demanded that physicians be thoughtful and careful when performing surgeries and autopsies. In addition to the case history, he also wanted each surgeon to state "*distinctly* his reasons for considering the operation necessary"; the description of the anatomical lesion; the nature of discharge, if treatment was successful; and, in the case of death, an additional note, in a separate blank, listing all postmortem observations.[24] A more careful and measured approach to studying patients and disease was encouraged in this context. What was most interesting about the Union's program of dissection was the new confidence with the dead body. In the reflections and case histories of the war physicians, one can detect the source of new ideas and the development of more innovative ways to understand, study, and manage the body.

The significance of this program was in fact vital for many physicians. For medical knowledge to change and develop through the war, physicians had not only to learn but to master anatomy. As noted earlier, W. W. Keen was tremendously inexperienced when he performed his first few dissections; however, as the war progressed, a very different Keen emerged. A case report prepared by Keen at Satterlee hospital illustrates, for example, the learning and teaching environment that the war physicians created.[25] As an example, John Shober, then a private in Company C, 14th New York, had been wounded at Malvern Hill during the Peninsula campaign on July 1,

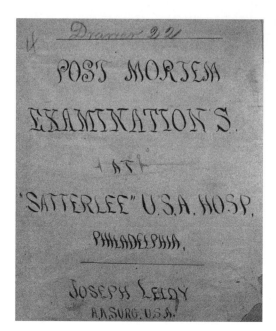

Postmortem examinations at Satterlee General Hospital, case histories of Joseph Leidy (Courtesy of the National Archives, Washington, D.C.)

1862. Shober was admitted to Satterlee hospital July 26, 1862, suffering from "diarrhea as a result of exposure." The patient was "very prostrate" and was brought to the ward on a stretcher and in almost "moribund condition."

At this juncture, Keen organized a consultation with the physicians then at Satterlee—Drs. Lewis, Hutchinson, Alter, Agnew, and Smith. This was in fact proper protocol and was common practice in the general hospitals. Together the doctors decided that a free incision should be made, the dead and loose bone removed, a single splint applied with a dressing of lint moistened in a solution of chlorinated soda, and a sling fitted to support the arm at right angles. They worried, though, about the patient's unpleasant chest symptoms, including a hacking cough and persistent pain in his right side. The Satterlee physicians ordered a course of beef essence, milk punch, quinine, and morphia. Within days, however, complications arose. The case report noted "abscesses formed, the quantity of pus was enormous," and "several pieces of bone were thrown off from time to time." The patient rallied and showed a slight improvement until December 15, 1862, at which point he became "very pale and suffers again from diarrhea." He died February 7, 1863.[26]

The postmortem was performed by Dr. Leidy in consultation with the physicians that admitted and treated the patient. Leidy noted, "The case presents several points of interest including the amputation when the patient arrived, the propriety of the exsection when performed, the cause of death and the value of the autopsy in showing the previous disease as well as proving that pyaemia did not occur. Amputation was at once laid aside by unanimous consent and the bodily disease seemed to indicate exsection upon arrival as unnecessary: but one can believe that as soon as the diarrhea and general health became better the bone should have been removed." Importantly, he concluded that the propriety of the exsection when performed was beyond a doubt. The cause of death was "undoubtedly pneumonia arising from the exposure to the cold. The autopsy renders all clear and is of assistance and value to the surgeon which otherwise would bury his skill and cause failure."[27]

The order to perform postmortems had a still more profound influence regarding how knowledge should be gained. Private James M. Loughlin of Wisconsin had been struck in the left hand on May 3, 1863, at Fredericksburg, and upon admission to Douglas Hospital May 8 it was noted in his case file that, along with the injury to his left hand, he also had a fracture of the left femur, but with no apparent external wound. It soon became evident that the knee joint was involved, and physicians decided that the femur might have been fissured into the joint.[28] The thigh became swollen and "fluctuated distinctly," and the pus accumulated to such an extent "as to disturb the integument from the hip-joint to the foot."

Assistant Surgeon Thomson believed the best course of treatment was to "leave the case to nature," feeling that life would be prolonged a few days by doing so. But the patient suffered tremendously. Thomson was concerned by the huge amounts of pus, but worse, the patient seemed "desperate, suffering profuse perspiration, dry tongue, rapid and feeble pulse," constantly and incoherently "muttering, delirious with diarrhea and a faint sickening of the breath." After "lingering until June 16," the patient finally expired. The case was of considerable interest to Thomson, and he thus performed a postmortem.

At first Thomson looked at the sheer number of openings through the integument under the surface of the thigh, which seemed to be communicating with the abscess. But after a closer look, he discovered a closed ball wound near the head of the fibula, which he suggested explained the "curious involvement of the joint." The bullet was found lying in contact with the femur. He thus determined that the ball must have passed near enough to the joint to involve it secondarily. He warned Hammond that this was a case that could teach surgeons at the field hospitals, those on the front lines of medical duty: "This case illustrates very perfectly the mode of death in wounds of the knee joint. The immense abscess in the thigh with some fluctuation in the joint was confirmed by tracing the track of the ball beneath it on its way to the point of fracture of the femur where the bullet was found. A careful examination and correct diagnosis in the field might have led to an early amputation which may have saved life." However, he cautioned that this would have been a most questionable procedure at the period when the case was received at his hospital because the patient was already suffering from severe infection.[29]

The postmortem reports reveal an interest in and a deeply intimate look at the internal body. As understandings of the body changed through the war, so too did the types of questions physicians were asking and thus the methods for managing these cases. Wartime medicine was anything but didactic; the emphasis, rather, was on developing practical knowledge. There was no single blueprint for change, but some physicians were no longer content merely to examine the dead body with the naked eye—there was increasing focus on a physiology of disease. Some physicians encouraged the study of the minute parts of the body and the fluids in an attempt to better understand disease processes.

In Satterlee hospital, Joseph Leidy recognized this opportunity. Leidy often positioned the practice of the postmortem as a "singular scientific endeavor," and it is not surprising that he so thoroughly embraced the wartime medical opportunities.[30] In the year before the outbreak of war, he suggested that medicine could not acquire the "dignity" of science "until it was based on an acquaintance with anatomy and physiology."[31] He had long been interested in microscopic anatomy and pathology and had studied in Paris with Pierre Louis. In 1861 Leidy was a professor of anatomy at the University of Pennsylvania, but anxiously sought a commission in the war so he could pursue further his interest in the body.

Yet a test of his existing medical knowledge could produce a reaffirmation of the wartime program of research—and it did. Leidy performed numerous postmortem examinations, and the general pattern of his case reports reflects his interest in both unfamiliar cases and investigative innovation. For example, in the case numbered 116 in Leidy's casebook, Peter Longheran, a private from Philadelphia, was diagnosed July 11, 1863, with tetanus due to an injury of the left ulnar nerve from a gunshot wound just below the elbow.[32] Leidy was curious to see whether his injury resulted in structural changes in the nerve itself and thus excised and examined the nerves microscopically.[33] He later submitted the nerves to the Army Medical Museum as per the order of Circular No. 2.

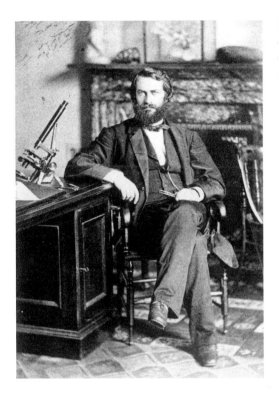

Joseph Leidy (Courtesy of the Academy of Natural Sciences, ANSP_Coll_457_Leidy_at_desk, © Academy of Natural Sciences)

In the case of Private Zach Banbier of the 136th New York Regulars, Leidy more extensively studied his body, which had been shot twice: in the right hand, which resulted in the loss of two fingers, and in the right arm about four inches below the shoulder, which was quickly attacked by gangrene. It was the gangrene that most interested Leidy. He concentrated on the pathological changes, and excised and studied the fluids in an attempt to delineate the cause of inflammation. It was common practice to focus first on the path of the missile. Leidy noted that the ball had struck the bone several inches below the head but did not fracture it at that point. The head of the bone was found detached from the shaft, and the neighboring parts extending downward to the orifice of the ball in the muscles and skin were found to be gangrenous.

He looked closer at some troubling aspects of the case, such as the upper part of the vein extending with the brachial, which was inflamed and contained pus, "which mingled with the blood, in the rupture of a slight pseudo-membranous or fibronous clot which had confined it." He also noted that for some reason both lungs were inflamed but especially the lower lobe of the left one, which contained a number of small abscesses. The fluids were of particular interest to Leidy: "The bowels were distended with air, and were agglutinated by recent soft yellowish, white pseudo-membrane from peritonitis. The cavity of the peritoneum also contained a quantity of thin pus." He commented on a "quantity of black fluid like matter in the stomach, and mucous, a similar fluid to which the patient had vomited." Finally, he mentioned that the spleen was large and flabby and contained several large abscesses. The liver, except for some inflammation, and the kidneys were deemed healthy.[34] He proceeded to microscopically study the fluids and preserved the spleen and lungs for the Army Medical Museum along with his case notes. He probably chose these specimens because of the abscesses, which Woodward also liked to study microscopically.[35]

The museum was important in supporting not only the work of the more experienced physicians but also the development of the next generation of American physicians. This structure was important for the production and reception of medical knowledge. For example, Leidy, like his contemporaries, noted at the conclusion of most of his autopsy reports what he preserved for the museum, thereby elucidating which specimens were important for showcasing specific diseases and wounds. Henry A. Fellows, a private in Company C, 12th New York Cavalry, received a gunshot wound of the right forearm, "the ball having passed obliquely, breaking the ulna." In his case file, Leidy noted, "The wound was extremely gangrenous; it was filled with a large recent coagulum of bilous from hemorrhage." While the organs of the chest were healthy, the spleen was "curiously mottled; in sections pale, comparatively bloodless and occupied by a great multitude apparently of bodies." He concluded this report noting that he had preserved and submitted "the bones, forearm and spleen for the museum."[36]

Hammond's directive that physicians preserve "interesting cases" for the museum was brilliant in its vagueness. Physicians usually found interesting that which they did not understand or had never encountered before—but with more than 12,000 Union war physicians, crossing all experience levels, there was a fantastic range of submissions to the museum. Keen, for example, found the case of Jacob Schlicher, age thirty-three, a soldier from Massachusetts, especially interesting. Schlicher was admitted to Ward No. 2 of Satterlee hospital on July 11, 1863, for a gunshot fracture of the superior maxillary and a wound of the internal maxillary artery that supplies blood to the face. Schlicher had been wounded at the Battle of Gettysburg on July 1, 1863, after being struck by a minié ball, which entered below the left eye and lodged just behind the upper molar, partially destroying the left palatine arch and knocking out the last two molars and portions of the alveolar process.[37]

Keen monitored the case closely, often checking on the patient three times daily. He noted that the patient suffered severe hemorrhage upon admission, and Keen had trouble arresting it because of the location of the wound. He tried to plug the wound but could not, so he decided, after consulting with his assistant surgeon, H. Schell, and several of his other colleagues, on a ligation of the common carotid artery. The *Medical and Surgical History of the War* shows that there were only eighty-two of these procedures performed during the war, with a success rate of 24 percent.[38] Arterial ligations were difficult (particularly because of the weak surgical background of many American surgeons). Through the war, more surgeons performed these operations out of necessity, but their doing so also reflects the developing confidence among surgeons.

Keen considered a number of factors before performing the surgery. He noted the efficacy of such surgery because, "the brain would be speedily supplied by the right carotid"; surgery would delay further hemorrhage; and it would "control the hemorrhage from the internal maxillary."[39] He noted that the "artery was found without the slightest difficulty" and was tied without injury. His goal was to stop the bleeding immediately; however, while the bleeding was arrested, the patient suffered "sudden loss of blood to the brain," for which Keen was prepared. The patient was treated with morphia, beef tea, milk punch, cold-water dressings, and brandy. Keen monitored the patient twice daily and kept thorough notes on the case. In addition to making physical observations in regard to pulse, temperature, appetite, and character of the wound, he conducted various tests on the patient's paralyzed side relating to his speech and intellect. The patient died forty-one days after the operation.

Keen performed the autopsy himself. He examined the lungs; the heart and its walls and valves; the abdomen, including the liver, gall bladder, pancreas, and kidneys; and the brain. He reserved his most careful analysis for the brain (which was his central interest). He used a microscope as a research tool and looked for the origins of pus and studied the role of inflammation. He cut through the dura matter, noting a significant quantity of pus (in the left hemisphere, anterior superior surface, arachnoid cavity) and studied the pus within the cavities of the brain. He examined both sides of the brain and the deposits of lymph that he found. He speculated that the anastomosis or joining of the arteries together "had undoubtedly been imperfect and the supply of blood insufficient in this (left) hemisphere."[40]

The next part of his report, "Substance of the Brain on Sections," is of particular interest because he focused almost entirely on the pus and cells, which were "ill-formed and irregular in their development of nuclei, under acetic acid." He then studied the fluids and abscesses hoping to understand their relation to the disease, and he concluded with an examination of the pus and nerves: "At the point of ligature a few drops of pus were found in a cup shaped cavity and throughout its entire consolidated portion, it appeared dark colored, as if degenerated and ready to slough away speedily. . . . The point at which the hemorrhage had taken place from the internal maxillary could not be found either by inspection or by injecting water into it, since the artery was rendered impervious probably by clotted blood. None of the nerves were injured."[41]

As required by Circular No. 2 Keen prepared and sent the specimen to the Army Medical Museum: "The specimen has been forwarded to the army medical museum along with the bullet. The specimen in addition to the previous points it will be noticed that the sympathetic nerve has been removed and the descenders noni cut at its middle. This was done in the dissection."[42] Of interest is the thorough analysis and clear desire to have familiarity with the internal body but also the use of the microscope in the hopes of understanding the role of inflammation, blood vessels and blood, pus, nerve and sense organs, and tissues, which supported the development of a medical model that involved the study of diseased structures in the absence of the living patient. Keen, like Leidy, was trying to ascertain fundamental alterations in the bodies, tissues, and cells using a microscope, an instrument with which he had had no familiarity until two years before this event. He was fascinated with the physical changes in the body, and his autopsy reports reveal how the postmortem was used to study and learn from the body but also how dissections became more sophisticated through the war.[43] He went on to publish this report in *Hays American Journal of Medical Science* for July 1864, as encouraged by Circular No. 5.

William F. Norris of Douglas Hospital was similarly interested in pathological physiology. He studied, among other aspects, the relation between fluids and specific disease states. In the case of Walter Davis, who had received a wound in the left ankle joint at Petersburg, Virginia, which led to the amputation of his left leg at the lower shin, Norris not only looked at the stump, including the arteries, veins, necrosed bone, knee joint, and cartilage and muscular space of the thigh, but also studied the heart, liver, spleen, and both kidneys and performed microscopic analyses of the fluid in the knee joint, the patches in the lungs of debris of lung tissue, and the tubes of the kidneys (and he sought albumen and casts in the urine).[44] He also studied the effects of pyemia, an unfamiliar disease for many Civil War surgeons and one that became easily recognizable because of the number of cases and autopsies.[45]

For Norris, it was an important objective to generate and integrate medical knowledge into wartime medicine. One particular interest for Norris was determining why pyemia spread so rapidly. Sergeant John Sproul of the New York Volunteers was wounded at Kellys Farm, Virginia, November 7, 1863, by a musket ball, which caused a compound fracture of the lower third of the left femur.[46] The thigh had been amputated at its middle within twelve hours after receipt of injury by Dr. Kimball of the 40th New York Volunteers. The patient was soon after diagnosed with pyemia. Sproul was put under Norris's care, and he reported that the patient was "blanched and suppuration was free." He was treated with "milk diet, stimulants, water dressing for the stump, flaps approximated by adhesive strips." This treatment continued for almost three weeks, until he died. Norris began his autopsy with a close examination of the stump: "There was firm adherence to the two flaps but no union of the skin. An incision was made in the thigh and the femoral artery and veins carefully dissected not from pouparts ligament or their termination on the stump." While the femoral artery and veins appeared healthy, Norris was perturbed by the "several icchymous patches on the muscles and in some places near the bone, small quantities of pus."

In fact, Norris was concerned about the amount of pus or pockets of pus that he found throughout the body: "The periosteum was thickened and easily separated between it and the bone was in many places small quantities of pus. It had also attached to the osteophyles mostly flattened pieces of bone forming to some extent a casing for the lower end of the femur."[47] He proceeded to study the thorax; the lungs, including dissecting them and microscopically studying the abscesses; the heart and the blood clots and fibrous clots; the spleen; the stomach and the large and small intestine; and the kidney, liver, and pancreas. He concluded with a microscopic examination of the "feotid material" found in the femur, hoping to find any aberration in body fluids caused by the disease, which he noted seemed to be "decomposing degenerative material; not pus." The desire to understand the body is clear, but as physicians searched for the origins of pus, inflammation, and fluids, they tried to ascertain whether these were pathological processes or the chemical signposts of disease. These types of investigations and questions paved the way for new paradigms of disease but also new ways to investigate disease conditions such as pathological chemistry (as discussed in chapters 3 and 6).[48]

The findings within the Civil War dead rooms were to be made available to all American physicians. For example, on September 14, 1865, Dr. H. Wood Jr. presented his paper "Synopsis of Autopsies Made at Lincoln General Hospital" for Assistant Surgeon H. Allen. His report was promptly published in the *Proceedings of the Pathological Society of Philadelphia*. He discussed 223 autopsies that were performed during 1863 and part of 1864. Wood performed all but 42 of the autopsies (the remainder were conducted by George McGill). He reported the autopsy results of deaths due to diarrhea, fevers, and purpura hemmorrhagica. He classed the diseases together, and each organ was dissected and compared. There were 41 cases of diarrhea, and the lungs, heart, liver, spleen, pancreas, ileum, and colon from each body were compared to create a picture of the diseases. The physicians were interested in the common features found in each case, such as the unhealthy condition of the ileum. Of greater interest, however, were the differences found in the cases, such as a presence of a strange and unfamiliar "exudation in the colon."[49]

There was in fact a keen interest in organs, tissues, and the structure of the body, and the order to perform autopsies validated this work as scientific interrogation that could legitimate the extensive analysis of the body or the body as the source of knowledge production. It was even common practice to inject the body with arsenic or some other preservative fluid so that it could be studied when time permitted. R. B. Bontecou, for example, found the case of Private W. A. Thacker "quite fascinating." Private Thacker was admitted to hospital number one, Beaufort, South Carolina, October 24, 1862, after being shot in the right side of the pelvis, "the ball entering at the left side of the coccyx, passing out of the pelvis through the great sciatic notch of the right side, and emerging from the integuments at anterior superior spinous process of ileum on the same side, having apparently traversed the bone at the whole distance."[50]

Bontecou began the normal course of treatment, which included wet dressings followed by cerate cloth dressings, a full diet, and rest. Things were proceeding well until November 3, when the patient called Bontecou's attention to a "pimple of his left frontal eminence" which was accompanied by "swelling, puffiness, which extended as far as the eyelid." Bontecou noted the appearance was not unlike "that which follows the sting of a bee."[51] He checked on the patient daily and noted that he steadily worsened. Bontecou observed that the "parts in the neighborhood of the pimple have a livid appearance; the swelling had extended to the left side of the neck, involving the face and closing the eye." The patient was treated with "antimony tartas" every three hours and low diet, and the poultice was continued. He was later given beef tea, stimulants, and anodynes for the pain. The patient continued to worsen, and Bontecou reported that "the swelling has extended to both eye-lids on both side of the face, it has never had the appearance of erysipelas but more like erythema, the skin not red but rather a translucent, edematous look." The patient became steadily more delirious even "quite wild all the time" and "cries out in the night, frequently coughing up sputa stained with blood." He died just nine days after the pimple had been discovered.

Bontecou made an incision down through the temporal muscle to the skull but discovered only blood and serum. After injecting the body with arsenic, in order to preserve it for study, he noted that the gunshot wound had healed (he traced the passage of the ball) and was content to leave the cause of death as erythema.[52] It was probably a correct diagnosis: erythema is a disorder characterized by redness of the skin and is caused by capillary congestion, which can be set off, for example, by a gunshot wound that may have caused joint inflammation or trauma. The nodules that Bontecou described as a pimple can indeed occur anywhere there is fat under the skin. The correct treatment is to focus on the underlying cause, and in this case he was right to prescribe bed rest, wet dressings, and proper diet, but he was, of course, ignorant of the probability of the bacterial nature of the disorder.

Postmortems during the Civil War were documented in the attempt to learn from bodies and diseases and were always descriptive and increasingly analytical. A master narrative emerged, which demonstrated that all physicians performing wartime dissections were learning by doing. Clinical material was relied on by some (in the attempt to confirm or reevaluate diagnoses); for others, clinical material was not always available, and bodies became a prized research tool, a chance to pursue previously underdeveloped areas such as the analysis of nerves or the brain or a chance to study the minute parts of the body microscopically. If Bontecou had used the microscope in the preceding case, for example, he might have been able to see a septal panniculitis with acute chronic inflammation of the fat and around the blood vessels. But Civil War surgeons had not yet been able to make the causal connection between what they saw under the microscope and the diseases under investigation. In the work of Keen, Norris, Wood, Bontecou, and the hundreds like them, we see American physicians with inadequate preparation seeking to apply science to the understanding of disease. It was, however, becoming clear to many physicians engaged in this work that the postmortem alone could no longer advance the science of pathology and reveal the cause of disease.

THE LABORATORY APPROACH IN MEDICAL STUDY

Historians of medicine generally agree that between 1870 and 1914 there was a fundamental change in the way in which diseases were investigated and understood. By the early twentieth century, organism after organism had been discovered for diseases that had plagued the world for centuries, such as tuberculosis, cholera, plague, pneumonia, and typhoid, as well as the vectors of malaria and yellow fever, which led to new ways of combating disease, including vaccination, public health measures, and preventative medicine. The story of medicine in the final third of the century has always been presented as dramatic and exciting, with words like "transformation" and "revolution" being commonly used to illustrate the dynamism of these years. The "great men" in the history of disease are always at the center of this narrative. Louis Pasteur, the father of the "germ theory," investigated fermentation and diseases of the silkworm, while Casimir Davaine conducted studies on anthrax. Joseph Lister later introduced antiseptic surgery, and Robert Koch's work on anthrax, cholera, and tuberculosis (and the development of his postulates, which gave shape to this new science) encouraged a shift in the way disease was understood: there was now a microorganism that could be identified confirming the presence of a specific disease.[53]

At the root of these new discoveries was a simple truth: medicine was no longer merely symptom-based; a disease could be identified even in the absence of a patient, moving medicine toward a science-based practice.[54] Yet this was initially a difficult concept for some physicians to accept. Proponents of empiricism advocated seeing each patient's symptoms rather than subscribing to a theory of disease that suggested that many individuals could be attacked by a single disease form. Not all physicians fully accepted the idea of specificity in disease. The debate centered on whether disease was a general disorder of the body or a distinct entity; and if the latter, how could proof of this be ascertained?[55] What was the role of the environment in relation to the individual? These larger debates, which existed between leading physicians in Britain, Germany, France, and elsewhere, were similarly present in America among physicians serving during the war.

And while it was not until the work of leading researchers such as Pasteur, Lister, and Koch became known in America (or encountered in Europe) that some physicians readily accepted the new doctrines, it was the diseases and the conditions caused by the Civil War that helped crystallize these debates for some American physicians. For hundreds of years, physicians had devised research programs in the hopes of elucidating the cause of disease. Different countries, branches of medicine, and even diseases had a long record of germ theories and practices. Debates over Lister's methods would dominate medical journals from the 1870s until the end of the century; however, Lister's discovery did not transform or overwhelm medicine overnight; rather, his was one of a range of germ theories in this period that helped shape the existing ideas.[56] Southern physician Joseph Jones, for example, became one of the "leading American exponents of the new science of bacteriology after being won over to the 'germ theory' when exposed to the work of Lister, Pasteur and Koch in 1870 while on a trip to Europe." He became an ardent supporter of germ theories and quickly "recanted his wartime stand [which favored a miasmatic theory of disease], now boasting of having been among the first to see gangrene bacillus and claiming credit for discovering the microorganisms responsible for typhoid fever as well."[57] Viewed in this context, recognizing only the "great men" in the development of laboratory medicine deprives us of a full understanding of the period, particularly in the American context.

THE MICROSCOPE AND CIVIL WAR MEDICINE

With so many soldiers dying of disease, perhaps medical research and improvements in medical science would turn things around in the Civil War hospitals. In particular, physicians were encouraged to use a microscope to study disease.[58] The more extensive use of the microscope during the Civil War represents the changing ideas about the cause and nature of disease and the body. As physicians cut open the body, studied lesions, and dissected tissues and organs, they saw that the process alone did not reveal much about *how* disease was caused or transmitted. One impulse among the war physicians, then, was to find different, perhaps more effective ways to study and understand disease. The microscope became increasingly important as an investigative tool during the war. It was used to search for the causal agents of disease in the attempt to elucidate better the diseases under investigation and to arrest them. The microscope promised improvements or, rather, new possibilities for medicine but also for the exercise of professional power.

The microscope furnished by the Surgeon General's Office was a Zentmeyer small-stand compound microscope, with an $\frac{8}{10}$-inch lens and an

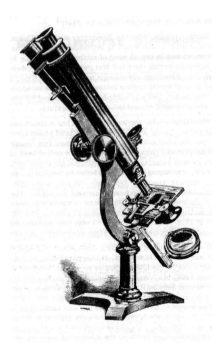

The Zentmeyer Army Hospital microscope (Courtesy of the National Museum of Health and Medicine, Washington, D.C.)

uncorrected ⅕-inch lens by the same make. Providing microscopes was part of the medical department's attempt to identify medicine with science and provide support for the emerging research culture. All physicians could apply for the opportunity to use a microscope in their investigations, but because of the cost and their relative scarcity in America, they were primarily restricted to those physicians affiliated with a general hospital or laboratory, those charged with the specific study of a disease, or those who wanted to contribute something to the development of scientific medicine. It was noted that "applications for microscopes by medical officers in charge of general hospitals will be favorably considered, provided the evidence be satisfactory that the officer will use the instrument for the benefit of science, and will report the results of his observations to the Surgeon-General."[59]

In March 1863 Hammond issued a circular letter detailing the conditions upon which the microscope was to be used and maintained.[60] Physicians were advised to keep the microscope "carefully in a dry place, as free from dust as possible," and when not in use, it should be "locked in a box to protect it from dust, and to prevent it being handled by improper persons." He went on to discuss proper storage, cleaning methods, and handling of the microscope, emphasizing that "each objective is to be preserved in its brass case, in manipulating the greatest pains must be taken not to injure or break the apparatus by hasty or inconsiderate movements."[61] Finally, he discussed the best methods for examining blood and urine, which again promoted careful study of the specimens and even more careful handling of the microscope. The instrument was clearly highly revered and expensive, suggesting once again the wartime medical environment was an important educational opportunity for those physicians who had never had such access.

This directive generated as much excitement among some of the war physicians as Circular No. 2. Woodward supported this enthusiasm by encouraging physicians in both field and general hospitals to use the microscope for anatomical investigation and practical work supporting the emerging relationship between science and practice.[62] He observed at the end of the war that "about two years ago, under my inspiration the Surgeon General's office bought a dozen microscopes, which were distributed to the general hospitals."[63] It was also common practice for physicians to order microscopes themselves so they could seize the opportunity of increased access to patients, bodies, diseases, and hospital work.[64] Some of the elite physicians owned their own or had had access to them in Paris, but essentially a new generation was introduced to microscopy.

As revealed by the letters to the Surgeon General's Office, physicians greatly desired a microscope, and it was common practice to promise the advance of medical science upon the receipt of one:[65] "I take the liberty of making application for the use of a microscope during the time I may be stationed at this hospital. I find it impossible to conduct autopsies and other pathological investigation without one in the thorough manner which is desirable."[66] Indeed, the use of the instrument was of much professional interest: "I have the honor to respectfully request to be furnished with a microscope for this institution. It will be used entirely for the benefit of science, and any interesting observations will be faithfully reported to you."[67]

The microscope was also used in the hospitals as a teaching tool: "I desire to make application to you for a microscope to be used in this hospital. My object in asking for one is solely to apply it to scientific purposes with the view of furnishing interesting and valuable pathological observations which I am enabled to make in this hospital. Such facts as I may gather, with the aid of the microscope, shall be promptly communicated to the Surgeon General. Personally, I am familiar with the use of the instrument, and I wish to give the Assistant Surgeons employed in the establishment an opportunity to familiarize themselves likewise with its use."[68]

It was, after all, wartime, and being equipped with a microscope was justified by its practical uses: "I have the honor to request that this hospital be furnished with a microscope. Many cases are constantly occurring in which the use of a microscope will not only advance the interests of science but materially benefit the patient enabling a more correct diagnosis to be made."[69] D. L. Huntington wrote Hammond from the Post Hospital at Fort Monroe, Virginia, asking for a microscope both to make "microscopial observations of value to science" and to "throw light upon the diagnoses of obscure cases."[70] The use of the microscope in diagnosis changed the way physicians thought about medical practice. Roberts Bartholow, for example, looked for clues in the bodily fluids and submitted his report on patients suffering from measles, which he treated in a general hospital in Chattanooga. He examined just over 100 cases and each day studied their urine microscopically, looking for "albumen and casts."[71] Microscopy encouraged physicians to think about the manifestation of diseases in a context other than its end stage or clinical symptoms, while imbuing physicians with new practical skills.

Middleton Goldsmith, who became superintendent of hospitals at Louisville, Kentucky, in 1863,[72] asked for a microscope that he said was necessary "for carrying out the orders from the Surgeon General in relation to the collection of morbid specimens."[73] Along with his request, Goldsmith outlined his plans for using the instrument, which provides an interesting view of how ideas about producing medical knowledge developed through the war. In 1862, before being charged with the extensive study of gangrene and erysipelas in his capacity as assistant medical director in Louisville,[74] he was fascinated with the collection and study of specimens and the diseases that attacked the troops: "I have the honor to transmit herewith an application for a microscope. . . . It has seemed to me that it would be well to institute a careful examination into the causes, treatment and morbid anatomy of three principle diseases among the troops in this department and treated in this hospital [diarrhea, typhus, and typho-malaria fever and pernicious intermittents including in the first and third dysenteric diseases]. . . . The object is to compare the results of treatment, fix the value of the diagnostic signs—ascertain the constant as well as varying morbid changes and present for the museum a complete series of specimens illustrating the morbid anatomy of the several diseases."[75]

Not every war physician would use or even see a microscope. But some did, and they went on to publish their case histories—which were made available to the many American physicians. In the process, newer methodological problems and practices were revealed, considered, and debated. While Civil War physicians did not make the larger connections between microscopic infusoria and diseases, the wartime research represents an important transition from the passive observer to the active experimenter. As physicians searched for more effective ways to manage, understand, study, and document both the destructive wounds caused by the minié ball and the fevers and septic diseases that often prevailed in the field and general hospitals, there was a new emphasis on lesions and delineating the relationship between inflammation and disease or the role that pus or "deficient blood" played in various diseases. And as some Civil War physicians engaged in their work with the microscope, they began to think about the manifestation of disease at the cellular level, further paving the way for the laboratory sciences to develop.

THE EUROPEAN INFLUENCE AND CIVIL WAR SCIENCE

Rudolph Virchow, professor of medicine at the University of Berlin, developed the idea that the cell was the primary locus of life and disease.[76] Virchow advocated what came to be known as cellular pathology,[77] which essentially suggested that diseased cells could spread disease to the rest of the body as cells divided (a process known as mitosis); thus all diseases could be traced as chemical or physical changes within cells.[78] Virchow was optimistic that cellular pathology would transform medicine, particularly through the physiological and pathological study of the body; arguing that all disease processes were ultimately cell processes, he encouraged physicians to begin using the microscope so that they could analyze structural change and disease processes such as inflammation and pus formation along with conducting chemical and physical investigations.[79] Cell theory, then, created a new way to think about and investigate disease processes and provided a model by which to distinguish between important and superficial characters in the description of tissues and cells.

As Virchow's work was being debated and studied by the scientific community in Europe, his work also gained a few converts in America. One in particular was Joseph Woodward. Woodward was particularly interested in Virchow's cellular basis of pathology (a summary of which Woodward had translated for the *American Journal of the Medical Sciences* in April 1861).[80] He was in a unique position as curator of the medical museum. He had not only an opportunity, an obligation even, to produce medical knowledge but also the institutional support to help develop the medical expertise of

American physicians. Thus, early in the project Woodward reached out to Virchow, and his decision to contact Virchow says much about how Woodward envisaged this project—it was a conscious attempt to enhance the scientific culture of the museum.[81]

Historians assign great importance to the German paradigm in the development of laboratory sciences, particularly, the reformed German universities and government-sponsored laboratories after midcentury. These institutions supported full-time scientists who did not have to (among other things) contend with antidissection feelings.[82] There was similarly a scientific dynamism in the Civil War hospitals and museum; both promoted a vast scientific enterprise that many physicians enthusiastically supported, and this influenced the direction that medical science went in the final third of the century. Military physicians did not have to explicitly deal with antidissection feelings, and the Army Medical Museum was specifically created to support developing ideas about research and medicine.

Recognizing this unique context and seeing firsthand the limitations of the Paris Clinical School, some American physicians consciously attempted to move medical study away from the tenets of the Paris School and toward the German ideology of "pure research" and the laboratory. This was one objective that Woodward articulated to Virchow: "It is not necessary for me to remind you that the eyes of thoughtful men in this country are turned to Germany as the fountain of scientific progress. Allow me also to add that we recognize in yourself as chief of men who in these modern times have succeeded in achieving a real medical breakthrough based upon the inevitable logic of facts."[83] Significantly, he also noted that he appreciated Virchow's *Cellular Pathology* so much that, at his suggestion, "the translation of your book (by Mr. Chance) has been reprinted in this country and distributed as a text book by the Union Medical Bureau to the surgeons of the medical corps."[84] Woodward went on to suggest that he made "these remarks from no desire to flatter you but because I wish you to understand that your answer to my present communication . . . cannot fail to exert an influence upon the progress of scientific medicine and especially of pathological-anatomical research in America."[85]

Virchow had long encouraged physicians to avoid a purely anatomical approach to pathology, and he reminded them that they needed to become pathologists and elucidate pathological processes rather than merely anatomical states.[86] Although by the twentieth century pathology and pathological anatomy were nearly synonymous in the United States, Woodward, in the tradition of Virchow, encouraged the development of independent investigation related to pathology during the war years. There was not an abandonment of the study of gross lesions, but one important message of the museum was to encourage the study of alterations in the cells (inflammation or degeneration) and their position in the body.

Woodward's specific reason for writing to Virchow, then, was regarding the microscopial section of the museum, in particular micropathological research.[87] Early in the war Woodward purchased 365 "fine injections" from Professor Hyrtl of Vienna.[88] However, Hyrtl only sold injections that were preserved dry, for study by reflected light, and were of limited use for Woodward. Thus, Woodward hoped that European investigators, particularly Virchow, would consider donating specimens to "aid an infant institution." From Virchow specifically Woodward asked for "specimens illustrating the minute anatomy of morbid growths" but, equally important, for advice on preserving specimens along with the most efficacious method of illustrating the minute anatomy of the soft parts, both normal and pathological.[89] He asked for information about the proper varnish for making cells and fluids for preserving microscopial preparations (so as not to alter the "soft parts"). He inquired about aniline for coloring microscopial specimens and degrees of permanency for the microscopial preparations of the soft parts.

Woodward was aware of the challenges of building a micropathological cabinet. Civil War physicians had to learn to master the microscope; they had to "see" the tiny particles, the minute units of cellular or biological activity; they had to think about function and disease states in a way that most had not done before the war.[90]

But, as Woodward noted, the microscopial series at the museum was crucial because "no intelligent efforts to prevent disease can be made without a reasonable comprehension of their nature, and this must rest upon a just knowledge of pathological anatomy."[91] Woodward continued, "Unfortunately in the United States pathological anatomy is but little studied. The few who pay any attention to the subject confine themselves to such course examinations as can be made with the naked eye alone, or if the microscope is called into requisition its employment is limited to the examination of scraps of torn fragments." He then explained that "the preparation of proper sections, with which only intelligent microscopial researches with tissue metamorphosis can be made is understood by but few physicians in America and practiced by still fewer. Under the circumstance there appeared little probability that an exact study of the pathological anatomy of our camp diseases would be attempted if it were not undertaken in the Army Medical Museum and it became therefore an imperative duty to make an effort in this direction."[92] The museum eventually had two well-prepared sets of microscopic preparations: the permanent ones, those preserved in Canada Balsam and those mounted in glycerine or various preservative fluids.

The reform and development of American medicine during the war then had deep roots—local, regional, national, and international. Civil War science was not a unique case of American exceptionalism but rather a chance for Americans to be on the same footing and engage in the same debates as European medical leaders. As one example, Woodward noted, "In a general way it may be said that the results of the museum are in accord in many respects with the comprehension of the modern Berlin school of pathological anatomy" and thus "contradictory of the doctrine of exudation taught so generally in the older medical text books in use in this country" but also "at variance in several particulars with the views of Dr. Lionel Beale, lately so favorably received in England."[93] In his correspondence with Virchow, then, Woodward described the unprecedented opportunity of developing the national pathological cabinet: "The innumerable wounds under treatment in our hospitals during the past year have furnished a rich field for collecting surgical materials, and about 2500 specimens have been placed upon the shelves, most of them of great interest, and accompanied by complete case histories, and these specimens are still rapidly accumulating."[94]

Of the medical section, Woodward's chief interest, he explained, "Medical specimens have been collected in considerable quantities, our difficulty having been less to find objects worthy of preservation, than to obtain funds for the purchase of glass jars of proper quality in sufficient numbers. . . . Though this difficulty will probably be remedied this year by the liberality of Congress."[95] He sent Virchow copies of some "circulars of general interest" and a copy of his recently published *Outlines of Chief Camp Diseases*, which as he explained to Virchow corresponded with the fundamental doctrines of *Cellular Pathology*.

In developing the Army Medical Museum, then, Woodward had two goals. First, he sought to create a new investigative framework in which to understand the nature of disease. Second, he wanted to become part of the international scientific community then composed of those engaging in microscopial work related to human normal or pathological conditions—and these interchanges helped shape Woodward's research questions. George Otis later remarked to Joseph Barnes about Woodward's work: "Under the direction of Assistant Surgeon Woodward the microscopial cabinet has received large accessories. Additional apparatus has been purchased and the means of investigations in this department are unquestionably of unsurpassed excellence. . . . For several months assistant Curtis has been engaged in experiments in microphotography and the results already attained have been favorably received by the scientific world."[96] To Woodward's delight, Virchow noted of the work at the museum, "Whoever takes up and reads the extensive publications of the American medical staff will be constantly astonished at the wealth of experience therein found." Virchow further observed that the particular strengths of the work included the "exactness in detail" and the "careful statistics" but above all a wealth of medical experience produced by numerous American physicians, which was then transmitted to "contemporaries in the greatest possible completeness."[97]

TECHNOLOGY AND CIVIL WAR MEDICINE

How did microscopic research develop at the museum? Woodward's commitment to developing microscopy intensified over the course of the war, as did his resolve to develop microscopy in American medical education. He had long been interested in developing microscopic tools.[98] His school notebooks show numerous notes and experiments on the use of heat, electricity, light (chemical changes that the sun can produce), the atmosphere, oxygen, hydrogen, carbon, and nitrogen, including ideas about how each could be variously used in microscopial experiments.[99] With the opportunity of the unique disease conditions then prevailing among Civil War soldiers, along with his position at the museum, Woodward concentrated on developing microscopic technique, including the use of aniline in histological research and photomicrography, particularly its uses for obtaining accurate representations of pathological histology.

As noted earlier, microscopic research was very new to most American practitioners. Moreover, cutting, staining, and mounting sections of diseased tissues and organs was tedious, time consuming, and difficult. Thus, not all physicians produced the same results in their preparations, which generated methodological and epistemological debates about the place of microscopy in medicine. These debates dominated medical journals for much of the nineteenth century; however, it was Woodward's objective to highlight the inconsistencies, teach new methods, and provide a forum in which microscopic findings could be debated. It was in fact the methodological problems, such as why contradictory representations of the same object continually appeared, which most allowed for the development of microscopic research in the medical museum. In the microscopial section of the museum, then, Woodward displayed thin sections of diseased tissues and organs, preparations exhibiting the minute anatomy of normal structures, and test objects. They were mounted in Canada balsam, in "such a way as to preserve their minute details" but also to secure "their indefinite preservation."[100] Woodward did not want the experience of the war lost, and he wanted the objects to teach.

By the second half of the nineteenth century, microscopic manuals, which explained the basic technique and function of the microscope, started to appear in the medical marketplace with greater frequency. A microscope, it was suggested, needed adequate lenses—color corrected or achromatic optical lenses were desirable—and the range of magnification was ideally between 30 and 300 times the diameter of the specimen.[101] Before Woodward developed the micropathological cabinet, then, his first goal was to improve the microscopic standards at the museum, in particular, to have better quality objectives. In the absence of a national framework for developing American medical education and microscopic research, Woodward once again turned abroad for motivation. For microscopy to be effective, physicians had to be able to "see" cells, tissues, infusoria, and "animalcules." Thus, first and foremost, Woodward spent an enormous amount of time trying to develop the best possible microscopes and lenses.

One particularly effective resource was his communication with the eminent physician Robin Leach Maddox. Maddox pioneered the use of photomicrography in London and had won awards for his microphotographs in 1853 from the Photographic Society of London.[102] Woodward wrote numerous letters to Maddox, in which he unselfconsciously asked for help in perfecting his technique, particularly regarding photography. They compared the results of their experiments with various lenses, accuracy of stage micrometers, lighting and magnification, and even favorite microscopic houses. Overall, Woodward and Maddox exchanged more than fifty letters on methodologies along with photomicrographs—and once again this collaboration helped shape Woodward's research at the museum.[103]

Woodward first created experiments designed to develop the basic apparatus. He wrote to the noted microscopist M. Zentmeyer in 1864 with detailed instructions about the type of apparatus he wanted constructed for photographing microscopial preparations. He also enclosed a drawing "based on some experiments made here which promise satisfactory results."[104] As test objects to check the quality of the lenses,[105] Woodward used the standard diatoms (pleurosigma angulatum, podura plumbia), a few parasites, anatomical objects, and some preparations from Civil War camp diseases, including the anatomy of the intestinal ulcers of camp dysentery and of the ulceration of the intestine in camp fever, along with a series on the small pox pustule.[106]

Most of the experiments in the museum related to the range of magnification and optical setup for the purpose of establishing the means to "amplify with the best distinctiveness." Woodward and Curtis experimented with a variety of lenses, including the ⅛-, ⅟₅₀-, ⅟₁₆-, ¼-, and ⅟₂₅-inch. They began by conducting trials with the "most difficult diatoms" to determine which lens offered the best results—or the best chance of "seeing" the image microscopically.[107] For example, he wrote Zentmeyer in 1864 to thank him for the "six microscopes recently furnished by you to this office," which were deemed "excellent" and "most credible workmanship." Most of the lenscs werc quite good, though the ⅕-inch object of glass was deemed "very inferior." The problem, as Woodward noted, was that upon examining the "anatomical elements, say, for example, the white blood corpuscles, of the mucous corpuscles in the saliva, it is impossible to get a satisfactory image of these objects."[108] Letters such as these are ubiquitous in Woodward's papers; however, what clearly emerges was his drive to improve medical technology, which, it was hoped, would lead to better understanding of Civil War diseases. He thus worked almost obsessively to improve the means of production, to be able to see and study the mechanisms producing disease.

Through the war and after, Woodward and Curtis continually compared and debated their findings with Maddox, which gave the researchers an opportunity to further develop microscopic standards.[109] Woodward was very pleased when Maddox validated the work being done at the museum: "I have had a private letter from Dr. Maddox in which he acknowledges the Army Medical Museum microphotographs to be the best made anywhere. You will see by the enclosed extract from the *British Journal of Photography* that Dr. Maddox and others do not hesitate to state this publicly."[110] The communication with Maddox was thus a great resource for Woodward but also for Maddox.[111] To show his gratitude for Woodward's and Curtis's time, Maddox presented the museum with a "beautiful set of photomicrographs," which Woodward had specially bound and promptly put on display.

As expected, the results of Woodward's collaborations were shared with Civil War physicians. Indeed, it is significant of the spirit of the project that he advised these physicians which houses produced superior lenses, such as Powell and Leasand, Ross, the House of Wales, or Smith and Beck.[112] And as medicine became more scientific in the postwar period, and medical schools were reformed along more scientific guidelines, students were encouraged to purchase their own microscopes. This work was thus validated, and Woodward continued his experiments but also his teaching.

Indeed, the wartime work laid the foundation for a new epistemological discourse about microscopy and photomicrography—both nationally and internationally. A. M. Edwards, president of the American Microscopial Society, wrote Woodward asking him to share his findings and methodology concerning the microscopic and photomicrographic work being performed at the museum. Woodward responded that it would be "[my] pleasure to communicate with you on any subject concerning microscopy or photomicrography"; he also sent a copy of *Circular No. 6* for members of the society, along with an open invitation to the museum's laboratory.[113] Edwards, in turn, presented Woodward with a number of specimens, which Woodward and Curtis photographed and later presented to the American Microscopial Society.

Woodward also wrote Heinrich Frey of Zurich, Switzerland, in response to Frey's recently published "Das Microscope." He experimented with some of Frey's methods and subsequently sent Frey three photomicrographs of the pleurosigma angulatum prepared with an English 1/50-inch objective, an enlargement of the first photograph to 19,050 diameters, and a third photograph taken with an American 1/8-inch objective. He explained his methods, described the quality of these glasses, and encouraged Frey to keep in touch and perhaps visit the museum.[114] Woodward similarly shared his findings with the physician T. Murmich of Vienna about his work in photomicrography. The two were interested in the methods of Joseph von Gerlach, whose work was of much interest during and after the war. "I have to thank you for your interesting letter with preparations from Gerlach. The photographs in color were a novelty to us. We have tried Gerlach's process and succeeded in it." Woodward then outlined some of his new experiments: "We have also been experimenting with transferring preparations through absolute alcohol to Canada balsam as in the preparations sent to us by Gerlach. . . . I enclose herewith a letter for Gerlach thanking him for his kindness in sending those specimens of microscopial matters. . . . I also enclose a photograph of cartilage to show our prospect of success in the photography of the soft tissues with high powers."[115] Indeed, Woodward found success with the methods of Gerlach, who was also one of the first medical researchers to use photomicrography in basic tissue research, and who only just published his handbook on technique in 1863.

While Woodward consulted and learned from the experts abroad, he in turn used his position at the museum to teach American physicians. W. W. Keen, for example, often wrote to Woodward asking for photomicrographic preparations to illustrate his lectures. Woodward typically replied, "I will endeavor to send you a few photomicrographs so soon as we print again which will be in a few weeks. Pardon me for saying here in the interests of the medical profession, if you are going to teach the microscope the sooner you learn to make your own preparations the better. No one is an accomplished microscopist who cannot make his own preparations." He also suggested further reading, "Extemporaneous preparations for each lecture are rapidly prepared by Beales method and the best of these put away in balsam by Gerlach's method from year to year, will soon lay the foundation of a good cabinet. Of course this implies labor, but no more than every European teacher."[116]

Woodward recognized that medical practice during the war occupied a new intellectual space: Americans were now producers of medical knowledge. As curator of the medical section of the museum, he aptly filled the role of educator. Even the most eminent physicians profited from the research at the museum. After the war, William Osler, as one example, often took advantage of the resources at the museum. His numerous letters to the staff contain requests for access to specific specimens, and he sometimes visited to examine, photograph, and make drawings, which were used to illustrate his own work.[117]

Woodward was elected an honorary member of the National Academy of Sciences in 1873 and of the American Microscopial Society for his "work and advances in the areas of normal and pathological histology."[118] He maintained his association with this society and numerous others as he worked to develop medical education and research during and after the war. As Woodward remarked, "I sent by today's mail two packages: one containing a dozen microscopial preparations, chiefly of the soft tissues mounted in Canada balsam preserving most of the structural appearances which could be seen in glycerine preparations. Also a package of photomicrographs of podura. I want to ask you to exhibit these preparations and photographs to the microscopial society and to any others in New York who are interested in such things. I should also be happy to hear the criticism of any points that may occur to you."[119] And it became standard for Woodward to close his letters with an invitation for society members to visit and tour the museum.

CIVIL WAR SOLDIERS AND DIARRHEA AND DYSENTERY

The fervent attempt to develop these standards was, above all, so that Civil War diseases could be better understood and investigated. Thus within this larger context there were important practical applications for the development of these new investigative tools—a clinical opportunity that Maddox and Virchow among others did not have, again highlighting the distinctiveness of the war's medical experience for American physicians. And here Woodward adapted the technological possibilities developed through the museum with the wartime clinical needs. Indeed, these new technologies reconfigured ideas about managing specific disease conditions—especially the most pervasive and challenging "diseases" in the Union army: diarrhea and dysentery. With more than 1,528,098 reported cases of acute diarrhea and dysentery, and more than 40,000 Union deaths, these were the two "diseases" most debilitating to the Union army.[120] Otis noted during the war that the "extreme frequency of diarrhea and dysentery make it important to understand these disorders . . . they were the chief cause of mortality from disease."[121] Soldiers reported repeated cases of chronic diarrhea, but as physicians noted, for some reason each case seemed to become more "formidable" as the war progressed. These diseases exhausted troops, took them out of the ranks, and thus were the subject of numerous investigations. And these investigations, so central to the development of physiology, were made visible through the museum.

Woodward's pathological work focused on the minute conditions of the mucous membrane of the intestine and the nature of the diseased structures and the morbid secretions. The objective was to find answers about causation, prevention, and treatment of diarrhea and dysentery.[122] As he observed of these studies, "The earliest detailed investigations into the pathological histology of the intestine in the camp fevers and diarrhoeas of our armies during the present war were made by me, at the Surgeon General's Office, in the fall of 1862, and a brief sketch of the chief points which I had up to that time established were published a year subsequently in my book on Camp Diseases." With some pride, Woodward observed that "these are the only observations of the subject which have hitherto been published, and so far as I have been able to learn they are the only ones which have been made, with the exception of the careful studies which have recently been carried on under my supervision in the microscopial branch of the Army Medical Museum, by Assistant Surgeon Edward Curtis."[123]

For Woodward, indeed for many Civil War physicians, microscopic research represented new ways to see, think about, and investigate the causation of these intestinal disorders and to differentiate between the normal and diseased states: What did the bumps, depressions, ulcerations, or enlargements found on the intestines, bowels, or colons mean? What role did they play in the formation, development, or seriousness of the disease? What could the fluids around the mucous membrane reveal about disease? Microscopy and photomicrography, Woodward argued, were scientific means to distinguish between important and superficial changes in tissue structure. Woodward's immediate goal, then, was to create a larger picture of these "diseases."

Civil War physicians in the field were asked to report on the relation of the environment and season on the cases of diarrhea and dysentery; to comment on treatments and symptoms; and, if possible, to microscopically examine the stools and study the body during autopsy. Once specimens were received at the museum's laboratory, Woodward went further in analyzing the microscopic appearance of the bowel, and he prepared gross and microscopic descriptions and pictures. These photomicrographs were intended to provide instruction on diagnosis but also reveal the nature of these diseases. Through these investigations, American physicians could also see the techniques of the new scientific medicine being produced at the museum.

With the use of the microscope and thus a deeper look into the disease state, the cases of diarrhea and dysentery were grouped into five sections in the museum: examples of follicular ulceration of the colon; the extension of follicular ulcers damaging the mucous membrane of the colon; ulceration of the bowel but displaying a yellowish or greenish-yellow pseudo-membranous layer; diseased small and large intestines; and tubercular ulceration of the bowel. The collection emphasized cellular, tissue, and fluid changes and was "illustrative of the normal histology of the intestine" along with the "changes they undergo in fever and diarrhea."[124] The objective was to show the different stages of diseases and the different manifestations as revealed through the examination of organs and tissues. Woodward put the series together in a way that would highlight the stages of disease, what he called the "most important phases of the anatomical lesions," such as the submucous connective tissues, ulcerative changes in the bowels and intestines, points of very active cell multiplication, and the various stages of follicular ulcers.

In trying to account for the spread and severity of these diseases, Woodward looked for answers in the cells. He studied, for example, the multiplication of the connective tissue cells or corpuscles and the role these cells played in the spreading of ulcers or enlarging follicles. Woodward closely examined the ongoing debates among leaders in the medical world surrounding cell multiplication in disease. For example, were the corpuscles that Woodward studied under the microscope "true cells, with distinct walls, as argued by Virchow and the Berlin School"? Or, rather, were they "mere masses of germinal matter without distinct parietes as Beale would have us believe"?[125] Indeed, one significant debate at the time among pathologists centered on whether, as Virchow argued, "inflammatory and pus cells had to originate from other cells" rather than from "amorphous substances," sometimes called blastema or germinal matter.[126] It was Woodward's opinion that through the "multiplication of these corpuscles by division that the greater number of elements is produced . . . not by the generation of new cells."[127]

But Woodward wondered, Did pus cells originate in connective tissue or rather in the blood? Why were abscesses formed, and what process allowed for their formation? What was the relationship between pus, corpuscles, and cells? Pus, as one example, was a common but little understood product of camp diarrhea and dysentery. While performing postmortems on the bodies of those that succumbed to either diarrhea or dysentery, case reports often commented on the existence of pus and blood in the intestines and hepatic secretions. Thus, in the drive to understand these processes, Woodward advised, in particular, to use a microscope for the study of tissues and bodily fluids.[128]

Woodward's emphasis on connective tissues and inflammation represents the shift in the museum from gross to microscopial anatomy in the pathological field. At their root, his inquiries concerned the role of the cell in pathological disturbances—to which there were no definitive answers during or after the war. Woodward's publications were mostly descriptive, but his work raised questions about disease processes and, most importantly, led to new paradigms of experimental medicine and new ways to investigate the body.[129]

DISPLAYING PATHOLOGY

But again, and to a remarkable extent, this larger project was about educating American physicians. "The best means of making the results of our microscopial studies available for the information of medical men in America," Woodward noted, "has exercised my most serious thought."[130] Part of Woodward's interest in developing improved staining methods and photomicrography was stimulated by Circular No. 5, which aimed to publish both case histories and photographic representations of the wartime cases in the *Medical and Surgical History of the War of the Rebellion*.

Before the war it was common practice to stain sections of tissues with carmine, the same method then used by Virchow. (Carmine is a natural dye obtained from the bodies of the insect *Dactylopius coccus cacti*, and the active coloring agent is carminic acid.) The use of synthetic aniline dyes became more common among histological researchers in the early 1860s because they allowed more visibility and greater contrast when microscopically studying or photographing tissues.[131] Woodward and Curtis, then, worked to improve staining and mounting methods.[132] In his first article on the subject, Woodward in detail explained the techniques developed at the museum. This was important. One of the reasons there were so many contradictory microscopic representations of the same images was because there was no one way to stain specimens, thus observers used a variety of staining procedures, which often produced discordant results. This undermined microscopic research and created continual conflict between opponents and proponents of microscopy. Thus, one of Woodward's objectives in the museum was to try to establish one common standard.

Woodward began by asking doctors in the field to preserve specimens from soldiers suffering from chronic diarrhea; they should "consist of as much of the intestine as is diseased even if the disease involves the whole. It should be taken out in one piece, the small intestine carefully preserved."[133] Once the intestine was received at the museum, it was boiled with dilute nitric acid in a porcelain capsule for two to five minutes, "pinned out loosely on a flat cork to dry," and then every trace of fat was removed.[134] Woodward then recommended taking a very thin piece of the intestine and using an ethereal solution of red or blue aniline for permanent preparations, soaking them for twenty-four hours, transferring them to turpentine, and concluding by mounting them in Canada balsam. Then the specimen could be placed under the microscope.

The permanency of these preparations was ideal for examining structural changes, including enlargement of the solitary follicles and ulceration.[135] He thus gave the structures different tints in order to examine each separately in the hopes of better displaying the disease process.[136] For studying preparations with the highest powers of the microscope, he again advised cutting the sections as thin as possible, soaking them in colored solutions of red, yellow, blue, or purple aniline in a dilute acetic acid, with the objective being to illustrate the presence of "flask shaped ulceration present in the mucosa." Sections were then mounted in liquor or glycerine, preserved and covered with thin glass, and displayed in the microscopial section of the museum.

These new staining methods greatly enhanced the microscopic structures then produced at the museum. Using the method as early as July 1864, Woodward observed, "I have made considerable use of aniline in my histological studies, and they have been extensively employed in the investigations carried on under my direction for the microscopial department of the Army Medical Museum."[137] Moreover, as Woodward observed, these methods "appear to be unknown in this country, and so far as I can learn from the journals accessible to me, is imperfectly understood abroad."[138] The work at the museum, in fact, allowed Woodward to develop "one of the great basic techniques" of the modern pathologist.[139] And thus it is significant in accounting for the emergence of histological research in the nineteenth century that the primary focus of Curtis and Woodward's first article was to explain the exact processes and results of their experiments and, perhaps more importantly, to state their objective, which was to "invite other laborers to enter the field."[140]

The second related way that Woodward attempted to establish an accurate record of the wartime preparations was through the use of photomicrography. Woodward and Curtis pioneered through experimentation new methods to photograph microscopic images, which could then be published. Photomicrography or photomicroscopy is a process in which an image is photographed through a microscope so that it can be magnified and studied. Thin sections of tissues were cut by hand with razors from frozen tissue mounted on the microtome;[141] they were then mounted on glass slides using an adhesive such as Canada balsam and photographed. The idea was to make available for study the stained histologic specimens then representing the various wartime camp diseases. During the war, photomicrography was primarily a means by which to *display* and *document* the results of microscopic analyses.[142] It was commensurate with how Civil War physicians produced knowledge: through the empirical observation of thousands of facts, cases, and observations, with photomicrography providing another means to see the internal body.

At first, Woodward employed artists to draw the specimens—the most noted of whom was Hermann Faber. "The arrival or recent specimens at the Museum has afforded good opportunities for making drawings representing the appearance of the preparations immediately after their removal from the body."[143] These drawings, however, were criticized by some physicians for being subjective: they showed not the true nature of disease but rather the disease as the artist saw it. Woodward explained that "such drawings have attached to them more or less suspicion of being at least in part ideal and for this reason numerous attempts have already been made both in Europe and America, to photograph objects as seen with the microscope."[144] Indeed, beginning in the 1850s numerous professional medical journals reported the varied efforts of the medical community in photographing specimens and organs in the hopes of better understanding histopathology.[145] The problem was that the representations were initially very poor. Thus, physicians continued to use engraving and lithography; however, some physicians of the era believed that photographing disease opened new possibilities for medicine—but again this was not without technical and conceptual debates.

For example, as Robert Koch developed his own microscopic research a few years later, he too was frequently plagued with the issue of "objectivity" and the claim that two observers "could not simultaneously view the same object and form a joint opinion."[146] Thus, a photograph, it was argued, was the only true way to fix an image. Koch brought these arguments to the forefront and argued that new standards had to be created and debated, and in the process he helped garner acceptance for photomicrography as a central resource in bacteriologic research. As Koch himself pointed out, the "photographic picture of a microscopial object is more valuable than the original preparation."[147] Objectivity of representation was similarly important to Koch's contemporaries, as seen in Woodward's efforts to improve microscopic standards, and in America many of these early debates were shaped and facilitated through the Army Medical Museum and Surgeon General's Library.[148]

Woodward and Curtis spent an enormous amount of time experimenting with different sources of illumination (first the sun and, by 1869, electric lights and magnesium lamps), along with various techniques for photographing histological specimens, including staining different sizes of soft tissues with different color aniline to see what photographed best.[149] They photographed normal anatomical preparations and thin sections of diseased tissues, and even the most "delicate microscopial preparations," showing the "most subtle markings," were displayed. Woodward explained that "reproducing microscopial objects can be employed with ease . . . a degree of success that had not previously been obtained."[150] And again, he invited other researchers to tour the museum and learn these methods. Importantly, these standards continued to develop through the museum with the next generation of war physicians, including George Miller Sternberg (the first American researcher to produce photomicrographs of the tubercule bacillus) and Walter Reed (leader of the group of researchers who confirmed the theory that yellow fever is transmitted by a particular mosquito species rather than by direct contact). And, in the tradition of Woodward, they advocated the use of microscopy and photomicrography for establishing "medical truths."

By 1869 the museum had just under a thousand pathological, clinical, and photomicrographic photos (of both test objects and histology), which were used to make engravings for the *Medical and Surgical History of the War of the Rebellion, Circular No. 6*, and the *Army Medical Museum Catalogue*, where Woodward observed that it was his intention to use these photographs to educate physicians on the disease conditions among the soldiers but also on photographic technique. Civil War physician William Thomson (whose photomicrographs had long been of interest to Woodward) also displayed his work at the museum, which included microscopic photographs of sections of femur, eyelid, kidney, ileum, colon, and skin. These representations were made at Douglas Hospital in the spring of 1864, with the purpose of demonstrating the value of photomicrography as an investigative resource, and its possibility with the compound microscope.[151]

Many of the museum photographs were subsequently used as teaching resources in medical schools. A volume of microphotographs was displayed at the Paris Exposition. In 1876 the United States celebrated its centennial with a huge exposition in Philadelphia, and numerous Civil War medical photographs were displayed in a volume entitled *Photographs of Cases of Consolidated Gunshot Fractures of the Femur*, along with a collection of photomicrographs (Woodward showed more than 200 lantern slides and photomicrographs). This exhibit brought the wartime medical work to the attention of the public, along with medical and scientific audiences.[152]

In 1873 John M. Toner instituted the Toner Lectures, which were held at the Smithsonian Institution in Washington. Select elite physicians were invited to present "memoirs or essays relative to some branch of medical science" that demonstrated "some new truth fully established by experiment or observation."[153] The lectures were specifically intended to "increase and diffuse knowledge," some of which had begun with the war. Joseph Woodward was invited to inaugurate the series, on March 28, 1873, speaking on the "Structure of Cancerous Tumors, and the Manner in Which Adjacent Parts Are Invaded."[154] The invitation was recognition of Woodward's status in the field of investigative medicine. Dr. Toner invited Woodward to "contribute something that would aid the general practitioner in the diagnosis of cancerous from other morbid growths."[155]

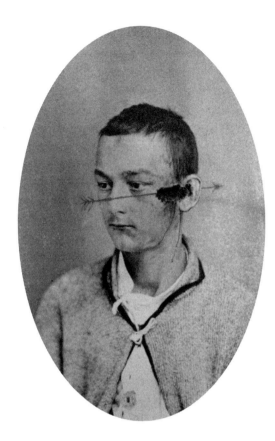

George Andrews, private, Company B, 39th New York Volunteers, age eighteen, was admitted to Harewood General Hospital, April 12, 1865, after receiving a gunshot wound of the face, the ball injuring the soft parts, at the Battle of Fort Stedman, Virginia. The photograph was taken by R. B. Bontecou and was used for teaching and research purposes. The hand-drawn arrow traces the path of the missile and emphasizes the discharge in the wound. (Courtesy of the National Library of Medicine, Washington, D.C.)

Woodward presented his work, which centered mostly on the histological representations of breast cancer, to an audience of more than 100 physicians.[156] He spoke about the anatomy of cancerous growths and illustrated his lecture with specimens from the collection at the Army Medical Museum, which he compared to preparations obtained from European histologists.[157] He projected the preparations on a screen with an oxy-calcium lantern and showed more than seventy microphotographs of selected preparations.[158] It was one of the first times that photomicrographs were used to illustrate a medical lecture.

After Woodward discussed mostly the anatomical facts and clinical phenomena related to his cancer research, in what became a common pattern for Woodward, he encouraged physicians to pursue their own research: "You will the more readily agree with me when I express the opinion that so far from this branch of the inquiry having been exhausted (anatomical facts) additional investigations are urgently needed and ought by all means to be encouraged."[159] In the process he was showing the efficacy of the new

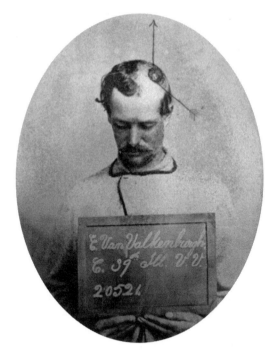

E. Van Valkenburgh, Company C, 39th Illinois, suffered a gunshot wound to the left side of the scalp, denuding the skull. The hand-drawn arrow shows the extent of the wound. This patient was photographed at Harewood General Hospital by R. B. Bontecou. The photograph was used for teaching and research purposes. (Courtesy of the National Library of Medicine, Washington, D.C.)

epistemological, practical, and technical standards that were pioneered and developed through the wartime investigations.

The Army Medical Museum was an important institutional foundation for the development of investigative medicine. Before medical school curricula were reformed, and while associations and journals were in their early stages, the museum provided intellectual support for some emerging specialties and scientific medicine.[160] Woodward believed in the efficacy of scientific photomicrography and displayed and documented the results of his wartime program of microscopic analyses. He studied the original preparations and the photographic preparations, but he was most interested in the methodological and theoretical considerations involved in developing this new means of studying and displaying the results of diseases—and in the process he helped usher in a new dialogue about standards.

In just three years, as Woodward observed, "the result of this effort is the microscopial series, which although small indeed when contrasted with some of the better European collections, is the only considerable micropathological collection in the United States."[161] With the high number of specimens representing the many disease conditions displayed at the museum, physicians could examine intricate structures of the human body and the process of specific diseases, which provided ongoing support for the changing conceptions of disease and the body that took shape during the war. Moreover, the use of new technologies exemplified the changing needs of elite medical practitioners. This differentiated medical study at the museum from traditional approaches to the study of disease, especially among the rank-and-file physicians, laying the foundation for a hierarchy of knowledge and a research ethic to develop in American medicine.

The autopsy, microscope, and photomicrography encouraged physicians to think differently about disease because they could see deep within the body in a way most had not before. It prompted very specific questions: What did certain manifestations mean? What could be learned by studying putrefactive substances? What might the blood reveal about disease causation? What were the "animalcules" or cells that seemed to either cause or result from specific diseases? Could certain therapeutics counteract a disease process? With the rise of the germ theory after 1870 the microscope would become ubiquitous in the medical world. But even before this change the war created unprecedented disease environments that demanded new investigative answers, and nowhere was that more evident than in the dynamic and spirited experiments precipitated by two of the most fearful diseases encountered in the Civil War hospitals: erysipelas and hospital gangrene.

CHAPTER THREE

Civil War Bodies and the Development of Experimental Method

Erysipelas and Hospital Gangrene during the American Civil War, 1861–1865

T he men are sometimes placed in wards already affected with hospital gangrene or with erysipelas and cases have come to our knowledge in which they have thus contracted these maladies . . . we fear that a good many have thus lost their limbs and their lives."[1] So noted Medical Inspector Frank Hamilton of the increasing incidence of gangrene and erysipelas as the war progressed. The Civil War saw both an unprecedented number of wartime amputations and the development of hospitals in which to treat and manage soldiers. These hospitals became a new source for septic infections like pyemia, gangrene, and erysipelas to develop—but also a new physical location in which to study the infectiousness of disease.[2] In late 1862 Surgeon General William Hammond issued special instructions to a select group of physicians to investigate what had become serious problems among the Union army: erysipelas, referred to as "St. Anthony's Fire" or the "Rose,"[3] and hospital gangrene, commonly referred to as the "typhus of wounds." These infections were responsible for significant wartime morbidity and mortality,[4] with a reported case fatality rate of 41 percent and 45.6 percent respectively.[5]

Gangrene and erysipelas are streptococcal infections,[6] generally the result of wound infections. The streptococci prevalent during the Civil War seemed to be of a much higher virulence than the strains commonly seen today.[7] Hospital gangrene was most prevalent in general hospitals, and once it appeared moved quickly among patients, a consequence of the imperfect understanding of aseptic technique. The bacteria did not directly attack the skin; destruction was caused as the bacteria released toxins into the skin and muscles. The infection spread rapidly through the body by the blood stream and continued to involve more tissues as it spread. As more tissues were destroyed, blood clots formed in the small arteries, stopping the flow of blood and nutrients, which was followed by further bacterial invasion and putrefaction.[8]

There were various types of gangrene reported during the war, including what was referred to as the traumatic and hospital types; but all cases were studied and recorded together. The authors of *The Medical and Surgical History of the War of the Rebellion* noted: "According to the conception or predilection of the surgeon, these terms, in many instances, seem to have been used indiscriminately, and it has been found utterly impossible to determine with accuracy the cases of traumatic gangrene, hospital gangrene, dry gangrene, etc."[9]

Erysipelas is a bacterial skin infection and today is often caused by infection with group A streptococci[10] or group A staphylococcus. It usually needs a break in the skin for the bacteria to gain a foothold. It can stay in one area or spread beneath the skin and, like gangrene, aggressively destroys tissues. Erysipelas generally attacked the legs, torso, and face, spreading peripherally. During the war it was noted that patients suffered from upward-spreading "hot, bright red, edematous, infiltrated and a sharp ulcerated tense hard feeling of the cuticle."[11] The skin was described as "smooth and shining but is rough to the touch due to the ulceration of the papilla."[12] The symptoms of the disease were "fever, delirium, constipated condition of the bowels, loss of appetite, headache, depression, pulse frequent and full"; when the disease was "deeper and seated among the cellular tissue these symptoms may be aggravated." Indeed, it was known that erysipelas involved cellular tissue and could be fatal if it spread to the lymph nodes and bloodstream, a condition physicians referred to as pyemia.[13]

The study of gangrene and erysipelas during the war was part of a pivotal debate over the origins of disease and how physicians understood the body. Within the new hospitals, physicians saw convincing evidence of the contagiousness of disease, which reconfigured ideas about disease causation but also ways in which to study and manage the infectiousness of disease. Three conditions allowed for the development of these investigations. First, there was support from the state—both technical and financial—and physicians were encouraged to develop effective methods for the management and protection of the soldiers suffering in the hospitals. Second, physicians found desperate subjects. The diseases were destructive and spread quickly—soldiers could literally see their limbs rotting as the diseases spread and thus cooperated with the hopes of improved treatment.[14]

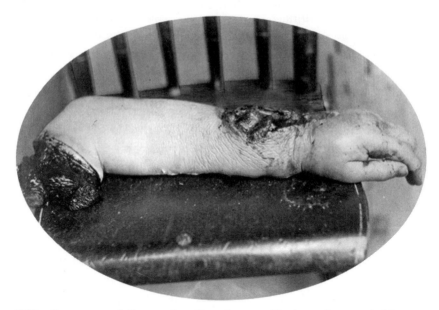

William Brown, corporal, Company, I, 1st Massachusetts, suffered a gunshot wound of the lower third of the forearm, injuring the ulna, with severe gangrene supervening. His left forearm, upper third, was amputated by circular incision. This photograph of the amputated arm illustrates the massive destruction of tissues caused by gangrene. The patient died three weeks after his operation. Brown was photographed at Harewood General Hospital by R. B. Bontecou. (Photograph courtesy of the National Library of Medicine, Washington, D.C.)

Finally, physicians found ample opportunity to create and conduct scientific experiments in the Civil War hospitals. The study of hospital gangrene and erysipelas also stimulated underdeveloped areas in American medicine, including the demand for hygiene and cleanliness in hospitals and medical equipment, the use of disinfectants to manage the disease environments, consultation about the management of disease, and practical demonstrations and the transmission of this knowledge.[15] In the process physicians developed a new set of guidelines for producing medical knowledge.[16]

Importantly, many physicians had limited experience with these diseases before the war.[17] When asked to describe the "peculiarities" in the local disturbance of hospital gangrene in his entrance exam, Joseph Woodward wrote that, "with regard to these, as my own personal experience in civil surgery has never showed me a single case for investigation, I shall be obliged to condense from my recollection of the graphic account of Rokitansky's Handbook of Pathological Anatomy."[18] There were, however, ideal conditions for the development of gangrene and erysipelas in the Civil War hospitals. Civil War weaponry was particularly destructive.[19] The conoidal (minié) ball, invented in the late 1840s and used in the rifle, was the central weapon of the Civil War and was responsible for the majority of wounds.[20] Easily shattering bones and causing ghastly wounds because the velocity was low and the metal could spread on impact, it created extensive surface wounds (often carrying clothing and other matter into the tissues), leading to ichorous wounds, amputations, and often severe septic infections.

STUDYING GANGRENE AND ERYSIPELAS

On March 14, 1863, as wartime hospitals overflowed with patients suffering from gangrene and erysipelas, Assistant Surgeon Middleton Goldsmith (acting on the orders of Hammond) issued a circular letter requesting that physicians submit all case histories of and recorded experiences with gangrene and erysipelas thus far and conduct special investigations into hospital gangrene. He instructed that "each observer should study the disease for himself as if he were observing a new disease, faithfully portraying the facts and appearances as they occur so that those reading his descriptions could see the cases as he saw them. When opinions or conclusions are expressed the facts upon which they are based should be clearly set forth."[21]

The circular asked physicians to study hospital gangrene's causes, transmission, pathology, and treatment. Because gangrene and erysipelas often appeared together, physicians would isolate these cases in the hospital and study the diseases together. Physicians responded to the circular by generating hundreds of case reports on both diseases. Goldsmith was aiming to determine whether they were "internal diseases" caused by a general disorder of function or developed in the body from a malfunction of existing cells, as Virchow's cellular pathology then suggested. Either of these explanations favored a physiological conception of disease—the idea that disease somehow rested in the body or bloodstream. Or, conversely, did an external agent, a separate disease-causing entity, enter the body from without to produce the disease, which would support an ontological conception of disease? Goldsmith asked physicians to consider "reference to a previous condition," the "solidity" of the tissues in the spread of the disease, the nature of the pus in the sores (both as it progressed or as it was arrested), and the role of putrefaction and decomposition.

The aim was to compile a complete picture of the diseases by addressing a range of issues: the introduction and development of the "poison" in the body, the expression of particular symptoms, changes in the sore at each particular stage, the role of predisposing causes, and the severity of the disease. Finally, Goldsmith requested that physicians suggest remedies on how to arrest the "gangrenous process," produce and maintain "granulation," treat the constitutional disorder, and treat the slough "when they have lost their poisonous quality."[22]

The common thread, when it came to these diseases, was that most physicians were simultaneously intrigued and shocked. The symptoms of gangrene in particular were unsightly and spread quickly within and between patients. Physician Silas Weir Mitchell observed, "There were things seen in the surgical wards which you will, I trust, never see, or only in jars in the surgeon general's museum. A slight fleshwound began to show a gray edge of slough, and within two hours we saw this widening at the rate of half an inch an hour, and deepening, until in some horrible cases arteries and nerves were left bare across a devastated region. It was what we called hospital gangrene. Instant removal to the open air of tents, etherization, savage cautery with pure nitric acid or bromine, and dressings of powdered charcoal enabled us to deal with these cases more or less well, but the mortality was hideous—at least 45 percent."[23]

Goldsmith was thrilled to have the opportunity to develop knowledge that might contribute to the larger understanding of these diseases. As he reported to Hammond, "These occurrences satisfy me of the great wisdom of your order detailing me for special duty in relation to this matter. . . . The surgeons were kind enough to express a wish to hear my views in the matter of pyaemia, hospital gangrene etc. Of course I was but too glad to gratify them and I took advantage of the occasion to enter fully upon the whole subject and distribute among the medical officers forms for the record of cases, from which I hope to get some reliable records of cases of pyaemia, resections etc."[24]

Sponsored investigations, it was hoped, might save lives and were thus begun with high expectations among all physicians. Some physicians adopted the traditional task of empirical observation, amassing information to be synthesized by the experts; others analyzed the diseases, patients, hospitals, and locales, trying to prove or disprove commonly held notions about the diseases; still others went further, adopting newer techniques such as chemical, microscopial, animal, and even human experimentation, adumbrating the importance of the laboratory for producing medical knowledge. Goldsmith observed in 1863 that "a series of investigations is now on foot seeking to discover the essential agent, if one exists, which sets up these diseases."[25] The chief debate centered on whether these diseases

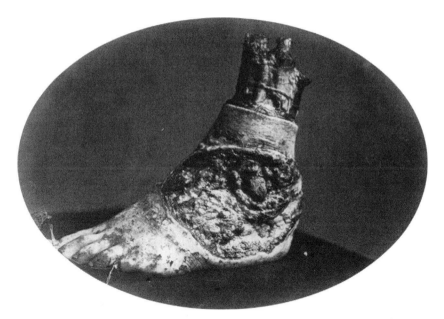

John D. Parmenter, private, Company G, 67th Pennsylvania Volunteers, suffered a gunshot wound at the Battle of Amelia Springs, Virginia, April 6, 1865, and developed a gangrenous ulcer on the left side of the foot. The foot was photographed at Harewood General Hospital by R. B. Bontecou. This photograph well illustrates the extent of tissue damage caused by gangrene. (Photograph courtesy of the National Library of Medicine, Washington, D.C.)

were "local affections" or had "constitutional origins." In order to understand how ideas about disease evolved during the war, it is necessary to take a closer look at how disease causation was understood at midcentury.

DISEASE IN THE NINETEENTH CENTURY

Joseph Woodward's *Outlines of Chief Camp Diseases* employs the same classifications as did the British Army in 1859 and 1860, which broke up the "zymotic theory" (decomposition or degeneration) into three groups of disease ferments: miasmatic (from air or water, soil and plant matter), enthetic or contagious (person to person or the result of inoculation), and dietic (related to constitution). He also mentions parasitic diseases (intestinal parasites and scabies) but suggests that they must stand in their own class of *Parasitici*, since parasitic diseases were no longer seen as a constitutional affection but rather an animal infecting the skin and intestines.[26] Some case reports refer to the diseases as septic ferments (meaning to rot) because of the massive destruction of tissues.

The chief conflicts at midcentury were between anticontagionists and contagionists. Anticontagionists generally believed in the existence of decomposing organic matter called miasma or miasms that would thrive in certain atmospheric conditions, including filth, in which a person with a constitutional predisposition was at greatest risk.[27] Miasms were thought to develop or arise from rotting vegetable or animal matter, including dead animals and feces, and would contaminate the air. Thus miasmatists often used the term "bad air" when describing disease conditions. Contagionists, on the other hand, suggested that the disease-causing matter was produced in the bodies of sick people, transmitted by exhalations, and inhaled by healthy people who then became sick.[28] Thus, each disease had a specific cause that was necessary for its development.

Many Civil War physicians were contingent contagionists and wrestled with the evidence of the cases they confronted. They generally believed that whether the disease was contagious was dependent on factors such as individual susceptibility, habits, filth, weather, diet, and virulence of the virus.[29] Physicians who were wedded to one cause of disease may have found their views challenged during their investigations. For example, those committed to the idea that disease was the result of rotting vegetable matter or "noxious effluvia" in the environment and depended on vulnerable constitutions may have had to concede that there was some sort of specific contagion that attacked indiscriminately.

Civil War physicians incorporated these ideas about disease causation into four general theories and used these specific headings to account for erysipelas and gangrene: constitutional, local, local and constitutional, and malfunctioning with regard to existing cells. The constitutional cause held that a debilitated constitution resulting from exposure, poor diet, fatigue, or impure water, along with a poison in the air or "miasmatic atmosphere,"[30] might lead to gangrene or erysipelas. Others believed in local causes—that direct contact with disease matter found on sponges, washbowls, or surgical instruments, especially in crowded, poorly ventilated conditions, would lead to an outbreak of disease. Finally some adherents of Virchow's recently published lectures on cellular pathology believed disease was spread from diseased cells to the rest of the body as cells divided; thus, all changes could be traced to chemical or physical changes within cells.[31]

But the process was complicated. Differing disease theories such as contagion (from person to person) or infection (indirect contact through water, air, or contaminated articles, with different diseases often erupting together) or miasma (putrid odors) were interchangeable and complementary for many physicians.[32] The case reports raised fundamental questions about the nature of disease, with which physicians had to wrestle. However, some sort of "poison" was causing serious infections in the Civil War hospitals, and this disease-causing matter was necessary for the disease to thrive and develop. Thus, in trying to determine the nature of these diseases, physicians were asked to think hard about what certain manifestations meant, including the pathological changes, degenerative changes, the role of inflammation, the nature of the pus, and decomposition, all of which demanded reflection about the fundamental nature of disease.[33] The approach to these diseases in terms of investigation, understanding, and treatment was highly individualistic—and the directive to study these diseases supported epistemological innovation.

Managing these diseases was a challenge, and contributing to the general understanding of them legitimized the physician's role as a producer of medical knowledge. W. W. Keen remarked that "hospital gangrene or the 'typhus of wounds' is in its most marked form, a fearful and unwelcome guest in any hospital; most of all in a military hospital. It claims many victims in its fierce attacks, and often puts to naught all the resources of the most skillful surgeon."[34] With his experience at a hospital post, Keen was able to offer some important insights on gangrene: "The question has almost uniformly been raised by authors whether the disease is constitutional or local. Without quoting particular authorities, suffice it to say that rather the larger number regards it as a local disease. 'Sometimes' in the language of Guthrie, preceded by and accompanied with, constitutional symptoms. But the concurrent constitutional symptoms are no proof of a similar character in the disease, for the removal of a benign tumor. An amputation, or a gunshot wound is followed by the same. No one as yet has ever seen the disease *originate* constitutionally, but *always* locally."[35]

The debate about local versus constitutional origins of the disease was important because it helped contribute to an understanding of causation. Did the disease rest in the body (perhaps developing spontaneously), or was there a specific contagion that traveled on fingers or sponges that was obtained externally and manifested locally? Was the physician or attendant somehow spreading the disease? Goldsmith's circular asked physicians to consider the "causes of the disease," whether local or otherwise, along with "how they operate" and if "any condition of general health predisposed the person to invasion of the diseases."[36]

Assistant Surgeon Daniel Morgan undertook an in-depth study of hospital gangrene and erysipelas in late 1862 and reported to Hammond and Goldsmith that on October 19, 1862, after three or four days of cold, rainy weather and the men being crowded together with little ventilation because of the rain, three cases of gangrene developed among the patients "all in the lower extremity." Also, about twelve or fifteen wounds, which had been healing, "stopped cicatrizing, and assumed an unhealthy appearance." He noted that the wounds "were red and punctuated in some small new vessels and they bled freely. On removing the dressing the parts already cicatrized became bluish, red and in the worst looking cases an inflammatory nature—red color with a hard base, was observed."[37]

Morgan reacted quickly. He removed the cases of gangrene to a tent with six beds and an allowance of space of 232 feet, and with treatment the patients rapidly recovered. Matters in the hospital progressed well until November 8, when the disease reappeared: "During the last an attempt was made to treat the cases in the ward without isolation, but it only ended in an utter failure and they were again removed. Four days before it made an appearance in barrack E the disease appeared in barrack B where its history was an exact counterpart to the one already related. From these two barracks the most over crowded, and by the way the only one in which erysipelas had appeared, the disease spread to all the others in most cases apparently by contagion and some clearly by infection."

Shortly afterward, Morgan left his post in Frederick and reported to the West Philadelphia hospital, where he continued studying gangrene and erysipelas: "One week after admission Dec. 30th 1862, I observed the cases of decided hospital gangrene, both of the thigh, in my own ward; and at the same time 8 of 10 of the other wounds began to look unhealthy." At this time he immediately and vigorously treated the gangrenous wounds with nitric acid, but he did not remove the patients from the ward; rather, he focused on preventing the further progress of the disease. "I ordered every other window on both sides to be lowered both day and night and put a reliable patient in charge of the matter. I obtained a sponge for each man; directed the nurses to dress the gangrenous and unhealthy sores and to wash their hands carefully in dilute chlorinated solution and to use no dressing or bandage a second time and soda freely used on the floor near those suffering from the disease."

He then compared what he had seen at Frederick and West Philadelphia in the hopes of painting a fuller picture of gangrene, and he found a marked contrast. In Frederick, for example, the gangrene was "noticeably contagious and spread widely" within the barrack, while in West Philadelphia, although "probably contagious it did not invade many wounds in the same wards nor did it spread mostly to adjoining wards." He attributed this apparent contrast to the fact that the patients suffering from gangrene were isolated in West Philadelphia whereas in Frederick they remained in the general wards. There were, however, some similarities between the two locations. He noted that both sets of patients improved with the use of nitric acid as an escharotic, that both attacks followed a "few days of bleak, cold and rainy weather, that both occurred where a number of wounded were collected together, that in individual symptoms both were precisely alike, and that they improved immediately on the setting of fine weather and under appropriate treatment."[38]

He evolved a concept of contagion and suggested the reality of a disease entity and a constancy of the disease from patient to patient; however, he also included older ideas related to miasma by placing a primacy on the environment. Indeed, Morgan subscribed to the view that the disease was local and constitutional; he believed that patients needed to be in some kind of debilitated state while exposed to debilitating local factors (e.g., atmospheric contamination or contact with gangrenous matter)—that is, a contingent contagionist environment. But what he proposed was a more scientific interpretation than merely a simple theory of toxic miasmas in filthy surroundings. Indeed, he emphasized the importance of antiseptics in hospitals, stressing that the surgeon had a responsibility to manage gangrenous wounds *before* they became septic and that the nurses must take precautions by washing hands before and after visiting patients, which had immediate clinical relevance in the management of these diseases.

In fact, ideas about disease causation became increasingly sophisticated in these investigations. In the summer of 1862, Goldsmith was sent to Nashville and Murfreesboro to conduct special investigations into both hospital gangrene and erysipelas.[39] His initial objective was to determine the epidemiology, pathology, and etiology of these diseases. While there, he traced the history of the causes of two outbreaks of disease, the first of erysipelas, the other of hospital gangrene. He noted that both disease outbreaks "were somewhat peculiar" and the "facts are pregnant with suggestions of scientific import." In tracing the cause of gangrene, he reported that it was of an "indigenous origin," meaning a "man having been brought into a ward with hospital gangrene imparts the gangrenous character to the wounds of other men." He proposed that it was produced by inoculation, that the "poison" spread through the "medium of the atmosphere and adheres with great endurance and tenacity to fomites, which spread through multiplication of gangrenous matter."[40]

In terms of erysipelas, he advanced the idea that it most often resulted "in the form of puerperal peritonitis from the infection upon the hands of the midwife, as in the historical German cases."[41] He was referring here to the brilliant findings of the Hungarian physician Ignaz Semmelweis. In the 1840s, Semmelweis noticed while working in the Vienna General Hospital the high number of deaths following childbirth. Semmelweis made a study of two maternity wards in the hospital—one of these wards was frequented by students who went back and forth between the autopsy room and maternity ward, and this ward saw numerous deaths, while the other did not. Semmelweis made the connection, then, that students were passing contaminated material from the dead bodies they autopsied to new mothers. As a result of his findings, he ordered all students to disinfect their hands in a solution of chlorine and water after performing an autopsy and before visiting the maternity ward. The number of deaths was immediately and drastically reduced.

Even so, in 1847 this was a radical theory. The root of the difficulty was the idea of a cadaveric particle that caused disease. In the decades before the Civil War, contagionism was politically unpopular; even the mere mention of contagion was contentious because of its association with repressive quarantine measures, which challenged both business interests and the individual liberty so prized in Jacksonian America.[42] Moreover, because a specific contagion for a specific disease had not yet been proved, the very idea was difficult to accept. Part of the problem too was that orthodox physicians were striving for legitimacy, and they did not want the public to think it was the physicians themselves who were inadvertently spreading disease.

The war years were different. Quarantine or isolation was no longer a political issue (at least in the military hospitals).[43] Soldiers needed to be effectively managed so they could be returned to the front lines. The soldiers were treated in large and sprawling hospitals where infections spread widely. It was an imperative, a social responsibility, that the medical department structure and secure these institutions to preserve manpower. But the Civil War hospitals also provided a model, a chance to research the underlying causes of these hospital infections. Goldsmith's reference to Semmelweis was based on his extensive research program in the Civil War hospitals and was significant in 1863. As one historian has pointed out, "In spite of a persisting tradition to the contrary, Semmelweis's work was widely known and frequently cited between 1865–1890 by many of the very persons who actively contributed to the etiological research programme—the programme that ultimately replaced *chimbuki*-medicine."[44]

Many Civil War physicians believed that erysipelas traveled through the atmosphere, was inhaled, and entered the blood through the respiratory organs. But Goldsmith wondered, If the poison acted from the blood, or rather had constitutional origins, why did the disease select the face as the beginning point? Furthermore, what could be learned about erysipelas by examining a woman during the "parturient state" and the relation to puerperal peritonitis? He reasoned that a woman giving birth exposed to the miasm would likely develop puerperal peritonitis, but during the "non-parturient state" or after giving birth many women escaped puerperal peritonitis. Why did the miasm affect women during labor? He determined, "Her uterus is stripped of its lining epithelium; the internal surface of the uterus is like a piece of skin stripped of its epidermis. After this epithelial covering is reproduced, the parturient woman is no longer any more liable to the invasion of erysipelas than she was before she became pregnant."[45]

He did not see how the disease resulted from the blood and then manifested local symptoms. He compared his theory with what he was then witnessing among Civil War patients: "Expose a hundred men to the miasm of erysipelas; a certain number will have erysipelas of the face, the disease always commencing in the eyelid, the alae of the nose, or behind the ear. The disease commences in no other part of the body; it does not attack the trunk or extremities. But if wounds or abrasions exist, the erysipelas no longer selects the face, but attacks with discrimination of region, the parts wounded or abraded—provided only that the parts thus wounded or abraded are uncovered."[46] He further found that men were more liable to attacks while in the crowded hospitals; but by protecting the face or open wound with remedies such as tincture of iodine or the frequent application of glycerin, simple cerate, or resin ointment, the tendency to new attacks almost disappeared.

In the late 1860s, as the noted British scientist Joseph Lister developed his methods for reducing infections in surgical wards, some physicians traveled to his wards to observe his methods: surgical instruments were soaked in carbolic acid, and carbolic-soaked dressings were placed on the wound (in 1870, he added a carbolic spray to treat the wound and surgical area).[47] Physicians found that by adopting these measures, the mortality from childbed fever fell drastically. Lister's measures were similarly studied and applied by Johann Ritter von Nussbaum in the early 1870s during the

Franco-Prussian War in his gangrene ward.[48] But these developments came after the Civil War, and it is of great significance that Goldsmith's work foreshadowed some of these discoveries.[49]

Goldsmith adopted almost the same idea that Lister would later advocate: keeping airborne germs away from open wounds. He suggested that, based on the facts, erysipelas must be a kind of contagion that acted "by contact with the skin" and that it floated in the atmosphere and attacked a face with an uncovered wound. The face was susceptible because here the "epithelium was thinnest," though he also suggested that wounds on the hand could engender an attack as well. Lister's "germs" were, however, living, and Goldsmith did not get that far (discussed further in chapter 6). But he did suggest that, when the material surface of the uterus was opened, the woman was also at risk of the contagion. He challenged Civil War physicians to reinvestigate the "accepted theory" that diseases were simply products of the blood and consider that perhaps there was some kind of influence that was caused and manifested locally.

As noted earlier, germ theories were complicated. Proponents of a physiological understanding of disease—namely, that disease was the response of the patient to a changed state or changed condition—always focused on the interiority of the specific patient. However, epidemics had always given some credibility to an ontological understanding of disease, supporting the notion that disease had a real existence separate from the response of the individual patient. It was thus difficult to resolve the debate with the physiology available in the mid-nineteenth century. Some data, such as the existence of tubercules in different organs, suggested the possibility of ontology, but the great variability of patients to similar stimuli suggested physiology. The discovery of a specific microorganism for a specific disease would stress ontology, but the variability of immune response would again raise physiological questions. During the war, Civil War physicians were seeing the complexities of medicine and disease and, as a result, thinking about disease and investigations in more sophisticated ways. Civil War physicians did not agree on a separate and distinct cause for gangrene and erysipelas yet, but their experience in the hospitals, particularly with wound and surgical infections, clearly paved the way for these new but complicated ideas about disease to emerge. Indeed, new ideas about the causation of puerperal fever was paramount in the development of bacterial theory.[50]

The key finding in these investigations, then, was that the diseases were local but that a local one could produce constitutional symptoms.[51]

Goldsmith encouraged physicians to focus not on the interiority of the patient but rather on the disease entity at the local level. Local applications were considered efficacious if it was a suitable substance with the "chemical power of decomposing the specific virus of gangrene so that it no longer exists, provided it can be brought in sufficient quantities in direct contact with every atom of gangrene matter."[52]

Pyemia proved more difficult to understand.[53] Pyemia was a serious infection. Cases of erysipelas could spread under the skin, into the blood stream, destroying tissues, causing inflammation and new sites of infection throughout the body. Goldsmith suggested that it was the result of a local wound that spread or had become infected.[54] He did not understand the behavior of the disease, so he suggested a simple theory of absorption, according to which, "in some diseases, THE GRAVAMEN OF THE CONSTITUTIONAL STATE, IF NOT ITS TOTALITY, IS PLAINLY DUE TO THE ABSORPTION OF THE PRODUCTS OF THE LOCAL PROCESSES. I say, absorption; for it is not possible to conceive of any other processes by which the whole organism could be involved to the extent noticed."[55]

The only other explanation may have been provided by the cellular theory of disease: "Adopting the coda of Virchow that all permanent infections have a permanent source of infection, I treat the source of the infection with remedies which tend to destroy or render innocuous the infecting matter."[56] Because the disease rested in the cellular tissue, physicians would have to use a syringe to inject a remedy into the cellular planes. But he encouraged other researchers to concentrate on the issue because the observations may have had a wider significance for the transmission of all diseases. Goldsmith's program of research well illustrates the climate in which Civil War medicine developed and why these years were important. There was an emphasis on mastering both the unfamiliar and familiar: "If the projected law is a true one, the effect would not be to revolutionize but to simplify; to give precision to methods now vaguely used; to give definite views and purpose to remedial measures; to draw attention to the completeness in the effect of traditional remedies; to supplant surmise with faith, and indecision and doubt with confidence."

Goldsmith concluded by noting that the "observations lead me to think [these findings will have] broader significance and wider application than is generally believed." He thus did not want to challenge beliefs but rather "invite investigation." He asked physicians, then, to think about new ways to study these diseases, in particular to consider the role of the "fluid products of the sores prior to the development of gangrene," during the "continuance of gangrene," and on the "arrest of the gangrenous process."[57] Specific manifestations such as "disorganization of the tissue, "vibrios," "globules," "animalcules," and "cells" were now studied at length, which changed the very nature of medical study during the war in America.

EXPERIMENTAL THINKING AND CIVIL WAR SCIENCE

On February 18, 1863, Joseph Woodward was dispatched to the Annapolis General Hospital "for the purpose of examining the microscopial appearances of hospital gangrene."[58] His chief objective was to determine how and why the disease spread with such rapidity. He made some clinical observations in his report but confined himself mostly to pathological histological considerations. He found two "diverse modes of extension" of the disease while in its "destructive progress," which was frequently combined in "different portions of the same excavation." He was referring to the spread of the disease and the damage to tissues (which involved the connective tissues and adipose layer). Physicians would often examine the first point of the disease, usually the point of entrance or exit of the wound, but the disease quickly spread to the tissues where the most damage would be wrought. Woodward examined the tissues immediately adjacent to the slough and noticed that they became slightly reddened without being increased in thickness and had a tendency to become greenish brown or black (as tissues were destroyed); the slough steadily progressed into the sound tissues "so long as it is not separated" and continued to extend by a "pus producing or ulcerative action."

The second class of the disease he examined was the slough invading the surrounding tissues deeper because the "thickened mass breaks down rapidly into a fetid yellowish ichor (signaling serious infection) and is quickly eroded in such a manner as that the subcutaneous connective tissue is more speedily destroyed than the skin which overhangs."[59] This variety was more serious, causing more tissue damage because it penetrated the "deep fascia," the "connective tissue septa," even the muscles and tendons, producing inflammation and often sepsis.

Woodward's methodology was to examine both "modes of extension" to try to determine how to arrest the spread and understand the pathology of gangrene—in particular, to determine at what stage the disease became septic and what changes could be observed along the way. Woodward suggested that gangrene was the result of degenerative and inflammatory action due to diseased tissues and cells. He believed the morbid changes were being spread from cell to cell and found these cases to be a good opportunity to study the "pus formation in the muscular tissue" and the role of the "muscular fibre" in the inflammatory process. He believed the "so called nuclei of the sarcolemma" contributed to the formation of the products of inflammation by enlarging, multiplying, and producing "broods which encroach upon the proper substance of the fibre." He considered that the pathogenic process causing inflammation had to be countered; when it was not, the wound took far longer to heal, or would steadily worsen, leading to sepsis. Woodward thus recommended local treatments, combined with improving the debilitated state, hoping to strengthen the patient from within and to counter the poisons.

Like many other cell theorists, he was opposed to any idea of an invading germ. Even when he saw the bacteria clearly, he failed to identify correctly their role in the disease: "An allusion may be made to the idea that the peculiar characteristics of this disease are due to the local presence of microscopial fungi. This idea is not borne out by facts. Accurate examination with a magnifying power of cases in every stage both where nothing but an ordinary water dressing had been employed as well as in cases in which various forms of antiseptic caustic washes had been applied utterly failed to demonstrate any cryptogrammic organisms except the ordinary bacteria which are to be observed in every decomposing animal substance."[60]

While his investigations did not lead to the discovery of the streptococci causing gangrene, his methodology was important. He studied "putrescent matter" and the blood ("scanty" red corpuscles and the increases in white corpuscles), trying to determine the internal manifestation of the disease; and most importantly, he studied sequences of the disease process (in the two stages he saw) and published his findings, including diagrams of his microscopic results and blood analysis.[61] While Woodward did not recognize the microorganisms that caused disease, he once again challenged the way in which disease was traditionally studied. The chief focus was on the diseased structures and morbid secretions rather than merely the symptoms obtained at the bedside.

The increasing emphasis on the bodily fluids and products of disease proved to be important in stimulating new investigative techniques, particularly pathological chemistry. The development of the basic sciences would help reshape understandings of medicine and disease. On March 19, 1863, Thomas E. Jenkins, assistant surgeon in Louisville, Kentucky, submitted to Hammond a report titled "On the Chemical and Physical Character of Sloughs Resulting from Hospital Gangrene." He was invited by

Hammond to conduct investigations into the nature and composition of the substances resulting from the actions of the morbid processes of hospital gangrene. He was asked to examine both the "poison"-producing gangrene and the products or chemical constitution of the decomposing mass that resulted from gangrene. This was an excellent way to incorporate chemical methods in medical research but also to explain basic functions such as digestion, respiration, and excretion, along with the role of blood and the products of disease in causation. Jenkins attempted to throw light on these diseases: "As there appear to be a fast gaining hope that chemistry is to throw some new light into or open the subject of pathology, especially in regard to diseases of an infectious character, I have undertaken these researches and commenced a series of experiments having for their object the accurate determination of all the substances resulting from the diseased action and their compositions, with a new view of discovering the agent or agents procuring such morbid action, or to find out some prophylactic or antidote for such materials as give rise to the disease."[62]

His experiments began with a physical investigation into the altered tissues involved in the "destruction produced by ulcerating processes of gangrene" and the new formulations resulting from such "destruction or alteration." He examined microscopically the products of the disease, including the pus corpuscles, pus mixed with sloughs, and pus treated with nitric acid. He found that the resulting matter of gangrene had special properties that were "solid, liquid and gaseous," but he could not explain the chemical changes produced by the disease. In particular, he could not understand why these chemicals initiated specific disease processes; he saw the bacillus but did not yet connect the bacteria with the disease.

His report was rather detailed. He discussed the solids contained in the tissues, diminished quantities of sulfur and phosphorus, and he searched for "lost elements" in the gaseous products of decomposition. He puzzled about "a minute quantity of $HSWH_3$ in the gases" and noted that "a portion of these elements exist in a much more complex state of combination and give rise to what I have reason to believe to be an alkaline body containing S & P as an essential constituent, a new body containing not only C, H, N & O, as most of the organic alkaloids are higher and much more complex than the alkaloids we are acquainted with as albumen is higher in its organization than sugar or fat." Since his first attempts at explaining the elements were unsuccessful, he promised Hammond that the "further elucidation of this matter is the subject of my future experiments. . . . In future communication I may be able to give you the exact constitution of this or these new bodies."

The chemical analysis of disease processes was a relatively new technique developed through the war in the hopes of better understanding gangrene. Jenkins assumed, like many doctors of this period, that the disease was the result of a chemical process. The new bodies he witnessed had some role in the disease, but what were they? Were they the cause or the result of the disease? As Jenkins noted early on, the full capacity of these diseases seemed beyond the knowledge of general physicians, but they did stimulate study, debate, and analysis—and new ideas about prevention and therapeutic management. For example, Jenkins reported that antiseptics would effectively combat the diseases by decomposing the organic body, abstracting water, forming with organic matter compounds less susceptible of decay by deodorizing the body or by destroying cryptogamic plants and infusorial animalcules.[63] The results were published in the *Medical and Surgical History of the War of the Rebellion* and a number of medical journals.

The physician Benjamin Woodward (no relation to Joseph) was similarly asked to report on the fluids of gangrene. Benjamin Woodward graduated from Rush Medical College in 1857. His thesis, "The Physician—His Qualifications and Mission," was well regarded by his peers, and just before the war he had begun some experimental work on iodine and its possibilities in medicine.[64] During the war he further developed his scientific interests and conducted experiments on the microscopic appearance of the ichor of gangrene and gangrenous erysipelas. Ichorous infection was associated with the putrid matter in the wounds, cavities, or gangrenous surfaces. It was common in the 1860s to differentiate between "good pus" (creamy, less foul smelling) or "ichorus pus" (malignant pus, the result of more serious infection).[65] Benjamin Woodward submitted his report entitled "Notes on the Pus and Ichor of Hospital Gangrene" to John Brinton early in 1863.[66]

Benjamin Woodward studied the two stages of gangrene. In particular he studied changes in the tissues and cells as revealed by the microscope. Woodward attempted to explain through his examination when and why "good" and "bad" pus would exist.[67] Why did some cases of the disease proceed to serious infection, pyemia, and often death, while other cases did not? He was particularly concerned with the "pus globules" and the transformation that created the globules. Were they the result of changes in the blood, for example? Or, rather, what process transformed "lymph cells" and "granulations" into pus? Why did pus globules exist in varying sizes? Moreover, the gangrenous matter seemed to "offer a nidus in which simple forms of animal or even vegetable life are rapidly generated." What role did these animalcules, then, play in the disease process?

He looked for answers specifically in the process of decomposition of the tissues, the debris of fiber—cell and blood discs, which he believed always existed in infectious gangrene. What he referred to as "cell and blood discs" never seemed to exist in "healthy wounds" or good pus. In gangrene ichor, on the other hand, what he referred to as "blood globules" were always found coming from the small vessels that "are ruptured and destroyed, but always in an irregular form." Cases in which only "good pus" existed tended to stay localized, and he also believed wounds would heal under good pus. By contrast, "bad pus" signaled a deeper wound and the inevitable invasion and massive destruction of tissues, tendons, and nerves.[68] The goal was "healing by first intention" (when tissues repaired with little inflammation),[69] which rarely happened in the presence of "ichorus pus." He also commented on the complications from sepsis (worsened by the sheer number of abscesses), which would aid the spread of the disease by invading more tissues and "putrefactive decomposition."[70] This was considered a process, and thus the goal was to arrest putrefaction in the wound by some kind of substance.[71]

But his work here did lead to some new ways to think about disease causation. Woodward was convinced that the disease had contagious properties, that it was the gangrenous matter, or a specific agent, spreading from wound to wound, that was responsible for the outbreaks. He informed Brinton that he would like to report an interesting finding. He conducted an experiment, taking a clean tube, filling it with filtered glycerin, placing one end of the tube close to a gangrenous wound, "which was a wall of putrefactive gangrene," and the other end in his mouth to draw "putrid gas through the tube" until he nearly "fainted with the stench."[72] He then closed the tube and left it for twenty-four hours, after which he examined it under the microscope. He used a ⅛-inch objective in his examination and discovered "numerable cells." He noted that consolidated glycerin developed around each cell in the tube and "then went to a man with a perfectly healthy wound and inoculated his wound with smeared glycerin from inside the tube." He placed the patient in a ward with no gangrene whatsoever, monitored the patient closely, and found within sixteen hours that "gangrene was well developed in the wound."[73]

He subsequently asked Brinton to consider another possible cause for gangrene: "Is cell matter thrown off from the gangrenous surface and floating in the air (contagious-miasma), and ichorus the 'morbus cause' (infection) in another case?" In trying to determine the cause he reverted back to familiar assumptions about poisons escaping from the body and carried by air to other bodies. However, he assured Brinton that in this case "gangrene was caused by contact" but also that "it is evident that the disease may be caused by 'cell matter' in the atmosphere and I think I see how disease can also be communicated in this way."[74] Of course, the two ideas were not unconnected. He did not abandon his initial ideas about disease; however, his experiments clearly challenged his ideas about causation.

It is important that Benjamin Woodward during the course of his investigation with gangrene patients confirmed that contact with matter from one wound could be spread to another. It is also significant that he thought about investigating disease in ways contemporary European elite physicians would understand. Woodward isolated the disease, cultured it and grew it outside the body, and inoculated it into a patient to produce the same disease, laying a foundation on which modern laboratory practice would build. While he did not yet understand the role of the microorganisms that he saw under the microscope, his experiments raised some important questions about disease: Did disease germs exist? Was the exciting cause of disease then actually a living "cell" rather than a chemical breakdown in the body? These findings were important to Woodward, and he looked for further opportunities to develop his research. He wrote to Hammond's successor, Surgeon General Barnes, just three months after his gangrene experiments, noting, "The reason why I wish a situation in a hospital is that I may be enabled to study the microscopic existence of pathological cell formation and proving the theory of cells in the air from various diseases."[75]

Perhaps most interesting, however, was his belief in the experimental method to produce knowledge about disease. Within the new hospitals and the development of the basic sciences came a confidence that allowed for the production of new ways to develop knowledge, which would support changing conceptions of disease. Civil War physicians did not have the luxury of, say, Louis Pasteur, who was at the same time publishing papers on the spoilage of wine and fermentation, hoping to prove that these processes were caused by distinct organisms. The immediate goal of Woodward and others was to restore the health of troops and prevent these diseases from ravaging the troops. Yet there was clearly a new outlook on studying disease that developed in Civil War hospitals. As physicians were forced to come to terms with the limitation of their own medical knowledge, they sought new, more scientific methods to produce knowledge about gangrene and erysipelas, including chemical and microscopial examination of morbid materials and even inoculation. As medicine moved from purely clinicopathological processes toward physiology, chemistry, and microscopy, physicians accepted the idea of the "experiment" for producing medical knowledge. The site of knowledge was moving away from the hospital and toward the laboratory for some physicians (although during the war these were inextricably linked). These newer methodologies did not yet translate into superior care for patients, but there was an obligation to advance medicine, which proved an important stimulus for therapeutic experimentation.

BETWEEN THE CLINIC AND THE LABORATORY:
Trials, Experiments, and Investigative Technique

As more physicians supported the idea that gangrene and erysipelas had a local cause, it strengthened the idea that the disease was a "thing" to be killed and influenced the course of treatment. Physicians were advised to clean the wound of all foreign material and then apply a remedy as soon as the wound showed signs of infection. The objective was to adopt a specific antiseptic that would "break up the putrescent actions either directly or indirectly."[76] An escharotic was applied to the slough (to separate infected and healthy tissue), the goal being to stop immediately the spread of the infection.[77] After the wound was cleaned and damaged tissue was removed, a disinfectant was applied in and around the wound. Finally, the wound was covered with dry lint soaked in a disinfectant, and the patient was ordered to rest. Numerous physicians actively and passionately debated various treatments, including the use of bromine, nitric acid, turpentine, permanganate of potassa, and iodine.[78]

These debates about the most effective management of the diseases proved important in stimulating ideas about body chemistry, and the "experiment" (which was generally planned but not controlled) became a valuable research tool.[79] Hospital positions afforded physicians the opportunity to experiment with different treatments, and for the first time on a significant scale some scientifically inclined physicians could conduct clinical trials with their hospital patients. Physicians justified the use of patients for clinical trials on the ground that the knowledge might save those still alive as well as advancing medical knowledge. The various findings were published in circulars and reports and widely distributed to physicians in the many military hospitals.[80] In some cases physicians were *ordered* to adopt

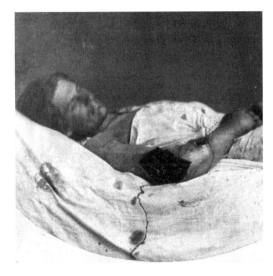

Frederick Pilgrim, private, Company D, 8th New York Cavalry, was admitted to Harewood General Hospital April 5, 1865. He suffered a gunshot wound to the elbow, and after a resection contracted erysipelas and then gangrene. The patient was photographed at Harewood General Hospital by R. B. Bontecou. This teaching photograph traces the path of the missile and the wound, debrided and ready for the local application of a disinfectant. (Courtesy of the National Library of Medicine, Washington, D.C.)

these new remedies, suggesting an important change in thinking: therapeutic information from one patient or one group of patients would work for another.[81]

Frank Hinkle, assistant surgeon at the Jarvis General Hospital, undertook experiments with permanganate of potassa to treat hospital gangrene. Dewitt C. Peters, the surgeon in charge of Jarvis General Hospital, noted of Hinkle's work, "I am firmly convinced that the use of permanganate of potassa will become general in the treatment of hospital gangrene. The experience here is decidedly in its favor, some cases have especially yielded to the treatment of the salt. Dr. Hinkle deserves great credit for introducing this valuable agent and thoroughly studying its properties. The remedy is highly popular with the soldiers, who don't dread hospital gangrene as much."[82]

Hinkle first became apprised of permanganate of potassa as an experimental remedy in the treatment of hospital gangrene when it was suggested to him by Professor Samuel Jackson of Philadelphia, who had been in communication with a French doctor who was also using the chemical compound as an experimental remedy. Hinkle, at his own expense, purchased a few ounces. This was relatively uncommon, but as he remarked to Hammond, "the investigations and study of hospital gangrene had for sometime occupied my mind." He looked at the American experience with permanganate of potassa as a remedy and found in the US Dispensary that the application of salt internally as a treatment had been used only for diabetes and as a "deodorizer in certain ulcers"; but "the information was too vague to be of use as a guide." He searched for other authorities but could find no one who had employed salt as a remedial agent and believed he was the "first to employ it generally in the treatment of hospital gangrene."[83] He introduced the compound to the Campbell General Hospital in May 1863 to experiment with cases from the second Battle of Fredericksburg. Once Hammond was aware of its efficacy, it was supplied by the government on requisition (being placed on the Army Supply Table as an "antiseptic with great power as an oxidizer").[84]

Permanganate is a chemical compound that takes the form of a salt and is a strong oxidizing agent. It dissolves in water, has a sweet taste, and is odorless. Hinkle conducted a study with fifty patients in Campbell hospital.[85] He used from "one to four grains in a solution of water" as a "tonic astringent to oxygenate the blood,"[86] applying the solution primarily locally as an escharotic (a corrosive substance which produced a scab), so that the tissue would die and begin regenerating.[87] He used a hair pencil (to avoid damage to surrounding normal tissue), extending the application over the cuticle four inches beyond the seat of the wound, after which he saturated lint with the dilute solution and applied it to the wound every three to four hours. Previous to the application, the wound was thoroughly cleansed with "castile soap and water"; in cases where the wound was too difficult to access, the concentrated solution was injected with a syringe two to three times daily. He found that, usually, with the local application of the solution, "the most aggravated cases of gangrene resulting from traumatic wounds were arrested" after the treatment was modified to "suit the state of the wound until healthy granulation ensued." His report noted that in most cases the gangrenous slough usually disappeared within five days, although simple dressings with a dilute solution continued to be applied until the wound was entirely healed. He found that using the remedy as both a simple dressing and a tonic astringent, "anti-hemorrhagic," and "vivifier of the feeble circulation in the flaps" for bed-sores and for the treatment of stumps after amputation "prevented sloughing" and helped "maintain a healthy tone in the parts."[88]

The idea of preventing disease outbreaks from erupting in the first place was an important development during the Civil War and added a new dimension to the physician's clinical responsibilities. In other words, they were not killing "germs" that were already present but rather preventing their development. Hinkle used permanganate as a prophylactic with great success. He treated gunshot wounds with a dilute solution before gangrene had the chance to appear: "I feel assured that gangrene would have attacked the wounded parts had it not been employed." He further used it as a deodorizer to "destroy all the offensive odors emanating from gangrenous wounds, which is a sanitary point gained in a surgical ward." In order to ensure that the ward was "properly sanitary," he employed it as a disinfectant, "placing tin saucers under the beds and used by the nurses after dressing offensive wounds."[89]

Hinkle was so fascinated by the properties of permanganate of potassa that he recommended it as a disinfectant after postmortems.[90] He also found its properties beneficial for preserving cadavers: "Acting on this theory I injected the femoral artery of a deceased subject with a concentrated solution of this salt and left the body unburied for seven days. At the expiration of that period, I with several other medical officers inspected the body and found it to be in a perfect state of preservation. . . . I consider the Permanganate of Potassa to be a boon to humanity in the treatment of hospital gangrene and that it compares favorably with the valuable properties of chloroform and ether."[91]

Hinkle's clinical trial produced favorable results. As one example, Private Charles McElroy of Connecticut suffered a particularly painful case of gangrene after receiving three wounds to the left leg at the Battle of Gettysburg, July 1863. He was admitted to the Jarvis General Hospital in Baltimore and treated by Hinkle. His case report noted that upon admission, "the limb presented a frightful appearance, the vitality having been destroyed far beyond the seat of the injury terminating all in extensive suppurative inflammation and sloughing." The patient developed gangrene on September 3, 1863, when he was "seized with violent constitutional disturbance, a high grade of fever, pain in his head, back and limbs with frequent chills." Gangrene set in, the wound was opened, "everting the integument and the pulpous variety of the slough was presented *en masse* elevating itself fully two inches above the level of the wound of a dark colored appearance apparently liquefying the flesh every hour as it progressed."

Hinkle then examined the pus, which was described as "highly pungent and very offensive in odor so much so that the nurses and those in attendance could scarcely remain a moment in his presence without experiencing sickness of the stomach." The patient was suffering, "sank rapidly under the disease," was monitored hourly "night and day," and treated with "nervous stimulants" and a healthy diet. Hinkle then began a course of treatment with permanganate of potassa, which was continued daily for a month, administered every hour for the first three days. Seventeen days after being infected with the disease, the patient began to recover; his appetite improved, and two weeks later the wound "granulated up beyond expectation and more than three-fourths of the wound cicatricized under this treatment."[92] This report is a good example of knowledge produced during the war that had an immediate and significant clinical relevance.

While some physicians had success with permanganate, others tried turpentine, also applied locally. In his study of patients at the United States General Hospital, Cincinnati, Acting Assistant Surgeon Roberts Bartholow found two varieties of gangrene: "true hospital gangrene," which was transmissible by "contagion from wound to wound," and a second "pseudo gangrene," which appeared once constitutional symptoms had been exacerbated by diet, fatigue, and exposure and thus lowered the reparative process in injuries. He commented on how quickly the damage was wrought once gangrene had spread through the connective tissue. He recommended using turpentine, immediately, as a local application, for, if the gangrene had time to spread, the rapidity of "destructive inflammation and subsequent death of tissues" was remarkable.[93]

Joseph Woodward spearheaded a number of experiments to treat pyemia, hoping to develop a means to help soldiers vulnerable to deeper infection. He asked a few physicians to conduct experiments on the therapeutic value of alkaline sulfites. Dr. Walter Atlee experimented with bisulfate of soda in purulent infection; M. Carey Lea studied the transformation of alkaline sulfites in the human system; and H. R. De Ricci examined the causes of excessive mortality after surgical operations and the therapeutic value of alkaline and earthy sulfites in the treatment of catalytic diseases, and he found bisulfate of soda particularly effective in treating "infections from animal poisons."[94] Woodward was most encouraged by Atlee's successful experiments and suggested to Surgeon General Barnes that sulfite of soda "be furnished for trial to such groups of general hospitals as the Surgeon General may direct."[95]

Carey Lea was also heartened by Atlee's findings, which demonstrated that the chemical-vital action of bisulfate of soda had the potential to "destroy or neutralize the poison" causing pyemia, and conducted a series of experiments with the agent.[96] But perhaps more importantly, in what had become a pattern in Civil War case histories and publications, he explained in detail his experiments, including what reactions to look for at what stage of the experiment, and invited researchers to devise their own experiments to help further elucidate both the physiological mechanism of bisulfate of soda and other potential uses of the agent.[97]

Through the war, it became more common for physicians to link their research programs with the advance of prophylactic and therapeutic remedies, which would give the wartime experiments immediate significance in the hospitals. In the *Richmond Medical Journal*, it was noted that "no sooner is any new substance . . . discovered, than experiments are made to investigate its physiological and therapeutic action on the living organisms of men and animals." It was further observed that "among the most important new remedies which science has bestowed upon medicine, may be mentioned in the preparations of the element bromine."[98] A chemical similar to chlorine and iodine and a powerful antiseptic whose vapors are corrosive and toxic, bromine was seen as something of a miracle drug in the treatment of erysipelas and gangrene.[99]

With imperfect understanding of causation, Goldsmith and other physicians of the era primarily focused on effectively managing these diseases—but less on ventilation and more on active prevention. Bromine was seen as an "antidote to the poison, whatever [the poison is] of hospital gangrene . . . and consequently [physicians] did not advocate the free circulation of fresh air" but rather on destroying the "poison" in the environment along with the diseased tissue so that healthy granulation could develop.[100] As Goldsmith noted, "It will be seen that the disease was developed in sores, small and nearly healed, as well as those which were extensive and recent; that in one case especially, it was developed at the sight of a purpurie extravasion, and that in another it invaded at a point almost cicatrized. It invaded wounds recent, wounds granulating, and wounds ulcerating. . . . That the disease, when developed was contagious is shown by the occurrence of several cases in the beds next adjoining those already affected."[101]

The strategies for managing these diseases, then, were developed within evolving ideas about disease causation. Physicians increasingly saw that gangrene and erysipelas often attacked indiscriminately, seemed to invade the body from without, and were contagious. Alex McBride, surgeon in charge of Camp Wallace, found that "the erysipelas prevalent here is very clearly contagious and idiopathic. . . . Nearly every nurse was taken down with the disease."[102] He further suggested that it "did not originate with wounds" but rather developed in any patient with an open cut or sore.[103] Goldsmith likewise argued that gangrene was a specific disease that "presented some constancy in most of their characteristics."[104] He suggested that the constitutional state, existing "at the time of the invasion, did not seem to have much liability to the disease; for the latter seemed to invade the strong and the feeble, the young and the old, the sick and the well with

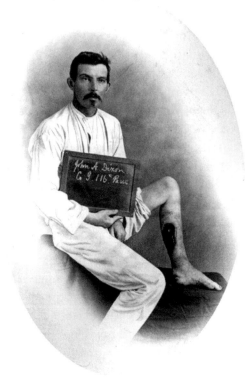

John A. Dixon, sergeant, Company I, 116th Pennsylvania Volunteers. at the Battle of Petersburg, Virginia, suffered a gunshot wound to the left leg, lower third, the ball injuring the soft parts. Gangrene later attacked the wound. The result was favorable. (Photograph courtesy of the National Museum of Health and Medicine)

equal facility." He observed that "the disease could in no case be said to have a constitutional origin," and he did not see one case in which the "constitutional symptoms precede the local disease."[105] With the use of bromine, Goldsmith argued that the specific character of any sore resulting from hospital gangrene or erysipelas could be destroyed, and cases so treated had a "rapid subsidence of the symptoms of infection."[106]

Goldsmith began with the "experimental use of bromine," as both a prophylactic and a treatment.[107] In November 1862, he ordered Benjamin Woodward to "procure bromine and use its vapors in all of the wards and watch its effects."[108] Woodward began by placing bromine in empty quinine bottles in all the wards, "enough to make its vapor very perceptible."[109] He repeated this daily and noted that "within 24 hours I saw a marked change for the better in all the patients since not one had died in the barracks from this disease except the one who was in the last stages of typhoid fever." He added that "no cases of erysipelas had originated in the wards since the bromine was used."

Benjamin Woodward wanted to confirm the results of the perceived value of bromine so he decided to "test the value of the article still further."

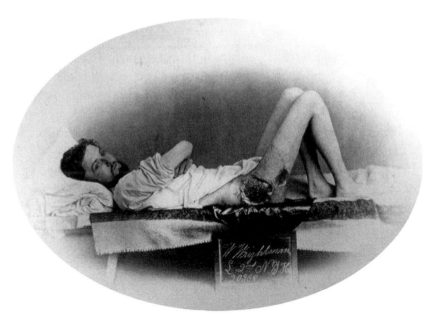

William W. Wrightman, private, Company L, 2nd New York Volunteers, at the Battle of Petersburg, Virginia, suffered a gunshot wound of the right hip, near the outer margin of the ilium, the ball injuring soft parts. While he was in the Harewood General Hospital, gangrene attacked the wound, destroying the soft parts extensively. Photographed and treated by R. B. Bontecou. (Photograph courtesy of the National Library of Medicine, Washington, D.C.)

He took a man who was suffering from erysipelas in the leg, "supervening in the wound and made him hold the naked limb over a chamber vessel in which was bromine and thus bathe it with the vapor." Benjamin Woodward continued this twice a day and noted in his report that, to his great satisfaction, "though sloughing was eminent, the disease was arrested and the man made a good recovery."[110] He concluded that, though the use of bromine in this way was new to him, he believed that its introduction into the wards of hospitals would be a "step towards the advancement of medical science."[111] It was common during the war to invoke specific ideas about cleanliness that had dominated in the prebacteriological era, such as opposing overcrowding, eliminating stagnant water and spoiled food, burying excrement, and isolating those suffering from infectious diseases; however, the study of hospital gangrene and erysipelas foreshadowed the importance of using antiseptics to kill germs in the hospital setting and in surgical rooms.[112] He recommended that in cases of "hospital gangrene, especially after amputating, and erysipelas supervening on wounds, the vapor of bromine brought in contact with disease may be the means of its arrest."[113]

Goldsmith similarly demonstrated the efficacy of bromine in the hospital wards.[114] He developed a solution (which was poured into deep vessels and empty quinine bottles in a dry room) consisting of one to two ounces of bromine, 160 grains of bromide of potassium, and enough distilled water to make four fluid ounces of the mixture. Bromine was released into the air, dressings were treated with antiseptics and patients were doused with them, nurses were ordered to wash their hands in chemical solutions, and hospitals were thoroughly sanitized.

In March 1863, Hammond sent Brinton to "the different general hospitals in Louisville and Nashville to examine the character, and incidence of the diseases and the different modes of treatment employed."[115] Brinton visited the principal military hospitals with Goldsmith and "carefully examined the various cases of hospital gangrene and erysipelas therein contained."[116] Brinton remarked that the gangrene was the same that he had studied while in Annapolis, though not as virulent, which he believed was likely due to the remedies employed rather than the "original character of the affection." Brinton, along with Goldsmith, also studied the use of bromine for the treatment of erysipelas while in Louisville.

Once again, there was generally little objection to these clinical trials because bromine promised a general therapeutic benefit and was framed as a part of the patient's necessary course of treatment. Patients did often complain of severe pain at the time of application; however, they had little choice between the treatment and probable death. Moreover, doctors warned patients that bromine was "very highly conducive to the welfare of the patient" and other patients, as it prevented "the spread of the disease."[117]

Hospitals 19 and 20 were set apart for these trials. Their locations were chosen because they were originally country residences, "located on rising grounds and well ventilated and once sent thither strict isolation is enforced." There were 228 cases of erysipelas treated in Louisville; 51 died, while 127 recovered. Bromine was used to treat the cases, and two different applications were employed: "first by action of the vapor of bromine in the affected part" and second "by a direct application to the erysipeletic surfaces of a solution of bromine of varying strength." Brinton later reported:

1. That the external employment of Bromine in the treatment of hospital gangrene has been attended, in Louisville, with the most marked and beneficial results.
2. That I have not observed that any injurious consequences, whatsoever, have resulted from its application, but the contrary.

3. That all the medical officers with whom I have conversed with in Louisville, Nashville, Murfreesboro, unite in testimony as to the valuable therapeutic powers of bromine in the treatment of erysipelas; my own observations confirm their views. And it is eminently deserving of further trial.[118]

Brinton also urged that "the results of the use of bromine in our hospitals are so marked and important that it would seem that they ought to be published or in some way brought to the knowledge of the surgeons in the service at an early period."[119] Thus, while not all Civil War physicians would engage in experiments themselves, they did have exposure to this research, which was an important part of medical teaching during the war. Goldsmith traveled to a number of hospitals where he was compelled to "take the surgeons to the bedside, teach them the disease, what to observe, what to record, what to investigate, how to apply the remedy and to teach them the pathological processes." He also took with him a man "who can make tolerable drawings of microscopic objects" to be included in his publications for the *Medical and Surgical History of the War of the Rebellion*.[120]

Indeed, Goldsmith agreed that these diseases provided an opportunity to train the "undergraduates" by members of the "senatus medicorum."[121] He noted in his report to Hammond, "Before the occurrence of any cases in our hospitals, I had directed the surgeons in charge to procure bromine, so as to have it ready for use when the disease appeared. Many of the surgeons had no experience in the use of the remedy. They were imbued with the idea, prevalent in the profession, that this agent is a highly corrosive and irritating one; and hence they almost uniformly used it, in the beginning, largely diluted with alcohol, water or ether. The inefficiency of this use of the remedy, comparably with stronger solutions, or with the bromine in substance will be seen in the case histories." Importantly, however, as surgeons gained experience with the remedy they gained confidence in its efficacy and learned that it was not to be the "corrosive and irritating agent which they had supposed it to be."[122]

By the end of the war more physicians were brought around to Goldsmith's viewpoint, because it worked.[123] G. R. Weeks, U.S. Volunteers, testified after examining the records of 115 cases: "Bromine has robbed gangrene of its terror, and shorn its power to stalk through the wards where the sick and wounded are congregated, spreading its contagious and pestilential influence in every direction. But, armed as the surgeon now is by the use of a remedy so certain in its effects, a feeling of security pervades the entire profession at this post."[124] Goldsmith, of course, concurred. "No cases treated in these hospitals are isolated; they are treated in the midst of other wounded men. When the bromine is promptly and thoroughly applied, the disease does not spread. In the beginning, and before the bromine was used promptly and efficiently, a few cases were produced by contagion, but not one after we got into the habit of using the remedy in the way we have now settled upon. . . . So strongly are our surgeons impressed with this application of bromine, that they have lost all dread of hospital gangrene spreading in their wards."[125]

This knowledge was widely disseminated. Goldsmith's first publication appeared in 1863 and was distributed to army surgeons, and state medical journals and associations routinely discussed the wartime findings. For example, Dr. Post presented a paper to the New York Academy of Medicine on May 20, 1863, discussing the use of bromine for the treatment of hospital gangrene. He observed that "local treatment seemed to have played the most important part in arresting the progress of the disease" and "the remedy used more than any other was [bromine] introduced by Middleton Goldsmith, Asst. Medical Director." Post went on to describe the properties of bromine, how to use the agent, and its overall effects. He concluded that the use of bromine in the "treatment of hospital gangrene is very conducive to the health of the patient" and "will prevent the spread of the disease." Post similarly relayed the "good effects claimed by surgeons for bromine in cases of diphtheria and erysipelas." These debates were ubiquitous. Similar testimonials were published in the *Buffalo Medical Journal, Army Medical Times, American Medical Times, Lancet,* and *American Journal of the Medical Sciences* between June and October 1863.[126]

The wartime management of gangrene and erysipelas was of considerable interest to American physicians generally. Part of the attraction was the relative unfamiliarity of the diseases but also the improved method for managing them. Also at the meeting of the New York Academy of Medicine on May 20, Dr. Parker observed that gangrene had "attracted a great deal of attention of late" largely because before the Civil War it was "but rarely met with, except now and then in our large hospitals."[127] He further noted that "very little had been written about the disease until within last few years," giving American physicians an enviable perspective on the manifestation and treatment of the disease. One of the subjects of the meeting was the contagious nature of the disease. Again he referred to the wartime debates about local versus constitutional causes. He suggested that, like smallpox, which "maybe developed either through vaccination or by direct exposure to contagion ... the very same thing is true with reference to hospital gangrene."[128] Parker referred to the recently published thesis of Dr. Ball, who, after having worked during the summer months with Dr. Weir in Frederick and studying forty-three cases of gangrene, demonstrated that it was propagated by "the promiscuous use of sponges, basins, and the like, and in a word, where the disease is prevailing."[129]

More interesting was the desire to test the wartime findings. Laboratory sciences such as physiology and pharmacology were inextricably linked to the clinic, which presented great possibilities of charting new directions for the future of medical education. After being exposed to a number of cases at the New York Hospital and Bellevue in the summer of 1862, Parker and his colleague Dr. Peck "made a trial of almost everything claimed to be useful in the treatment of the disease, and we came to the conclusion that what is called there the disinfecting powder, composed of percarb. of iron, pulv. cinchona, and opium, was the most grateful application." For the constitutional treatment of patients, they found success by "scattering the patients, the plentiful supply of fresh air, a clean skin and generous diet." Dr. Detmold suggested focusing on a local remedy of nitric acid. He discussed the investigations of a "distinguished German writer, who maintained that the deposit on the surface of hospital gangrene consisted of a multiplied cell growth, which immediately on being formed, underwent destructive assimilation." Thus, he advised using local applications immediately and favored nitric acid or bromine.

Again, Dr. Post, who traveled to Nashville, Louisville, and Murfreesboro to observe Middleton Goldsmith's work, told the academy that, on the basis of what he had seen, "the application of [bromine] in the treatment of hospital gangrene is very highly conducive to the welfare of the patient, and I think it will prevent the spread of the disease." He then outlined for the members of the academy an interesting case of hospital gangrene of the leg, "where in the course of the disease, the posterior tibial artery became involved and hemorrhage occurred." He went onto to note that the interesting feature was that the "Surgeon in charge tied the artery at the bottom of the sloughing surface, and applied the bromine immediately over it." Within one week "the case was doing remarkably well."[130] He found this a subject worthy of further investigation. He observed that "the general result of tying arteries in the midst of sloughing parts is that hemorrhage takes place very soon again. .... If bromine has the power of arresting this sloughing process, it is a fact well worthy or our investigation." Perhaps more interesting, Dr. Edward Jarvis of Massachusetts, also present at the meeting, replied that he followed up on the case himself and within twenty-five days the patient was "perfectly recovered."[131]

The use of bromine to treat and prevent gangrene and erysipelas was considered one of the most significant scientific achievements of the war. But was it really the miracle drug it was purported to be? As physicians read the glowing testimonials, some were prompted to experiment with the agent to see why it worked so well. In March 1863, the use of bromine was the subject of debate at the annual meeting of the Cincinnati Academy of Medicine. Dr. John Davis inquired if any physician "had any experience in the use of bromine according to the plan suggested by Dr. Goldsmith of Louisville." The matter under consideration was Goldsmith's assertion that bromine "would destroy what produces erysipelas, or renders it contagious; believing that erysipelas depended upon some principle that was contagious, and that bromine would destroy this." Dr. Murphy noted that at the Third Street Military Hospital patients benefited from bromine. He reported that "when putting the mucous near the vapor of bromine you destroy the pavement cells, and it was reasonable to suppose it has the same effect on the fluid of gangrenous wounds. It destroys the toxaemic matter."

Dr. Davis conducted experiments at the Home of the Friendless Hospital and found that bromine in conjunction with the muriatic tincture of iron was "much more satisfactory than with bromine alone." Dr. White found that bromine had "done no good" and suggested that chlorine in similar cases was "worthy of a trial."[132] Others suggested that the effect of chlorine was negligible while "one ounce of bromine in a gallon of water . . . poured in small vessels and placed throughout the wards" was more efficacious. Dr. White recommended a more controlled trial with bromine because in the Civil War hospitals it was commonly used in conjunction with other agents and thus the "results were inconclusive."

In November 1865 physician Roberts Bartholow attempted to throw light on these questions and published the results of his experiments, which were designed to discover if and why bromine worked so well. He examined bromine alone, and some properties of bromine including bromide of potassium. He investigated the chemical properties, physiological effects, and therapeutic uses. He recognized that bromine could (and had been) studied from both "the rational and empirical view" since its uses were "derived directly from its chemical and physiological actions" and that other uses had been discovered by its "empirical employment." But Bartholow was explicit about the objectivity of his experiments: owing to its "scientific accuracy . . . rational therapeutics is preferable to a blind empiricism." He first described in detail the chemical properties of bromine, including its specific gravity, solubility, properties, and effects when mixed with other chemicals. He then conducted experiments on bromide's physiological effects (there was at that time a number of physicians engaged in experiments designed to ascertain the efficacy of bromide for treating hooping or spasmodic coughs, or bromide as a sedative, or as a treatment for nervous and heart disorders, which Bartholow also wanted to build upon).

He used his own body for the first series, which involved ingesting twenty grains of bromide of potassium.[133] He "experienced a sense of fullness of the head, became drowsy and had some confusion of ideas . . . dryness in the throat, and a metallic taste in the mouth." He examined his urine and noted that it took four hours for the agent to pass into it. Five hours later he took another twenty grains of bromide of potassium and became drowsy, fell asleep, became restless, and suffered headache. As he continued taking the agent internally his symptoms worsened. On the following day, he ingested forty grains and suffered a "frontal headache" and irritation of the "schneiderian mucous membrane with increased flow of mucous and sneezing." He also experienced "confusion of ideas, intoxication, evidenced by impaired locomotion and trembling of the muscles." He concluded that bromide taken this way is an "irritant in large doses to the mucous membrane of the stomach; it is rapidly absorbed into the blood, and may be detected soon after in the urine," and finally it acts "upon the nervous centres, producing sedation, sleep, reduces the action of the heart and arteries, lowers the temperature and diminishes the retrograde metamorphosis tissue."[134] To ascertain the long-term effects of the bromide he selected two hospital patients.[135]

One was an enlisted man, the second a private patient, both being treated for spermatoorhoea. He noted of these experiments, "The subjective sensations of the patients were, however, not readily drawn from them. Somniferous effects were experienced in each case. One of them slept soundly in the afternoon who was not in the habit of doing so, and complained that he could not keep awake. Loss of sexual appetite occurred after a variable period, but in neither instance until the remedy had been administered from five to ten days. In both cases a papular eruption appeared on the face and forehead. . . . Muscular weakness, shortness of breath, dizziness and diminished mental power were produced. All of these symptoms disappeared in a short time after the discontinuance of the drug." Bartholow used his own body for just twenty-four hours and three doses of bromide of potassa ingested internally. In contrast, the experiments that he conducted on his patients lasted at least ten days. And yet the findings were almost the same: taken internally bromide of potassa "diminishes and ultimately entirely, neutralizes the sexual appetite; it produces weakness of the muscular system; is an irritant to the stomach"; and it "interferes with the secondary assimilation, lessening the retrograde metamorphosis of tissue."

Bartholow then turned to an examination of the local uses of bromine. Could bromine treat disease and its properties, as well as be effective as a hygienic agent and a curative agent in certain constitutional conditions? Through a chemical analysis of the properties of bromine, Bartholow determined that while its physiological effects were "not very decided," as a therapeutic action it was an "effectual disinfectant and deodorizer." He also found that, as a deodorizer, bromine diluted with alcohol and water could be injected into the cavities of the body and treat "offensive vaginal discharges" and "foul abscesses." He further suggested that bromine was effective in treating sloughing and gangrenous ulcers. He cautioned that it was a powerful agent and had to be prescribed and applied carefully and judiciously. But he determined that, when used on true gangrene, it was effective as a deodorizer and escharotic.[136] This finding was significant. The mostly empirical knowledge generated during the war was tested in a controlled experiment, proving that the wartime findings were generally correct. However, Bartholow recommended further controlled experiments to fully establish bromine's efficacy and other potential uses. For example, he discussed some experiments then going on in which dogs were injected with rattlesnake poison, and he suggested that bromine seemed to be efficacious as an antidote to the poison. Thus, the war experiments demonstrated the potential of bromine in treating gangrene and erysipelas; however, it also encouraged other physicians to think about why bromine worked and other ways it might be effective in civilian and hospital practice.

Like Bartholow, J. H. Hollister, professor at the Chicago Medical College, examined some of the wartime investigations of gangrene and erysipelas. "The testimony of Surgeon Woodward, 22nd Regiment Ill. Volunteers, to Surgeon Goldsmith," he wrote, "is very decisive, as to the effects of the vapor of bromine in wards devoted to the treatment of erysipelas. Others speak so decidedly in its praise when used in its volatile form to prevent the contagious effects of erysipelas, that I confess a desire to see their experiences more fully verified." He then noted that he too wanted to test it, which he did "by liberating a moderate amount of its vapor in all confined rooms where contagious or even pernicious diseases are to be treated, with the view of determining to what extent it has power to neutralize the miasm which is productive of contagion."

Hollister agreed that the efficacy of bromine was due to the fact that it exerted a perfect "neutralizing effect upon the poison producing hospital gangrene. . . . It has seemed in many instances, an absolute specific against the ravages of this disease, controlling the progress of the sloughing, and changing the wound to the condition of a healthy ulcer in which, granulations springing up readily, the recovery was rapid." Like many of the physicians who either saw the benefits of bromine or experimented with its properties, he did not understand the physiological mechanism of the agent. He said, "Of the manner [in] which it exerts its beneficial effect, both upon living and decomposing molecules, I am not able to speak," but the fact remains "that when, in its full strength, the solution of bromine has been applied to a gangrenous ulcer or wound . . . the fetor disappears, the rapid decomposition of tissue is arrested, the wound soon puts on favorable appearances, the patient demands food, improves strength and soon rallies from his critical condition."

He concluded his paper by requesting that any physician who had conducted a trial with bromine report the results of his experience and comment on bromine's efficacy in the prevention of erysipelas and the cure of gangrene.[137] Perhaps most interesting of all, physicians began to use and administer bromine within the hospitals and as a remedy in private practice after the war. In a controlled study from 1865 and 1876, gangrene, erysipelas, and other hospital infections were managed with bromine and drastically reduced.[138] Physicians carefully recorded the results of their experiences with the agent, and again this knowledge was transmitted for all American physicians.

This is the climate in which scientific medicine developed during the war. The war created the conditions to support a vast increase in the number and range of clinical trials that transformed both research and clinical practice. There were clear standards for these trials, which were designed, published, and debated by a larger body of physicians. As for the specific causes of the diseases, these were still vague. Civil War physicians had not made the larger connections between cells, organic matter, chemical processes, and the resultant diseases, but they investigated concepts of disease, management, and treatment, and these findings were shared and debated, as they built on each other's work during and after the war.

The wartime program of research revealed the importance of prevention and hygiene in the hospital setting both to keep hospitals clean and to prevent the eruption of disease in the first place, which supported the scientific discoveries. In what became routine, Assistant Surgeon R. Weir, General Hospital, Frederick, Maryland, listed a common set of precautions for preventing the spread of hospital gangrene. "Hospital Gangrene the typhus of wounds may be regarded as a species of moist gangrene," he explained, "characterized by its contagious and infecting nature and due to a peculiar poison of as yet unknown origin." To manage the disease he instituted strict rules: "No dressing or bandage was permitted to be used a second time but was taken from the wound. Oakum [treated with creosote as a preventative] was also largely used; and to each patient was given a new sponge which was frequently and thoroughly cleaned and always kept in view at the head of the bed; and nurses were required to wash their hands frequently in sol sodae chloride before visiting any other patients."[139] The prominent physician Henry Hartshorne similarly noted that "attendance in delivery by a physician who is visiting at the same time a case of puerperal fever or of erysipelas, is at the risk of the patient; if the danger of conveyance of the disease be removable, it is only so by the most careful and thorough cleansing and disinfection. The clothes should be changed and the hands washed in strong solution of chlorinated soda before visiting others."[140]

Just a few years earlier, in response to the criticism from anticontagionists about his assertion about the contagiousness of erysipelas and puerperal fever, Oliver Wendell Holmes Sr. was compelled to retreat from his earlier position: "The first thing to be done, as I thought when I wrote my essay [in 1843] was to throw out all discussions of the word contagion, and this I did effectually by the careful wording of my statement of the subject to be discussed. My object was . . . to show that women had often died in child-bed, poisoned in some way by their medical attendants."[141] Experiences with these diseases allowed a significant development of ideas related to both the management and nature of disease. Considering that Joseph Woodward had never seen a case of gangrene two years earlier, American physicians had come a long way in a very short time.

The wartime investigations reveal a dynamism and complexity, with many ideas emerging about gangrene and erysipelas: they appeared to be contagious, individual patients suffered common symptoms, and common features were established about the pathology of the diseases, though both could vary in virulence from one person, campsite, and locale to another. Different factors, such as the constitution of the patient, his attitude, the conditions in which he was wounded or transported, the climate, and the food he consumed, figured into creating a picture of these diseases suggesting that the transition toward purely ontological conceptions of disease was complex. But the very setting in war raised questions about the nature of disease causation and transmission.

Ideas about disease were no longer primarily about "filth." Conceptions about disease causation and transmission were more medically and scientifically sound. The application of chemicals to the body was consistently reinforced, the use of chemicals or antiseptics to prevent "putrefaction" or destroy "poisons" was considered crucial in the management of these diseases, and physicians conducted clinical trials. Moreover, the findings were published and tested in more controlled experiments. The "experiment" pointed the way. More importantly, many Civil War physicians accepted the authority of those who produced knowledge about these diseases, creating a hierarchy in American medicine. Finally, there was strong evidence in favor of some sort of contagion being involved in the transmission of these diseases, which would support emerging work in bacteriology. These various threads were not pulled together until years later when the laboratory work in Europe helped give shape to the investigations, but the way to study medicine and disease developed for many physicians.

Some physicians requested microscopes to detect specific "vibrios," "cells," "fungi," or "animalcules." This led to new worlds related to disease. Most importantly, though, diseases were studied away from the patient, changing basic assumptions about how to investigate disease processes. Other physicians found their niche in testing and experimenting with therapeutics, a relatively new method for producing medical knowledge. The work of still others laid a foundation for developments in public health. Perhaps most important of all, the government recognized the value of medical research and offered both financial and technical support. The idea of specializing and becoming an "expert" in these investigations was an attractive prospect for many of these physicians. New intellectual frontiers were encountered, and identities were formed in these investigations. As Goldsmith remarked to Hammond, "I have to thank-you for the abundant opportunities which you have given me for pursuing my investigation into bromine as a treatment to their present fruition."[142] He also remarked to Brinton of his observations into erysipelas and pyemia that the work was "striking and important."[143] Goldsmith was not alone in being able to position himself as an "expert" on a specific class of disease or area of medicine during the war; with the opportunity to pursue specialized areas of study, physicians could achieve a new type of professional dominance.

CHAPTER FOUR

Medical Specialization and Specialized Research

The Civil War provided unparalleled opportunities for a physician to develop an expertise in a specialized area of medicine. Physicians were often challenged by the patients under their care, particularly since the range of unfamiliar diseases and cases manifested peculiar and often devastating symptoms, thus allowing physicians seeking the distinction of specialist a chance to develop specialized knowledge. Medical specialization, once associated with anti-intellectualism and quackery,[1] now had a new intellectual dimension: becoming an expert could save lives, conferring a measure of status and identity on the physician who could successfully diagnose, manage, and treat these challenging cases. Indeed, Silas Weir Mitchell hoped that his work and research at Turner's Lane Hospital would "become a means of aiding a neglected class of sufferers."[2]

While those physicians who had benefited from foreign travel, particularly to Paris and Vienna, had seen the efficacy of specialization or found support for specialized research, it was with the emergence of a new medical context in America that the possibilities of specialization in medicine could be seen but also accepted by the larger body of general practitioners. Before the war, physicians may have come across a specific type of case or class of disease only infrequently; thus, trying to forge a career in treating just the brain or heart disease, for example, would have been very difficult and not financially viable. This changed during the war, and specialized hospitals were introduced for practical purposes: the separation of specific diseases could streamline medical practice during the war.

Civil War physicians treated thousands of young men in blue with many identical health problems, and most of these men were anonymous or unknown to the practitioner. The focus increasingly became the disease or the condition rather than the individual patient or the individualized care that had dominated before the war. Those physicians interested in or adept at managing a particular class of disease often earned the appointment of surgeon in charge, or a post at a specialty hospital, and through the process physicians were able to display new forms of professional competence and authority.

Circulars No. 2 and 5 converged in an important way to support the development of medical specialization. In addition to emphasizing the new pathological conception of disease and the use of new technologies, the circulars helped to create a new intellectual space in the circumstances of war. By requesting physicians to research and produce knowledge related to various diseases and specific conditions, two things happened. First, as some physicians wrote their case reports as required by Circulars No. 2 and 5, there were some diseases far beyond their medical knowledge, which the numerous letters to the staff at the Army Medical Museum asking for advice about diagnosing specimens or unfamiliar diseases reveal. In turn, Woodward and Brinton replied, correcting misdiagnoses or consulting with a specialist in the study of that particular disease during the war. This created a hierarchy; as some physicians felt their limitations, others carved out fields of investigation, interpretation, and intervention in the management of particular diseases. This chapter is concerned with a very early stage in American medical specialization, particularly the conditions created by the war, which proved an impetus to specialized study. As more Civil War practitioners embraced medical science, it became easier to introduce specialties into Civil War medical practice. The following pages explore how specialties took shape, the specific conditions and cases that led to demands for the specialist, and the patterns that were established in the process.

Specialization in medicine was not a fully formed professional category before, during, or even immediately after the war.[3] Specialization, until the middle of the twentieth century, actually meant many things, and at least three kinds of specialists existed. The first type comprised specialized knowledge seekers or rather physicians who studied particular problems or groups of problems, and so enjoyed a reputation in the associated diseases. The second was represented by GPs who held expertise in a particular field and so were preferentially consulted by their peers and patients. These specialists were usually mature practitioners who evolved into a special consulting role but could be younger practitioners with opportunities for advanced study. One example here is S. D. Gross (he noted in his autobiography that part of the reason he accepted the chair at Jefferson Medical College was to leave Louisville and shed his family practice responsibilities). Finally, there were the "exclusive specialists," who confined their practice to a limited field and took only referral patients, which would be the dominant form in the twentieth century. The GPs with special expertise, from the second group, were both the most feared and opposed by the masses of the profession because they competed "unfairly" for the same patients as traditional GPs. The first type was at some level essential to the other two groups, and it is this group that the Civil War hospitals most encouraged.

There were certain benchmarks generally associated with the emergence of specialization that did not develop during the war—including standardized training programs, regulation boards, university-based teaching, formal associations, and the line between observation and experimentation. And these new specialists for the most part maintained dual roles as general practitioners and specialists. There were, however, some important features of wartime medicine that did support medical specialization and the move toward professionalization in American medicine, including specialty divisions within the Civil War hospitals, government-sponsored research projects, resources for specialized study, a published record of experience, and the sheer growth of the medical profession. It is important, then, to think of specialized study during the conflict as the attempt of some physicians to respond to the challenges that demanded specialized expertise and intervention while also profiting professionally from the opportunities that were presented. Moreover, this intellectual foundation extended to the public. With sons being treated in Turner's Lane Hospital for neurological disorders by Silas Weir Mitchell or for heart conditions in Jacob Da Costa's ward, some members of the public were exposed to medical specialization as a new professional category full of scientific promise.[4]

CIVIL WAR MEDICINE AND SPECIALIZATION

At the outset of the Civil War, Union medical professionals were forced to utilize churches, factories, barns, and even large private homes for the wounded because there were very few permanent hospitals and certainly not enough to care for the mass casualties. Deserted barracks were used at first to treat the wounded, and eventually immense pavilion hospitals were constructed. Silas Weir Mitchell recalled that these hospitals each held from "one thousand to six thousand patients and they sheltered thirty-thousand beds in and around Washington, and that near to Philadelphia we had twenty-six thousand, about twenty-thousand of these being in neatly constructed pavilion ward hospitals."[5] He recognized the value of so many patients and suggested that "the American physicians, quick to learn, profited by their vast clinical opportunities."[6]

The hospitals in fact revealed the limitations in medical knowledge and thus encouraged knowledge production: "I have the honor herewith to forward for your approval my special requisition for the books which are italicized on the supply table. I am confident that the works asked for could and would, be used by the medical men here to the great advantage of the service. . . . The works more particularly desired are those treating the specialty of the eye, ear, skin and venereal."[7]

At first, though, the development of specialty hospitals was a very challenging undertaking. As Silas Weir Mitchell observed in 1864, "Many difficulties and embarrassments naturally arose at the outset of an undertaking so novel as that of a special hospital meant to receive only a limited class of cases. As the Surgeon General increased the number of such hospitals, creating distinct wards for various classes of diseases, these obstacles soon disappeared, and the good results of the system became apparent."[8] Physicians designated "specialists" were revered for their expertise in a way they had not been before the war.[9] Indeed, the competition among general practitioners and the wartime specialists before and, to a lesser extent, after the war was not so profound during it, largely because specialists helped to manage the diseases and disorders many doctors had little familiarity with or desire to treat. In an already overwhelming medical situation, specialty hospitals and doctors were instrumental in helping to manage the medical challenges. As Mills Madison, Medical Directors Office, St. Louis, noted, "I have the honor to request that a surgeon who has experience in the treatment of diseases of the eye be sent out here for the purpose of taking charge of a large and increasing number of cases occurring in the hospitals of this department."[10]

Medical Inspector John LeConte,[11] a well-known naturalist and entomologist was among the war physicians instrumental in creating an infrastructure in which wartime specialization could develop.[12] Though LeConte (like many professionals) initially viewed the war as a distraction to his work and an annoying political controversy, he rallied to the cause of the Union and proved extremely valuable in his capacity as medical inspector. He was first elected an associate for Philadelphia of the U.S. Sanitary Commission, but later secured a rank of lieutenant colonel and the position of medical inspector of the United States Hospitals in Philadelphia.[13] He was particularly effective in improving hospital record keeping. He noted to Brinton that "my object was to produce a series of hospital records from which the nature of treatment of the cases could be learned and from which a student desiring a monograph on a particular subject could procure satisfactory information to dispense."[14]

As LeConte worked to streamline medicine during the war, and as he studied the variety of diseases, he also saw the efficacy of specialists for the management of them. He proposed specialized hospitals "for certain classes of cases" and, where possible, "placed under the *right kind of man*."[15] He noted that "in the case of gunshot fractures it appears to me that the medical director can easily ensure better success by sending all such cases to a *particular hospital* to be healed by some *particular surgeon*."[16] There was even debate about the efficacy of having all specialties in one specialty hospital or rather separate hospitals (ultimately some were housed in the same hospital in separate wards, while others had a separate hospital designated).[17] Indeed, it soon became necessary to employ an executive officer in the general hospitals whose duty it was to "assign new patients to the wards" and also "transfer the cases in the specialties such as the eye, nervous diseases, and injuries etc. to the special hospitals."[18] By 1863, special wards "had been appropriated by order of Hammond in several hospitals for the treatment of special diseases," including heart diseases, nervous diseases, injuries of the eye and ear, and skin ailments.[19] These special wards proved useful for managing patients but also for small groups of physicians and researchers.[20] As Mitchell recalled of his work on neurology, "Thousands of pages of notes were taken. There were many operations, many consultations, and toward the close we planned the ultimate essays which were to record our work."[21]

Historians tend to take for granted that, though change was a long time coming, the 1870s ushered in striking new novelties in American medicine, including the rise of new institutions, specialist societies, and new ideas about the laboratory that allowed for larger medical reforms to occur.[22] Perhaps most striking of all, because the idea had been so contested, was the new support for the medical specialist. William Rothstein writes that by 1869, members of the American Medical Association (AMA) passed a number of resolutions that would define a new relationship between general practitioners and specialists. He further notes that "considering the hostilities of so many general practitioners to specialists these resolutions were surprisingly mild and even sympathetic." What accounted for this apparent transformation? After all, it was just a few years earlier that members of this same body sought to disassociate themselves from specialists altogether. According to Rothstein, the change in perspective was simply because by the late 1860s these new specialists were "powerful men in the profession," who controlled medical societies and had prestigious posts at hospitals and medical schools, with a wide array of wealthy clients.[23] Moreover, many elite physicians supported specialization, and by 1870 there was increasing support for the development of research universities that would naturally support curricula reform in medical schools.[24]

By 1869 specialists had carved a niche for themselves in American medicine. But what processes allowed for this shift in thinking or the larger acceptance for specialization? And how did this work become known to the general public? There is no denying how important the clinics, laboratories, and model of European science was for the development of American medical education and professionalization in the post–Civil War period. But the medical developments during the Civil War established patterns, attitudes, ideas about disease, and above all a new foundation for the medical sciences. The way medicine was structured during the war, in fact, prepared physicians, the government, and the public for a social transformation in medicine. Very simply the medicine of 1860 was vastly different from the medicine of 1863, and the medicine of 1866 was vastly different again.

Silas Weir Mitchell provides one such example of this transformation. After graduating from Jefferson Medical College and studying in Paris for a year with the eminent physiologist Claude Bernard, he returned to Philadelphia with fervent desire to develop the basic sciences. He was part of a small group of American physicians who wanted to make "greater efforts to expand man's knowledge of his body, his environment, and the universe" and was thus part of a "network of American scientists who wanted to introduce the research ethic into American higher education."[25] One noted historian suggests that Mitchell's focus on clinical research during the Civil War limited the time designated for laboratory work and thus Mitchell's "scientific productivity declined."[26] This assertion stems in part from Mitchell's own desire to obtain a physiological chair, and his apparent failure to do so has often overshadowed his contribution to clinical specialization.[27] However, Mitchell's interest in physiology did not decline during the war, nor did his scientific productivity. In fact, by 1860 specialization in medicine was one of the most dynamic areas of medical science. Taking a closer look at Mitchell's career highlights the unique but also important opportunity that the war years offered an individual physician.

In the 1850s, Mitchell began a series of varied physiological investigations, employing chemical and microscopial methods in his work. He examined uric acid crystals and their alterations in highly acid urine and looked at relations of the pulse to fixed statistics of deep inspiration or expiration, blood crystals of the sturgeon, and the muscular phenomena following a blow on the muscle from a percussion hammer (a lab experiment on the contraction and secondary, local or hump reaction). With his friend and colleague Hammond, he undertook experimental studies of poisons from the Rio Darien and demonstrated they were powerful cardiac poisons. The two studied the toxilogical effects of sassy bark, the alkaloids of corroval and vao, and the venom of the rattlesnake and investigated the anatomy and physiology of the respiratory and circulatory organs, the toxicology of arrow, and ordeal poisons and snake venom, later described as "a perfect model of what investigation into the physiological action of a poison ought to be."[28] They also examined the circulation, physiology, and respiration of the chelonian and the treatment of rattlesnake bites.[29]

Mitchell was clearly interested in scientific investigation before the war, but these pursuits had not allowed him to make real strides in the larger development of American medicine. As Mitchell observed two years before the war, "Considering the adventurous ingenuity of the national mind, as well as the solid character of its achievements in other lines of scientific research, it is not easy to see why a science so eminently experimental as physiology, should be able to boast so few active laborers and so small a number of conspicuous results."[30]

A chief problem, as noted earlier, was the lack of sufficient external support for medical science and research, along with the resistance from the rank and file for developing or even reforming American medicine. In fact, by the 1850s some general practitioners, in fear of losing patients, went so far as to suggest that specialists in medicine be denied entry to the AMA.[31] To protect their own status and positions in the field, the rank and file argued at the time that practicing physicians only needed to understand general medicine and that focusing on one organ or one area of the body was simply unacceptable for a well-rounded physician. Circular No. 2 would change all of this. The very directive of the circular required that physicians focus on specific organs, tissues, lesions, and specific disease conditions. For some rank-and-file physicians this revealed new possibilities for medical practice, but for the elite physicians the increase in scientific knowledge provided an unprecedented opportunity to develop specialties in medicine while establishing identities as specialists.

NOSTALGIA, NEUROSIS, AND NERVE DISORDERS:
Turner's Lane Hospital and the Development of Neurology

Thomas Carroll of Company D, 3rd New Jersey, had been injured by a pistol ball while seated on a fence rail, suffering paralysis and atrophy of the arm muscles, likely owing to a lesion of the spinal centers. One of the interesting characteristics of the case was that his left shoulder muscles were "fearfully atrophied," prompting Mitchell to make casts of both shoulders, which were then sent to the medical museum to illustrate the "deformities" caused by the disorder (classed as a wound of the nerve center).[32] Throughout the war and after, the Surgeon General's Office encouraged and fostered such contributions and soon expected doctors to publish their findings for the benefit of military medicine: "The attention of medical officers in charge of USA General Hospitals is invited to the importance of preparing illustrations of the results of surgical operations. . . . In selecting the proper subjects for representation, it would be well to choose not only cases in which results have been favorable, but also those in which they may have been unfavorable. In a collection like the National Museum truthful representations of both good and bad results are alike instructive and valuable for future reference and study."[33]

Brinton too noted the developing collection: "It is practical and has already powerfully influenced for the better the treatment of the wounded soldier. . . . I would simply recall to your mind the lessons to be deduced from the study of the specimens on the shelves, of injuries of the joints from conoidal balls; a class of injuries previously almost unknown and the treatment of which at the commencement of the war was unsettled."[34] There was, then, a national recognition of the extensive damage that was wrought by gunshot wounds, but more specifically, disciplines such as neurology became visible through the Army Medical Museum and the new specialty hospitals.

Turner's Lane Hospital in Philadelphia was a pavilion-style hospital opened in August 1862 for the study and treatment of neurological disorders and wounds of the nerves.[35] Surgeon Alden of the regulars was in charge of Turner's Lane (primarily handling administrative matters); other prominent staff members consisted of George Morehouse, W. W. Keen, Silas Weir Mitchell, and Jacob Da Costa, who was assigned his own ward for the study of "exhausted hearts." Mitchell was also assigned as contract surgeon to Filbert Street Hospital (where he first became interested in the nerve wounds resulting from war injuries) and Christian Street Hospital, opened June 1861 (first organized for the treatment of nervous diseases). It was during his tenure there that he began to develop his expertise in the nervous diseases that he observed in the soldiers.[36] According to Mitchell, this "so pleased the Surgeon General that a hospital for neural disorders was created at Turner's Lane in August 1862 and pavilions were built for four hundred men."[37]

During their time together at Turner's Lane Hospital, Mitchell became a mentor for Morehouse and Keen. They were able to create a small "medical society" (where they were not impeded by the AMA),[38] and the interactions there set all three doctors on a new professional course.[39] Keen later recalled that it was "the most fortunate event of my professional life that I came under [Mitchell's] stimulating and elevating influence. . . . I was stimulated at once into authorship."[40] Mitchell demanded meticulous research and case reporting: "He taught the important art of elucidating the case histories of patients; the importance of little hints which were often the insignificant surface out-croppings of a rich vein of facts; the importance and methods of cross-examination to ferret out the truth, and above all the ability to interpret these assembled facts in making a diagnosis."[41]

The first significant study based on the research from Turner's Lane was on reflex paralysis (*Circular No. 6*), which focused on cases of sudden palsy as a result of wounds in remote regions of the body. As Mitchell noted of these injuries, "paralysis of a remote part or parts has been occasioned by a gunshot wound of some prominent nerve, or of some part of the body which is richly supplied with nerve branches of secondary size and importance." He was particularly interested in how these injuries "differed from paralytic affections which result from disease of organs." If a minié ball, for example, passed above any large nerve, there was a corresponding destruction of function as if the bullet severed the nerve fibers.[42]

They examined, in particular, how the effects of shock and gunshot injuries both variously affected the medulla oblongata (which regulates several basic functions of the nervous system) and the possible interruption of reflexes at remote nerve centers.[43] Another study, *Gunshot Wounds and Other Injuries of the Nerves*,[44] was based on 2,000 pages of notes taken over a year.[45] These first wartime publications on how to diagnose and treat nervous wounds outlined in detail the methodology pioneered at Turner's Lane and were illustrated by numerous Civil War case studies.

In the course of fifteen months, statistics of Civil War nervous cases were compiled and the immediate effects of nerve wounds were studied and compared. Classifying, diagnosing, and treating these disorders were of equal importance in these first investigations. It seemed to Mitchell that in all European hospitals, particularly military hospitals, there were those rare cases of nerve diseases. In various publications, military physicians in the Crimea or other wars of the period often commented on the existence of these types of nervous cases, but they were not described at length or in helpful detail in the existing textbooks. There was thus no guide for treating nervous cases during the Civil War. In fact, these maladies had previously been treated with curiosity rather than any real medical efficacy. Mitchell noted, after a "long and large experience" in the Civil War hospitals, that the "indications for treatment grew to be well defined" and therefore needed to be published.[46] And some Civil War physicians clamored for what Mitchell described as his "novel symptomology for nerve injuries."[47] Surgeon R. Weir, for example, wrote the Surgeon General's Office in 1864 requesting 100 copies of *Circular No. 6*, which was subsequently distributed among medical officers.[48]

Mitchell, Morehouse, and Keen divided their time between their general practices and Turner's Lane Hospital. Their day usually began with a visit to the hospital by seven o'clock, then a stop in at their own practices, followed by a late afternoon and evening visit to Turner's Lane.[49] Before being assigned at Turner's Lane, Morehouse worked as an assistant surgeon at the general hospital at 16th and Filbert Streets and performed a number of surgeries, including trephining to treat an abscess of the brain following a gunshot wound.[50] Morehouse was extremely interested in injuries of the brain and thrilled to receive an appointment at Turner's Lane. Keen had worked at various hospitals during his first sixteen months of service and was also the Army Medical Museum's representative in Frederick and Philadelphia, where he gathered and forwarded specimens to the museum. He was ordered to the Christian Street Hospital and then Turner's Lane, where he pursued his interest in diseases and injuries of the nervous system.[51]

It was a period in their careers they clearly relished: "Several nights each week" Keen stated, "we worked at note taking often as late as twelve or one o'clock in the morning and when we got through we walked home a couple of miles talking over our cases. . . . The opportunity was unique and we knew it. The cases were of amazing interest."[52] The physician William H. Welch later recalled of the work at Turner's Lane: "One is reminded of the almost feverish activities of the young Bichat in the Hotel Dieu by the work, until the late hours of the night, of these three ardent investigators, minutely observing and recording in thousands of pages of notes phenomena often both new and interesting, analyzing, conferring, apportioning to each his share in working up the results. The opportunity was unique and they seized it with full realization and utilization of its possibilities."[53]

The team examined "every conceivable form of nerve injury"—from shot and shell, from saber cuts, contusions, and dislocations, and most of the men were "worn out from fever, dysentery and long marches." The general approach to the treatment of gunshot wounds to the extremities or major nerves was generally through a primary amputation, if possible, or by restoring function to the limb, as opposed to surgically repairing the nerve.[54] The three also studied epilepsy, palsies, reflex paralysis, singular choreas, and stump disorders. They were interested in injuries of nerve centers, injuries of the sympathetic nerve, wounds of the fifth and seventh nerves, injuries of nerve trunks or branches—and they studied alterations of motion, lesions of sensation, lesions of motion, alterations of calorification, and the treatment of nerve lesions.[55] Mitchell and his team also examined a number of changes in the muscles, including paralysis as to will, loss of tone and firmness, loss of electromuscular contractility, loss of electromuscular sensibility, atrophy, and contraction. Mitchell looked at what he referred to as "diseased muscles," the ability or inability for volitional movement, and the effects of electricity on the muscle.[56] Thus within the new specialty hospital very specific divisions or categories were created to study Civil War nervous conditions.

These conditions proved a constant source of interest and learning, such that "if urgent calls took us into town, we returned to the hospital as if drawn by a magnet. In fact it was exciting in its constancy of novel interest."[57] So complete was the field of study "that it was not uncommon to find at one time in the wards four of five cases of gunshot injuries of any single large nerve. It thus happened that phenomena, which one day seemed rare and curious, were seen anew in other cases the next day, and grew commonplace as our patients became numerous."[58] Thus, while Mitchell acknowledged that "the years from 1862–1865 left a busy Army Surgeon small leisure for lab work," he also recognized that "the organization of the Christian Street Hospital for nervous diseases and later that of Turner's Lane afforded a chance for study unknown before."[59]

Mitchell's wartime experiments and publications reflect his new opportunities, but his approach to neurology was clearly influenced by his training as a physiologist.[60] Most of the disorders at Turner's Lane were functional[61] or psychological, which laid the conceptual foundation for Mitchell, Morehouse, and Keen's program of research.[62] Mitchell did examine various organic symptoms related to brain and spinal injuries, such as congestion, meningitis, hydrocephalus, hemorrhage, tumors, softening, atrophy, myelitis, and hyperaemia, but more of his cases exhibited functional disturbances, such as headache, trance, hysteria, delirium, chorea, reflex spasms, and tetanus, which is where the initial focus lay.

Neurological study was so new to the examiner that it was often the patient's complaints that allowed for the development of a larger body of knowledge. Thus the high volume of patients in the Civil War hospitals was beneficial here and central to the development of this specialty. As Mitchell remarked, "Should it be asked how so full a knowledge of these early phenomena was attainable off the battle-field, we reply, that the utmost care was exercised in ascertaining from the patient the state of his functions, and that it was common to find that wounded men who are not weakened by loss of blood or excessive shock have a very natural curiosity as to the condition of the wounded part, and are apt almost immediately to handle it, and to try to move it." It was also helpful that "the large mass of our patients being Americans, they were usually possessed of at least some education, and often of considerable intelligence and power of observation, which was certainly not dulled by the interest with which some men regarded their own cases."[63]

Martin Anz of Company B, 68th New York Volunteers, was shot with a musket ball in the back side of the left leg at the Battle of Bull Run on August 30, 1862.[64] It was determined that the ball must have injured the head of the fibula and then lodged in the head of the tibia. After the initial case history, a clinical picture was soon established and generally included "the first impressions of the individual so injured, the nerves wounded; the amount of shock, and the extent of primary derangement of the functions of motion and sensation."[65] The patient informed Mitchell that he fell upon being hit and was unable to walk, but, on trying, found that he could flex and extend the foot. Anz was sent to Ebenezer Hospital in Washington on September 6, where he underwent several operations to extract the ball, which was finally removed in December. His leg lay in a fracture box for six weeks, during which time a surgeon united the wounds of exit and entry by an incision, which, according to Mitchell, "probably implicated the tibial nerves"; because of this intervention or perhaps the changes in the ball track, after some weeks "he had lost all power to extend the foot."[66]

After Anz was sent to Turner's Lane, it was observed that it was the pressure on the "muscular cutaneous nerves" and on the "front of the tibia below the wound" that caused shooting pains in the foot. The patient suffered "great pain walking," and there was burning and swelling in the foot. Anz was diagnosed as suffering an injury to the tibial nerve leading to "paralysis of extensions of foot." The diagnostic test, prognosis, and treatment employed by Mitchell was electricity, which he used for the purpose of exercising muscles in persons at rest.

European neurologists began the development of medical electricity in 1849 when famed French neurologist Guillaume Duchenne used the induced "faradic" current and in 1856 when Polish German neurologist Robert Remak used the primary "galvanic" current. Their publications became the source of much interest during and after the Civil War among those interested in neurology.[67] Very few physicians understood the use of electricity as a form of treatment, which supported the development of the specialist or rather a physician who was familiar with both the treatment and the equipment. The use of electricity had previously been associated with quackery until it was determined that "electricity has deservedly won a position in legitimate therapeutics."[68] This was in large part because the "value of the remedy had been tested and proved by men whose motives are beyond mistrust, who are as thorough clinicians as they are accomplished scientists."[69] It was once again an opportunity to orient medicine along the same lines as in Europe because of the new environment in which to experiment and test certain theories and therapeutics but also to demonstrate new types of professional competence.

Mitchell was extremely pleased, for example, to be able to undertake "numerous and elaborate researches" to "test and verify" Duchenne's views.[70] As Mitchell observed in regard to electricity, "as respects its value in traumatic lesions of nerves, we feel constrained to state that it has been understood and rightly appreciated by M. Duchenne alone. . . . After a year of great experience in the use of electricity, we are still satisfied of the essential correctness of almost every proposition on the subject which the distinguished physician has laid down."[71] In addition to adopting a more widespread use of electricity, Mitchell also advocated some newer treatments based on his Civil War experience, including a combination of rest in conjunction with massage[72] and overfeeding.[73] By the 1880s Mitchell was in fact renowned for his "Weir Mitchell" cure.

In the case of Martin Anz, Mitchell prescribed the electric test to stimulate the nerves and muscles. In particular, Mitchell wanted to exercise the muscles with the least amount of pain, and to do this he used an induction current, with interruptions as slow as one every two to five seconds.[74] He studied both electromuscular contractility of the muscle (a diseased muscle may be capable of volitional movement but not exhibit the least tremor under the most violent shocks of a battery) and electromuscular sensibility (which gives rise to pain when the muscle is faradized). By restoring or testing the function of the various muscles with electricity, the physician could determine whether neural connections could be remade (thus, "recall to functional life the muscles"),[75] what muscles could recover, or whether muscles had lost all ability to respond to electric properties. The use of electricity helped to determine both the extent of the damage and the course of treatment. It was, however, complicated, and Mitchell advised that it should be done by a "clever operator who knows his anatomy well" and who "may need experience to manage them so as not to shock and disgust the patient by inflicting needless pain."[76]

It was found that Anz suffered slight sensibility on his calf and extensors, but on the front of the leg and on the outside, "dry conductors gave burning pain on the skin."[77] By July 15 the patient was "much better," and by January 12, 1864, it was noted the patient had been acting as ward master, had been on furlough twice, and was finally placed in the invalid corps. On his last visit, Mitchell measured Anz's calves and checked the sensation of the leg and the motion of the foot, in which he found "full extension of the foot, but not flexion, no extension of the great toe, and no adduction."[78] He further found after performing an electric test, "absence of muscular contractibility in the f. annicus and p. congus," the "electrical sensibility lessened" but with "excessive muscular contractility in the calf muscles, which are liable to painful cramps at all hours, and on using electricity."[79] Mitchell found the amount of contractibility under faradization to be a good test as to the condition of the muscle (which he compared to healthy corresponding organs); if it appeared similar to the healthy organ, the chance of future volitional control was more likely.[80]

The work on reflex paralysis due to indirect lesion of the nerve substance classed as "spinal commotion," pioneered by Mitchell, Morehouse, and Keen, was considered their greatest contributions to the field.[81] The symptoms of reflex or indirect paralysis closely mirrored injuries to the spine, which led to detailed clinical symptoms for each affliction.[82] For example, did the ball pass over the spine causing loss of motion or shock, or were large nerve trunks or sensory nerves encountered? They found in their research that if a ball passed the sciatic nerve and palsied the limb, even at a distance of an inch, the immediate effect could be the same as if the nerve itself had been hit. The delineation of this similarity actually helped Mitchell, Keen, and Morehouse better understand nerve disorders within the context of the pathological-physiology of the body by revealing some very specific limitations in their knowledge. For example, when the ball had gone through the neck (back to front or front to back), which is so rich in nerves, could that cause the spinal column to be concussed at the side? Could paralysis of the arm result from the shaken spine or concussion of the spinal nerves at their exit, or were nerves in the lower tissues of the neck causing the paralysis? They did not know fully the damage (temporary or permanent in the body) that would be caused by the destructive minié ball.[83]

Mitchell, Keen, and Morehouse thus recommended that Civil War physicians adopt a specific methodology to try to answer these questions, which were deemed of "much clinical interest." First, they advocated a "careful study of these singular cases in field hospitals, with special reference to the parts implicated in the wound, and by an anatomical examination of recent wounds in men who have been slain."[84] With this examination they advised physicians to "minutely ascertain, by ocular and microscopic examinations, how far around the ball track there is injury of tissue," including examining the damage to the "bone, nerve, and muscle" to which the ball may have come into contact. They further advised, if possible, that physicians should conduct experiments and elucidate the facts that would help to "clear up a subject that has never yet been rightly studied, and would probably lead to most valuable results."[85] Physicians were also advised to complete thorough clinical histories through the "careful communication" with the patient. Thus, in developing neurology as a specialized discipline, physicians were advised to equally examine the pathological conditions and the complaints of their patients, and this approach laid the foundation for clinical neurology to develop.

On December 13, 1862, Jacob Demuth, a Swiss immigrant of Company D, 108th New York Volunteers, received a shell wound to the right thigh at the Battle of Fredericksburg. He was marching double quick when a fragment of shell as large as a musket ball struck his right thigh at the junction of its upper and middle third directly over the femoral artery.[86] The fragment did not enter deeply, but lodged in the leg and was removed a day later without injury to the vessel. The patient reported that he felt a burning pain in "both feet and the right arm in front of the right chest and in the right thigh above the wound," and while the power in his left arm slowly returned, he was "paralyzed as to motion in his right arm and both legs."[87] The loss of voluntary control and sensation generally followed all "grave wounds of nerves."[88] These were considered to be direct nerve wounds probably caused by the passage of the ball. When there was no possibility that the nerve was touched, the loss of function was attributed to local shock.[89]

Mitchell found the condition of local shock "very curious." If the ball passed *near* the sciatic nerve, for example, the limb would be instantly paralyzed, with volitional control returning after about a week.[90] But Mitchell was perplexed about the relationship between loss of motion and loss of sensation, which did not equally damage motor and sensory fibers.[91] This apparent contradiction directed his research, which examined whether "the fibres of motion and sensation may be grouped in bundles, and thus be liable to insulated disturbance" or whether of the "two orders of nerves some difference in constitution or sensitiveness to foreign impressions, makes one more liable to suffer than the other."[92] Thus, their wartime experience revealed the limitations in their knowledge and the need for further research and experiments.

While Demuth's wound was healing, it was observed that he had a headache, which lasted for about four weeks; he did regain the power to move his right arm, though feebly and slowly, but could not stand on his left leg. By January 25 Demuth was sent to Washington where he was able to walk with the help of a cane but soon suffered a relapse in which the paralysis increased. On June 4 he entered Christian Street Hospital, to be treated by Mitchell, who conducted a number of tests, including checking his nutrition, sensation, tactile sensation, and range of movement. Mitchell examined Demuth's movement and found that the patient had some power to move the thighs when lying down but could not lift his legs from the bed. He had no motion below the knee, with the exception of some movement in his toes. Pressure on the cicatrix caused "feeble twitching of the anterior muscles of the right thigh," and both legs were "subject to cramps and twitching which increase at night."[93]

Mitchell then turned his attention to sensation. It was found that the patient suffered from "shooting pains" at the seat of the wound, "darting from the thigh to the knee," with a burning sensation in both feet; pressure or pinching of the muscles gave him "more than the usual pain," causing Mitchell to believe he had hyperaesthenia of common sensation. Lastly, he measured nutrition and found no special atrophy of individual groups of muscles, but both legs were "slightly wasted," the legs below the knees were congested but not swollen, and the muscles of the legs were "irritable to induced electric currents."[94] After these tests, the patient was diagnosed as suffering from reflex paralysis and was first ordered to have rough fricheons with cold to the spine and to take a twentieth of a grain of strychnia three times daily; however, under this treatment the cramps and twitching increased so that, after three weeks, the strychnia was "finally laid aside as useless or worse."

About the middle of August, Mitchell placed a blister on the cicatrix with the "effect of greatly relieving the burning in both feet." At the same time, the patient was ordered to use the hot and cold douche to the spine alternatively. Electricity was continuously employed during the two months, and a month later he was also treated with iron and quinine. It was observed that the electric treatment caused a "rapid amelioration of his case" and that he "soon left his bed and began to walk on crutches"; however, by early November the treatment was abandoned after the patient ceased to improve. At this time it was observed that he could use his right arm well and walk unaided, although with a little unsteadiness of gait. In early December, Mitchell once again performed a thorough examination of the patient's motion and sensation and, this time, also checked the level of pain.

Mitchell's interest in pain as a symptom of nerve disorders affirmed his commitment to the production of new forms of scientific knowledge. He learned that the immediate effects of shot injuries to the nerve were pain "not generally felt locally, but at some point in the distribution of the nerve—in completely divided nerves; total loss of sensation in the parts supplied by it; shock more or less profound, proportionate to the reflex disturbance; and paralysis of motion and sensation, complete or partial."[95] He recognized that it was not the most important symptom, but because it was reported upon so frequently and prominently, he made special examination of its phenomena.

He classified three types of pain: neuralgic, aching, or burning, noting that they sometimes mingled. Pain was found to be caused by either the scar or the nerve tracks and was treated with "frictions over the cicatrix, with moderate exercise of the part," the use of leeches placed over the nerve, the application of blisters or cautery, along with hypodermic injections of morphia.[96] Burning nerve pain resulted after a partial injury to a major nerve (later called causalgia), which was the more "formidable symptom" and forced Mitchell, Keen, and Morehouse to exhaust their "ingenuity in devices for its relief."[97] This eventually consisted of isolating the starting point of the pain, which was found to lay in some "altered state of the ultimate nerve fibres and connected with the defective nutrition of the part."[98] They treated burning pain by blistering the seat of pain with Granville's lotion,[99] followed by a cantharidal ointment or cantharidal collodion, water dressings, avoidance of air and heat, and morphia injected once a day. Mitchell later observed that although cases of burning neuralgia had been received in England with critical doubt, he did not doubt the validity of this reaction, noting that it was often so intense that in one year "over forty thousand injections of morphine were used."[100]

There was a more practical story, however. These were soldiers, it was war, and they had to be returned to their regiments. In some cases of causalgia, the pain was so intense that it could be greatly aggravated by something as innocuous as the vibrations caused by music or even the rustle of dry paper. Men often took to pouring water in their boots to "lessen the vibration which the friction of walking caused."[101] Mitchell recalled after the war that he had never seen such intense cases and such suffering. Thus while part of this research was developed to create a fuller picture of nervous diseases, at the root of his wartime research projects was a soldier who needed the type of treatment that few physicians at the time were qualified to give.

In the case of Jacob Demuth, Mitchell noted that there was an "absolute loss of sense of pain in the right leg, belly chest, and arm"; so complete was this "analgesia that the most intense use of the nails on the right hand or the right nipple caused not the least sensation." As was standard practice, Mitchell measured the patient's temperature in the leg and foot and found that "higher heat caused reflex movements which did not tend to remove the limb from the irritant, but were merely convulsive in their character," while intense cold also gave rise to these irregular movements.

The importance of communicating with the patient in the development of treatment is evident in Mitchell's final note. As he employed the electric test, he found some difficulty in determining the state of the muscles as to their electric sensibility, "owing chiefly to the want of intelligence on the patient and to the fact that he spoke an impure German patois which made it no easy task to obtain from him a clear statement of his feelings."[102] Mitchell was always pushing his patients, particularly when using electricity, to try to distinguish between "prickling pain which the current causes in the skin" or rather the more important "deeper muscular pain." In the final note regarding Demuth's case, Mitchell observed that the electromuscular contractibility was found slightly diminished in the right leg and arm, and it was much impaired in the extensors of the toes on both sides. Everywhere the muscles responded slowly, but active and passive movement was restored and with the douche, iron, quinine, and liberal diet, the patient was "relieved" and discharged on December 14, 1863.[103]

Some of the prescribed treatments were clearly painful—thus one question to answer, then, is did patients simply refuse treatment? In one revealing case Chas. A.P. of Company G, 88th Pennsylvania Volunteers, was injured at Cedar Mountain, July 12, 1862. He fell and struck the right ulnar nerve causing numbness and tingling. He progressively lost power in his fingers, thumb, and wrist. He was described as "feeble" and "unable to write." Electromuscular contractility was reported as diminished in most of the muscles, and electromuscular sensibility was lessened. The patient went through a series of electric tests to the flexors, and leeches to the ulnar nerve track, but his treatment was stopped when he deserted on August 10, 1863. However, he returned November 19, 1863, looking for further treatment for his flexors, which during his time away had "greatly shrunken." His limbs had become "atrophied and contracting," and he had very little motion. The patient, however, had a drinking problem, which Mitchell found difficult to contend with. But even so, the patient was treated for another month after which time the case was laid aside as incurable. Before he was discharged, casts of his two arms were submitted to the Army Medical Museum, and he left the hospital December 12, 1863.[104]

The interesting point is that this patient, like numerous others, returned seeking further treatment from the doctors; some, of course, stayed and endured the treatments. Mitchell later noted how gratified he was in the great number of soldiers "who came to us, despairing cripples, and have left us eased of pain." These men either left the hospital either "entirely well" or at least had some use of their limbs. There is a sense in these case histories that the patients had high hopes that this research program might materially "cure" them.[105] On a larger scale, specialization was becoming a more visible medical and social category—one that promised innovation through medical research, which translated into acceptance and even demand for these treatments from some of the soldier population and, by extension, the larger public.

The cases at Turner's Lane, then, provided a unique opportunity not only in the number and range of cases but also in the unrestricted way that research questions could be pursued and the unrestricted access to willing patients that informed these questions. Mitchell found the case of J. L. Calvert particularly compelling because of the unusual symptoms. Calvert had been shot July 1863, one inch to the left of the fifth dorsal spine, while loading his weapon and was admitted to Turner's Lane in February 1864. Immediately after being shot, the ball "passed downward, between the bones and superjacent tissues, crossing the spine and emerging three and half inches to the right of the tenth dorsal vertebra."[106] The patient suffered great pain in his back and shoulder, which eventually passed. The more interesting symptom was that "an exquisite hyperesthesia of the shoulder muscles on both sides" developed early in the case. The condition was described clearly by the patient and was found to affect the subcuticular tissues and muscles, so as to limit motion, owing to the pain it caused, and even a "light pressure on the skin gave pain."[107] The patient regained normal range of movement in his right arm, although "feeble in power," but he was returned to duty.

This case baffled the doctors at Turner's Lane. Mitchell remarked that "this case was so interesting that we were at pains to satisfy ourselves of the verity of his symptoms," and in trying to do so, they asked the patient (without sight) to "mark the limits of the hyperaesthetic spaces when tested by drawing a pencil point across the boundary between healthy and over-excitable regions."[108] They also found numerous contusions on his lower spine, which were also found to be a symptom of muscular hyperesthesia. The physicians at Turner's Lane were trying to establish a pattern of symptoms or behaviors that could be linked to specific nervous disorders. They took thousands of pages of notes and compiled statistics using the symptoms of the patients to direct their focus. They were thus able to determine in this and other cases, for example, that both cutaneous and muscular hyperesthesia, or the extreme increase in sensitivity or pain, was not uncommon in wounds of nerve trunks or spinal injuries.[109]

There was an immediate benefit to these experiments. As one example, the treatment and management of spinal cord injuries progressed and developed through the war. Physicians learned to immobilize patients with spinal cord injuries before moving them to prevent further or more serious injury. Physicians also learned through experience when and how to operate on a patient with a spinal cord injury. Finally, physicians learned that patients with spinal cord injuries needed active rather than passive treatment to aid recovery.[110] These findings and experiments were used as a guide until Sir Ludwig Guttmann and others instituted even more effective treatments for dealing with paraplegics during the Second World War.[111]

EXPERIMENTAL SCIENCE AND THE CIVIL WAR BODY

Mitchell, Morehouse, and Keen also embraced newer forms of experimental and physiological science, which evolved from their work on neurology during their tenure at Turner's Lane Hospital. One series of experiments, and a subsequent article, concerned the antagonism of atrophia and morphia.[112] Before this article, very little had been published by American physicians on the "therapeutical conception of the doctrine of contraries."[113] As Roberts Bartholow later observed of their research, "In 1865 an admirable paper, based on clinical and experimental observations made at the military hospital for wounds and injuries of nerves, and embodying the results of an immense experience, was published by Drs. Mitchell, Morehouse and Keen."[114] This particular subject represented the developing importance of physiological science during the war. Once again the larger goal in this series of experiments was to produce knowledge that would be practically beneficial for the soldier-patient.

Mitchell and his team were in fact hoping to answer questions about the physiological antagonism of atrophia and morphia. Both atrophia and morphia had been used widely to manage pain in Turner's Lane Hospital (especially for causalgia). If the antagonism of medicines (meaning opposition of actions) could be correctly established, it might also better elucidate the subject of remedies and diseases. What could the disturbance of function caused by a drug tell physicians about the disturbance of function caused by a morbid process? Bartholow pointed out regarding these kinds of experiments that "as disease is a pathological physiology, so far, at least, as related to function, the derangements produced by disease may be opposed by other derangements set up by medicinal substances."[115]

The hospital as a site of clinical research during the war provided an opportunity to stabilize somewhat the conditions of the experiments; in this case it was by confining their study to "the use of the agents by injection only" and because "they were studied by more than a single observer."[116] The team suggested that they were uniquely qualified to offer important insights regarding the results of the experiments because "the information which our notebooks give in regard to the comparative value of remedies used to allay pain, is the result of an almost unexampled experience."[117] They conducted trials with various pain remedies, including conia, atrophia, and daturia but found morphia, a preparation of opium for subcutaneous use, the most efficacious. They also found that it could be injected anywhere in the body to alleviate pain, the exception being cases of burning neuralgia, which were relieved only when the morphia was injected near the site of pain.

The physicians were in fact concerned about the "incessant use" of hypodermic injections to manage pain. It was observed that the "the resident surgeons made every day from twenty to thirty subcutaneous injections."[118] They thus formed experiments on soldiers who were being treated for painful neuralgic diseases or other afflictions causing pain. After subdermal injections of the two medicines were tried, sometimes conjointly, sometimes in succession, they reported that "the results of these observations [were] so interesting and so puzzling, that we finally entered upon a deliberate course of experiments with the attention of ascertaining in what respect and to what degree and through what periods of time, the two drugs in question were antagonistic. While the final conclusions thus reached by us have served in a measure to strengthen the belief in the mutual power of these agents to counteract one another in the economy, they have also brought to light a range of very curious facts, which we think are novel, and which could certainly not have been learned from any course of experiments upon animals lower than man."[119]

Once again the team elucidated the importance of having live patients who could reveal all of their symptoms, not just the visible ones, which could truly be ascertained only "by the statements of the person who feels them." In late 1865 Claude Bernard published his *Introduction to Experimental Medicine*, which suggested that experimental studies made in the laboratory with animals could reveal information about the pathological state of a human. But the wartime experiments on live humans were performed before Bernard's influential work. Having live patients for certain experiments (such as the clinical trials with bromine) was seen as both unproblematic and a rare research opportunity—as long as physicians emphasized that the goal was to produce medical knowledge that would preserve the health of the troops or to return men to service. Moreover, bacteriological science, in which researchers relied extensively on the use of laboratory animals, was not yet well established in medicine.[120] Mitchell did inject morphia into dogs by way of comparison and found the symptoms did not "correspond accurately to those which occur under like circumstances in man."[121] Mitchell's publication built on the previous works of Charles Edouard Brown-Séquard and William Norris, assistant surgeon at Douglas Hospital, who had separately conducted studies on the antagonism of atrophia and morphia. The questions Mitchell, Morehouse, and Keen addressed, however, were unique as they were constructed on the basis of having living patients as a resource for their inquiries.

They examined whether the two agents had different effects on circulation and, if so, did one neutralize the other?[122] After injecting the two agents subcutaneously into the patient, they studied the eye (looking for pupil dilation), then the effects of the drugs on cerebral function (looking for headaches, spasms, visual defects, partial deafness, drowsiness, and nausea), and finally the effect of the agents on the bladder and to what degree each of the agents controlled pain. They emphasized the following conclusions as a guide for physicians: conia, atropia, and daturia have no power to lessen pain; morphia was the most effective agent for relieving neuralgic pain, especially when injected near the seat of pain; morphia had little effect on the pulse, while atropia lowered the pulse a little and then raised it within a few minutes; and as regards to circulation they did not counteract one another: both agents were mutually antagonistic to the eye with atropia acting much longer than morphia.

After studying each drug alone and the two together, the doctors noted that the "antagonisms were made clear" and also their "agreements in action" (as in the common tendency to "enfeeble the bladder").[123] The most important finding was that the "narcosis of morphia is lessened by the presence of atrophia, but its analgesic power is unaltered." Thus, as a remedy for pain, morphia would not be counteracted by atropia. In treating painful cases of neuralgic suffering, it was of great practical importance for them to determine this fact. "If atropia lessens or destroys the unpleasant influence of morphia on the cerebrum, but does not alter its power to allay pain," they observed, "there seems to be no reason why we should not use them together so as to obtain all that is best from morphia with the least amount of after discomfort."[124]

This detailed description of their experiments illuminates the environment in which both medical specialization and specialized research evolved. There was a practical concern: the soldiers who were fighting for the Union were suffering, and Mitchell, Morehouse, and Keen could help alleviate this pain by finding answers in their research. By publishing the work, this knowledge was transmitted with the intention that it would be used by those working in the general hospitals, and the many patients (or perhaps subjects) under their care enabled the physicians at Turner's Lane to conduct controlled and thorough clinical studies incorporating a broad range of research questions. This research provided unfamiliar medical knowledge to general practitioners but also allowed these new specialists to claim an unprecedented type of specialist expertise.

NEUROLOGY IN THE POSTWAR PERIOD

A particularly interesting aspect of this work was the ongoing relationship that was formed between Mitchell, Morehouse, and Keen and their Civil War patients. These relationships helped form one of Mitchell's postwar research projects: the relation of pain to weather. But at the core of his interest was how patients fared in life after losing a limb. The ongoing association with these patients represented one of the earliest longitudinal studies on neurological disorders in America. Many of the former patients were scattered across the country after the war, which prompted Mitchell to examine the effect of weather patterns on nervous injuries and stumps, and he compared clinical and experimental results. This project first took shape when a number of his former patients sent him letters complaining about "darting" pains in wounds that had been sustained during the war.

After contacting the meteorological office, he conducted a study in which he tried to reconcile his patients' symptoms of pain with various weather patterns. He looked specifically at waves of rain and found the rain area and pain to be concentric, thus linking symptoms of pain with climate disturbance.[125]

Mitchell also examined the influence of nerve lesions on local temperatures, again with the aim of comparing clinical and experimental results. He found that nerve sections cause "fall and then rise of local temperatures, so also does thorough freezing of a nerve."[126] To know if the rise after section was due to the "direct influence of nerves" or to the "vasal dilatation," he emptied his "own arm of blood by a bandage, put on a tourniquet and then froze my ulnar nerve at the elbow." He found no rise of temperature, and when the blood was let back in, "the thermometer rose above the normal in the ulnar territory."[127] In the relation of pain to weather, Mitchell studied the relation of traumatic neuralgia of the stump to air, temperature, and humidity, showing that storms were responsible for a large percentage of attacks of pain and discomfort of the stump.[128]

He also conducted, with his son, John K. Mitchell, assistant physician at the Orthopaedic Hospital and Infirmary for Nervous Diseases, Philadelphia, and lecturer on physical diagnosis at the University of Pennsylvania, numerous follow-up studies of Civil War patients who had suffered nerve injuries or lost limbs. In the years following the war they sent letters to Mitchell, Keen, and Morehouse's former Civil War patients and also placed an advertisement in the *Washington Post* looking for potential subjects. They inquired about the "date of wound, amputation of limb, character of wound, interval between wound and amputation, symptoms during this period, operation: nature of flaps; symptoms following operation including shock; pain, character, extent and seat of pain (this answer as fully as possible); the extent, duration and recurrence of suppuration; healing when complete; when the artificial limb was first worn; general health; alteration of pulse; body temperature; digestion; intellectual powers; and finally, general disposition."[129]

The elder Mitchell directed that should patients have any trouble answering the questions, they should show a physician his letter and "ask him carefully to go over your case. . . . I am so well known that I'm sure any one will do me this kindness, because I desire in the interests of medicine and science to get an exact account of your case, and if you desire it, you too could have a copy of the paper when it is printed."[130] Clearly some of his former patients were willing and eager to contribute or receive medical treatment; John Shaw Billings later remarked that "many would go by the medical museum with their addresses for Mitchell."[131]

A number of very fascinating letters from soldiers who had apparently suffered nerve injuries during the war were sent to Mitchell and his team. For example, L. S. Benton wrote Mitchell in October 1892, "Learning that you take somewhat of an interest in soldiers I write you regarding myself. I understand you have paid considerable attention to nervous diseases. I was shot through the lungs and my spine was fractured at Antietam. For many years the wound was kept open and I cough some and that lung is very susceptible to cold. My greatest trouble however is nervousness and insomnia for which I have suffered extremely for the past 17 years. I have been treated by all the specialists in Chicago where I formerly lived and though I am much better, I am far from well. I have called on you on two different occasions in years past but you were abroad. Will you advise me when I can find you, and of your charges."[132]

Richard D. Dunphy, who had lost both arms seven inches from the shoulder in 1864, as another example, provided the following history of his case: "During this period felt burning sensation of the nerve and weakness, unable to urinate for 2 days after operation, flaps good covered bone, extraordinary pain and burning for about three weeks in the stump, great quantity of pus and twelve pieces of bone or splinter came out in three months. Now red at end of stump, feels like a prick of a pin to touch the stump, more sensitive than other body parts, worst sensation is in winter when they feel chilly and cold; summer weak and faint sensation, can raise both stumps back to the back of my ears, wears an artificial limb but it makes me sweat, twitch and the limb feels shortened."[133] Similarly, Wesley Jones of Talking Rock, Georgia, who had lost both of his arms during the war responded, "Severe pain at the time, circular operation, suppuration severe. Now, general health weaker, hearing impaired, stump is tender, bothered by cold, sensitive to touch, sensibility to heat and cold, can flex and rotate what remains of stump, twitches involuntarily since directly after amputation, feels the hand but it feels like the fingers grew out at the wrist, limb feels shortened."[134]

John K. Mitchell later observed that "the matter is one which has never been investigated, and the only extensive material which exists for its study is among those who were unfortunate enough to lose limbs in the service of their country."[135] The first collaboration was a monograph entitled *Remote Consequences of Injuries of the Nerves and Their Treatment: An Examination of the Present Condition of Wounds Received in 1863–65* (1872). This was followed by *Clinical Lessons on Nervous Diseases* (1897). According to his father, John

K. Mitchell had "with inconceivable trouble recovered the present histories of some 40 of the survivors of our great conflict, thus giving my own cases with these added records, a history covering nearly thirty years," which "added a valuable chapter to our knowledge of nerve injuries."[136] The responses provided excellent material for advancing the knowledge related to both the continuing symptoms and the various manifestations of nerve disorders—but also identifying further research projects.

It was in fact remarkable for the development of neurology to have the former patients as a resource in which to expand the knowledge relating to nerve and stump wounds. For example, with these follow-up studies, the Mitchells learned that the elder Mitchell's former patients suffered common and lasting symptoms, including pain, sensitivity (particularly to weather), and twitching. They learned of the psychological effects of suffering wounds of this nature, helping to establish a foundation in which theories and treatment of posttraumatic stress disorder (PTSD) could develop. For example diagnoses like "traumatic neurosis," "nervous shock," "physical shock," and "neurasthenia" were associated with ideas related to PTSD and were commented on frequently in both the original case reports and follow-up studies.[137] Through these questionnaires, Mitchell was able to explain, somewhat, how his patients fared after the loss of a limb and reflect on the ongoing physical and social challenges of living without a limb. For example, in 1875 Mitchell published "Stumps and Spasmodic Disorders: Chorea of Stumps."[138]

In the postwar period, Mitchell continued to develop his expertise related to nerves and nervous diseases, becoming so well known for this work that he was able to pursue neurology as a full-time specialty. He is largely to be considered the father of neurology, but most importantly, his clinical approach to the discipline and detailed methodology chiefly directed approaches to the new specialty.[139] In 1867 Turner's Lane Hospital became the Philadelphia Orthopaedic Hospital and Infirmary for Nervous Diseases, where Mitchell was appointed in 1870 (and it became part of the University of Pennsylvania Hospital in 1938). He discovered new diseases (erythromelalgia, or Weir Mitchell's disease), he expanded his famous "rest cure" for hysteria and related disorders, and he continued to publish widely on nervous diseases.

Not every physician who read the wartime and postwar publications on neurological disorders would become an expert; rather, the Civil War nervous cases helped ensure that neurological study would perhaps engage physicians who encountered these disorders by providing instructions on how to understand nervous diseases, or rather reveal the limitations in the knowledge of the general practitioner and thus the efficacy of the medical specialist. This larger recognition by American physicians would later translate into drives to reform medical school curricula and create other forms of institutional support for neurology, such as the Philadelphia Neurological Society and the American Neurological Society, which was founded in 1875 with Silas Weir Mitchell as the first president-elect.

CARDIAC DISEASES AT TURNER'S LANE HOSPITAL

When Turner's Lane was established in August 1862, one of the wards was assigned to Jacob Da Costa, an appointment that "afforded him a chance for a study of exhausted hearts and for other valuable papers."[140] Da Costa's work has been considered elsewhere in further detail, but it is worth briefly reviewing his achievements in the field of heart disease in this discussion of the Civil War and medical specialization.[141] Da Costa was a graduate of Jefferson Medical College and received graduate training in Paris and Vienna, where he first became interested in pathology and internal medicine. He wrote to Hammond on May 9, 1862, offering his services as an "attending physician by contract for one of the military hospitals in Philadelphia."[142] He reported to duty on May 14, 1862, as an acting assistant surgeon at the Filbert Street Hospital.[143] He took an interest in the heart diseases of soldiers while at Filbert, and it was noted that he "is the only acting assistant surgeon connected with the hospital who is now performing special duty, and has charge of the ward containing cases of heart disease, his compensation is 80.00 per month."[144] Even after he secured a post at Turner's Lane Hospital, he continued his association with Filbert Street Hospital, where his duties were deemed "necessary to the interest of the service."[145]

Jacob Da Costa's first significant wartime publication, partly based on his research at Turner's Lane and Filbert Street Hospitals, was an 1864 treatise entitled *Medical Diagnosis*, written "to furnish advanced graduate students and young graduates of medicine with a guide that might be of service to them in their endeavors to discriminate disease."[146] He recognized the opportunity to present a study of the prevailing diseases encountered during the war, and as some of the case reports relating to Circular No. 2 revealed, this was an area in which some American physicians desperately needed further training. Da Costa hoped that his treatise (which was reissued through nine editions) would help general practitioners and young physicians with their medical diagnoses.[147]

In this first publication, he included a section related to his wartime work on cardiology, which was just under a hundred pages. He produced a general guide on heart disease, which included an analysis of anatomy and physiology, different methods of physical diagnosis (measuring palpitation, percussion, and auscultation), and symptoms of heart disease including functional and organic diseases of the heart. He included illustrations and graphs to accompany his descriptions. He built upon this work more fully with his postwar publications, which were based on the investigation and analysis of at least 300 cases of heart disease seen at Turner's Lane Hospital.[148] Although he used Civil War case histories to explain heart disease, Da Costa noted that it was equally "interesting to the civil practitioner, on account of its intimate bearing on some obscure or doubtful points of pathology."[149]

Da Costa's wartime research resulted in two significant publications and a number of lectures. The first publication traced the passage of functional valvular disorders of the heart into organic valvular disease and in particular explained the "real value and meaning" of murmurs as signs of organic valvular disease.[150] The second article concerned "irritable heart," a form of cardiovascular disease associated with stress, anxiety, cardiac exhaustion, and debilitation. Da Costa began calling the heart diseases he diagnosed in soldiers "irritable heart"[151] in 1862, which was very important for the development of this specialty.[152] With this designation, he identified a common but largely undiagnosed problem among soldiers. He wrote to the War Department to call attention to this "form of cardiac malady," particularly as he observed it after the Peninsular campaign. This had the important effect of having the medical department formally recognize this problem among soldiers, which it did by sending numerous cases to Da Costa's ward, allowing him "to study the affection on a large scale."[153]

Before the war, Da Costa's chief understanding of the heart diseases among soldiers came from reading the British Blue Book of the Crimean War in which sixty-two cases were classed as having various heart diseases.[154] He looked for cases of heart disease during the Civil War and found that "irritable heart" was "encountered in every army of the United States and attracted the attention of many of its medical officers."[155] These instances of irritable heart baffled physicians who had never encountered these symptoms. The physician A. J. McKelway of the 8th New Jersey noted after the Battle of Williamsburg, May 5, 1862, that "disease of the heart appears to have developed in several cases from overexertion preceding the battle and excitement and effort during its continuance. In these cases the pulse remained for days at 110–120 beats per minute. Some fifteen cases, which have been discharged or sent to the hospital, originated at that time."[156] During episodes of cardiac exertion, soldiers variously fainted, coughed up blood, or found it difficult to breathe on exertion. As the war raged on, then, it was a problem that had to be understood and managed to preserve the health of the armies.

Though these cases proved challenging to existing medical knowledge, some physicians were also aware of the great opportunity that these cases represented: "To this day, nowhere, whether as the result of ordinary duties of the soldier or of actual war, has the subject so far as I can find, been made one of careful clinical investigation. It is very possible that from inherent circumstances our war furnished more material of the kind than is likely soon to be met with again; for so many men called, by the tap of the drum, from civil pursuits, and sent without previous training into the field, is not a state of things likely often to happen."[157]

Da Costa's case histories and subsequent publications wonderfully il-lustrate how heart disease as a specialty took shape. In explaining the di-agnostic signs or symptoms of heart disease, Da Costa emphasized first and foremost the importance of accurate clinical histories. He was able to determine that heart disease generally affected men who had been in the service for at least a few months and that the patient usually suffered from diarrhea, fevers, scurvy, and sunstroke, along with the more common hard field service and exigencies of a soldier's life. Patients often complained of "cardiac uneasiness and pain, headache, dimness of vision, and giddiness."[158] After being diagnosed, a patient may have had a short stay in a hospital but, after returning to his regiment, would continue to show symptoms such as shortness of breath, dizziness, palpitations (sometimes violent), and pain in the chest (sometimes severe, sometimes dull).[159] Da Costa noted at this juncture the patient's heart would pound quickly, causing "irritation"; and while sometimes the heart could be brought back to its normal condition, it was often difficult to control, and the soldier was usually discharged, sent back to the hospital, or placed in the Invalid Corps.[160]

Along with the physical symptoms of the patients, Civil War physicians were also advised to examine palpitation; cardiac pain, often described as sharp and cutting or dull and heavy; where the seat of pain was; abnor-mal pulse; respiration; nervous disorders; digestive disorders; and urine. Da Costa's articles also detailed the results of his experiments with various remedies, including tincture of gelsemium, veratrum viride, belladonna, or tincture of digitalis, to reduce the pulse. Sometimes oxide of zinc followed by strychnia or digitaline granules would be prescribed along with rest (often for months). The efficacy of the remedies varied from patient to patient, and Da Costa kept case notes on the remedy used for each; however, he seemed to have had the best results with Morson's digitaline.[161]

Initially, most physicians studying irritable heart focused on the functional disorders of the heart rather than organic affections, a distinction that was thought to be one of "practically of the highest importance."[162] The *Medical and Surgical History*, for example, noted that, "of 4,901 men discharged for disability . . . during the early part of 1863, 2,323 cases were certified on the ground of heart disease: 1,123 are said to be organic and 1,200 functional."[163] Surgeon Sanford B. Hunt explained the differences between "disturbance of the function of the heart dependent upon causes foreign to the organ itself" and organic disease, which manifested as a "valvular murmur, a diffused impulse, an enlarged area of percussion and a friction sound in the pericardium."[164] Hunt observed that "so far as organic disease is concerned the diagnosis of the mere fact is not difficult. . . . It is only when we come to sub-classify, that diagnosis becomes nice and difficult."[165]

Civil War physician Henry Hartshorne also discussed these difficulties in his 1863 study of heart disease in the army.[166] He wrote about "muscular exhaustion of the heart," which, he noted, was little understood by the medical officers, inspectors, and pension surgeons.[167] His objective, then, was to delineate between the different types of cardiac affections that affected soldiers. Hartshorne was thorough in his discussion. He drew out the varieties of heart disease that he saw in soldiers, including acute endocarditis and pericarditis, which were "the most rare." Dilatation of the heart, without "the signs of thickening of the walls," occurred in a number of cases, "especially dilatation without evidence of true muscular hypertrophy." There were also the cases of valvular disease—some were pericarditis, others were dilatation with hypertrophy and with attenuation, but he also found numerous cases of palpitation or functional disturbance of the heart's action, which he attributed to nervousness, tobacco, exertion, anemia, and the most debilitating, cardiac muscular exhaustion.

Like Da Costa, he agreed that what he classed as "cardiac muscular exhaustion" was a problem that had to be managed in order to maintain the overall health of the Union armies. The symptoms of the exhaustion as elucidated by Hartshorne were "rapidity with comparative feebleness of the pulse while the patient was at rest" and "great acceleration of the heart's movement on the slightest exertion." Most of the men that Hartshorne treated were soldiers serving in the Army of the Potomac, and before the war they had been in good health. Hartshorne was puzzled because when the men were at rest their pulse was 85–90 beats per minute (BPM), but after walking only a few yards slowly, the pulse would race up to 120–130 BPM. On percussion he found men had a "short jerky movement" rather than the "heaving movement of concentric hypertrophy." Most cases were free from murmur, and anemic murmurs were also quite rare. Instead, he found a comparative deficiency in "duration and loudness of the first sound and an approximation of it in character to the second sound." These sounds were more pronounced if the patient was suffering from intermittent diseases.

Most of these patients did not die from functional heart disease, so autopsies were rare; however, if the patient died from another complication and was suffering from heart disease, physicians were careful to perform an autopsy. In some of these cases, Hartshorne found the heart "attenuated, flabby and pale," but specific degeneration of the heart was absent, which led him to the conclusion that functional heart disease was atrophic in character and degeneration was a common attendant. The soldiers traveled great distances, exerted themselves tremendously, and often lacked clean water and proper quantities of food. The heart, then, was forced to work hard enough to provide for the overtasked body, which, Hartshorne suggested, led to weakness of the heart. But why did "soldier's heart" develop in some soldiers and not in others? And what was the relation (if any) to organic heart disease?

Da Costa, the leading researcher in heart disease, recognized the difficulty the war physicians had in differentiating between functional and organic heart, and these difficulties directed his research.[168] In his 1869 article "On Functional Valvular Disorders of the Heart," he recognized that within the "light of generally existing knowledge," physicians, when making the distinction between organic and functional cardiac affections, "will often be led into error."[169] But Da Costa studied his patients over a course of seven years and found that, in waiting to publish, he had the "opportunity of ascertaining the sequel to many of the cases recorded" that he found to be of "particular value."[170] In waiting to publish, he was able to reveal a much more comprehensive picture of cardiovascular disease (since heart disease develops slowly), which up to that time had been little studied and was not well understood by his contemporaries.

At first, Da Costa assumed that organic and functional organic affections were "widely separate."[171] But it was not long before his investigations revealed that cases of irritability (rapidly beating heart) could develop into hypertrophy of the heart (increased organ size, caused by inefficient valves or hardening of the heart muscle forcing the heart to work harder), generally accompanied by a slow and labored pulse and in marked contrast to the rapidly beating irritable heart.[172] In an analysis of 200 patients in Turner's Lane Hospital, 136 were diagnosed with "irritable heart" and 28 with hypertrophy, and 36 were classed as functional passing to hypertrophy.[173] He was at first shocked at this discovery, but as his patients multiplied, he "began to trace the connection; and observation showed me . . . the links connecting the disorders."[174] Thus, on the basis of his Civil War cases, he demonstrated the transition from irritability to hypertrophy.

One study concerned Edward K. of the 114th Pennsylvania Volunteers.[175] The soldier was reported to be a heavy tobacco chewer and had repeatedly suffered from constipation and dyspeptic symptoms. In September 1863, after just six months with his regiment, the patient was suffering extreme and frequent attacks of palpitation and was sent to Turner's Lane. Da Costa noted that he was "weakly-looking" and ill-nourished; his gums were "spongy and bled easily," and his pulse was 92 BPM, "extended and abrupt," and the first sound was "decidedly deficient." The patient was given ergot, gentian, and nitrate of silver, and he was able to work as an orderly. By March 1864, his pulse was 84 BPM, less extended, and the "first sound was of a much better volume," and though he still had "cardiac pain and palpitation on exertion," he was recommended to the Veteran Reserve. Interestingly, in July 1870 Da Costa again treated the patient and found that this somewhat mild case of irritable heart had become a "decided one of hypertrophy." The physical symptoms were shortness of breath with palpitations, but Da Costa noted that "the transverse diameter of cardiac dullness was 4½ inches; the pulse extended and forcible, the apex beat lowered; the first sound was indistinct, prolonged, murmurish."[176]

Through his research with his Civil War patients, Da Costa was able to demonstrate that irritable heart could develop into cardiac enlargement and functional heart disease could be transformed into organic heart disease.[177] In order to differentiate between functional and organic heart disease, he placed a premium on correct diagnosis, in particular the "value and meaning of cardiac murmurs."[178] As one example, he demonstrated that "non-transmitted apical systolic murmurs were significant" and that these murmurs were caused by "unusual forms of mitral regurgitation."[179] This work was pathbreaking and highly significant. As one historian has demonstrated, Da Costa's observations "transcended the cardiology of his era as well as that of his twentieth century interpreters."[180]

Once again this research produced immediate and significant knowledge that could potentially benefit the soldiers. Da Costa observed that from a military point of view there were lessons to be learned from his program of research. He cautioned that "it is important not to send back soldiers just convalescent from fevers or other acute maladies, too soon to active work . . . their equipments be such as will not unnecessarily constrict, and thus retard or prevent recovery; that recruits, especially very young ones, be as far as practicable exercised and trained in marches and accustomed to fatigue before they are called upon to undergo the wear and tear of actual warfare."[181]

But the chief value of demonstrating the connection and intermediate steps between "functional derangement and organic change" was "to the practitioner of medicine." After all, like Mitchell, Keen, and Morehouse's, this program of research was a "contribution, based on trials made on a very extensive scale."[182] Da Costa established information that could help other physicians understand what different murmurs (or the presence or absence of murmurs) meant when diagnosing a patient. He cautioned physicians not to ignore functional disorder of the heart or assume it could go away, for if left untreated, it could very well pass into an "incurable malady."[183] He explained the techniques established at Turner's Lane Hospital and emphasized the importance of accurate patient histories, record keeping, and long-term studies for producing new forms of medical knowledge. In the process, he established a research pattern and a hierarchy of specialty knowledge, and his association with Civil War patients as an ongoing resource gave his original research added dimension, enabling him to investigate the long-term effects of heart disease. Through his wartime work, like Morehouse, Mitchell and Keen, Da Costa was financially successful and advanced himself socially, but above all this work provided a body of knowledge, which detailed the wartime advances in the study of the heart and heart disease—and a foundation for this medical knowledge to develop.

PUTTING A NEW FACE ON WAR:
Reconstructive Surgery and the American Civil War

Challenging cases, the growth of hospitals, the need to manage the soldiers after battle, the opportunity to develop specific expertise, and the wealth of clinical material all had a tremendous effect on the development of surgery and surgical specialties. Two conditions allowed for the development of improved surgical technique: physicians were making strides on preventing infection in the surgical wards, and pain was now controlled through anesthesia. Chloroform, ether, or a mixture of the two was administered for a number of conditions or operations, including amputations, excision of limbs or bones, and, before the administration of bromine or nitric acid, gangrene and erysipelas, eye surgeries, tumors, dental surgeries, some nervous diseases, and facial reconstructions.

Introduced in 1847 by Sir James Young Simpson, chloroform was first used, though very rarely, during the Mexican-American War (1846–47).[184] Physicians began using it in civilian practice in the late 1840s and 1850s, and it was extensively used during the Civil War.[185] Though surgeons used anesthetics before the war in the public hospitals or private homes where surgeries were often performed, few kept detailed records or statistics.[186] The use of anesthetics was very new to some Civil War physicians, though many had read about their use in the Crimean War. In his manual on military surgery, Samuel Gross remarked, "In the war in the Crimea, the British used chloroform almost universally in their operations; the French also exhibited it very extensively, and Baudens, one of their leading military surgical authorities, declares that they did not meet with one fatal accident from it, although it was given to them during the Eastern campaign, thirty thousand times at least."[187] The Union records show that of more than 80,000 operations performed, only 254 were done without some kind of anesthetic allowing for the performance of difficult surgical procedures.[188]

One of the most interesting new surgical interventions was reconstructive surgeries, largely pioneered by Dr. Gurdon Buck, a member of the U.S. Sanitary Commission.[189] A central objective of "plastic operations" was to repair the facial wounds of the soldiers so that they could return to their prewar lives or rather have a productive postwar life. While the loss of a limb was associated with heroism and a physical representation of their sacrifice to the war effort, facial deformities were more difficult to accept. Surgeons were aware of this contradiction. Case reports often comment on the "improved appearance of the patient" upon successful reconstruction, and "saving" these men from potential ostracism in part guided the desire to develop this area of expertise. As Gurdon Buck's son recalled:

> In one of these cases the greater part of the nose, upper lip and
> adjacent cheek had been destroyed, and the poor fellow presented
> such a repulsive spectacle that everyone shunned him. For a period
> of about two years, as nearly as I can recollect, father persevered
> in his efforts to reconstruct the missing parts. Operation followed

operation at intervals of 2 to 3 months . . . finally, all his efforts were crowned with success, the man had a new nose, full upper lip, and an entire cheek. At the time he was dismissed to his home his face presented a very lumpy and uneven appearance; in fact, he was anything but attractive looking. But in the course of the next 2 to 3 years, all these grosser irregularities disappeared, and it could then be seen how marvelously well Father had succeeded in solving the difficult problem presented to him. In the meantime, the man had married and was leading a happy and useful life as a farmer.[190]

It was thus the patients who sometimes urged surgeons to fix their appearances: "Distressing deformities prompted surgeons to yield to the solicitations of the patients, and to intervene with but slight anticipation or hope of success."[191] But with few options after being shot in the face, patients were very willing to take their chances with these experimental operations.

A total of thirty-two "plastic operations" were recorded in the *Medical and Surgical History of the War*.[192] Many men suffered gaping wounds and destroyed chins or jaws as shell fragments tore through their faces. These cases were grotesque, unfamiliar, and difficult to treat and manage. Circular No. 2 asked that doctors submit specimens and reports of cases that were deemed "interesting" or "important," and reconstructive surgery fell well into these categories.[193]

Reconstructive surgery consisted of removing the disorganized parts and paring and approximating the sound tissues by twisted sutures. And while in some cases favorable results were achieved, the deformities following gunshot wounds of the face were usually accompanied by extensive loss of tissue or chronic disease of the osseous structures, which tended to decrease the rate of success in these reparative surgeries.[194] The challenges and difficulties, however, were in fact epistemologically productive because they emphasized the need for more varied educational and research opportunities and perhaps a group of researchers who could collaborate and develop this branch of surgery.

Dr. Gurdon Buck, a pioneer in military plastic surgery, responded to the challenge of treating these cases but also of training American physicians. Like Da Costa and Mitchell, he was an agent of change, a pioneer in the development medical specialization. He graduated from the College of Physicians and Surgeons in 1830, and prior to the war he studied in Paris and Vienna before being appointed visiting surgeon at the New York, St. Luke's, and Presbyterian hospitals, a visiting surgeon at the New York Eye and Ear Infirmary, and a founding member of the New York Pathological Society. His work was considered highly successful and provided a model for plastic operations to develop. The *Medical and Surgical History* noted, "Dr. Buck's operations must be reckoned among the chief triumphs of modern plastic surgery."[195]

One reason his work was revered was that his approaches were so innovative. *The Medical and Surgical History* observed that, while most surgeons followed Jobert's method,[196] Buck's "extraordinary operations abounded in original expedients." In particular, he detailed specific methods for "advancing tissue through the use of relaxation incisions," the "outline of pedicles by pattern," and the "rotation and advancement of flaps of soft tissue."[197] His medical experiences during the war profoundly affected his development as a surgeon. It was in the wartime hospitals that he developed the operative method for correcting congenital deformities, including harelip, alveolar clefts, macrostomia, and macrocheila. He also described for the first time the "pachydermatoceles of von Reclinghausen's disease," in which he "sectioned the body of the mandible for reconstruction of the nose,"[198] and, finally, he developed innovative treatments to treat and manage burns.[199]

Buck was cognizant of the importance of these new methods and techniques. As one physician noted, he helpfully "contributed to the museum a number of casts and photographs illustrating the remarkable operations that he has accomplished for the repair of deformities from shot injuries of the face," and he provided "instructive descriptions that he has published in the journal, of the steps of these difficult and ingenious surgical achievements."[200] Hammond too recognized the value and uniqueness of these cases and ensured that they were submitted for the museum.[201] Indeed, of one particular case it was noted that "this horrible deformity appealed to the Surgeon General who saw the case . . . and also to Dr. Buck, who had a large experience in plastic surgery and in the remedying of severe facial defects."[202] As a result, Buck's work was prominently displayed at the museum: "I enclose herewith the history of the case requested and it is accompanied by a photographic liking of the patient. The record of the case is up to the time of the first operation performed at the hospital. I have since operated three times and kept an accurate record, which I design to embody to a complete history at the termination of the case and to furnish it with full illustrations, photographs and a plaster model for the national museum in Washington."[203]

Buck also contributed to the development of this specialty by a number of case histories for the *Medical and Surgical History*, and he published twenty-one articles. In 1876 Buck published the first reconstructive surgery textbook in the United States, *Contributions to Reparative Surgery*, illustrated with his

Civil War case studies, which was considered his most influential publication in the development of this specialty.[204] The book consists chiefly of a record of operations, focusing on the remedy of deformities either congenital or the result of burns, gunshot wounds, or other accidents. He classed his cases into three categories: loss of parts involving the face and resulting from destructive disease or injury, congenital defects from arrest or excess of development such as harelip, and cicatrical contractions following burns.[205]

One of Buck's most interesting cases originated at St. Luke's Hospital, where he reconstructed the face of Elbert Hewitt, a private of Company C, 6th Vermont Volunteers, who had been wounded at Winchester, Virginia, on September 19, 1864. A fragment of shell that struck his mouth carried away his front teeth above and below, lacerated the under lip at the right angle of the mouth, and laid open the right cheek from the mouth to the jaw. The nose and lip were also split vertically and damage to the face was extensive.[206] Buck waited almost six months to operate. When he performed the first operation, at Central Park Military Hospital, he noted that the "injured parts have all cicatrized and the upper lip is drawn in and adheres to the lower jaw overlapping its alveolar border from which the teeth have been carried away."[207] Because this adhesion produced a "notch capable of lodging the fore finger, which permits a constant escape of saliva to the great annoyance and discomfort of the patient," Buck resolved to reconstruct Hewitt's face in the hope that he would be more comfortable.

The operation took only three hours and was carefully documented. He began by removing the disorganized parts and pared and approximated the sound tissues with sutures to reconstruct the face. The patient suffered some swelling and discomfort immediately following the operation, but within a month the sutures were removed and "union by adhesion had taken place in every part of this extensive wound."[208] The patient was up and about, moving through the ward and "regarded his condition as very materially improved." Buck restored Hewitt's articulation and mastication and stopped the saliva from passing through his mouth, and he was discharged from service on July 25, 1865.

Interestingly, a few months later, the patient searched for Buck. In late 1865 he asked Buck to perform a second operation to improve his mouth. Buck complied, and the operation was performed under ether, at the New York Hospital in January 1866. Once again Buck pared and adjusted the sound tissues and secured them together with sutures, and Buck noted that "everything went favorably after the operation, and was highly satisfactory to the patient as well as the surgeon."[209]

On January 19, 1866, the final sutures were removed. Though the patient could not "close his lips," he declined further operations "being satisfied with the improvement." Buck sent three casts of this case to the Army Medical Museum, all representing different stages of the operation. The first was taken before the first operation (number 265 of the Surgical Section of the Army Medical Museum), the second two months after the first operation (number 485), and finally the third cast was taken after the second reparative operation, along with photographs of the case (282 of the Photographic Series of the Museum), proving once again the value and importance of having ongoing relationships with the Civil War hospital patients in the development of these new specialties. Some patients were examined at "periods from three to seven years after the reception of their injuries," which allowed a broad clinical picture of these surgeries to be established, but also reinforced the importance of keeping careful case histories.[210] The new technology of photography allowed these patients to be photographed in various stages of recovery. And the postoperative photographs demonstrated the possibilities for scientific medicine by providing a visual record of new specialties such as plastic surgery.

Buck performed these operations in a specialized ward in the New York Hospital, the surgeon general and the staff at the Army Medical Museum actively sought the results of these operations, and Buck reacted by allowing a body of work to be established in this area. There was now a record of publications, once again detailing with precision the conditions under which to operate, the exact way to perform such operations, and how to treat the postoperative patient. Buck's work was considered particularly useful because he outlined in detail his understanding of pedicle flaps, different methods of skin transfer, his technique for performing cheiloplasty for harelip, and the results of his experimental treatments for discoloration of the face caused by burns, providing a model in which to further develop reconstructive surgery. Physicians took pride in being able to restore the faces of these men, thereby helping their reintegration into postwar society, and they themselves formed an identity and gained a certain status in working to develop this new, and difficult, specialty.

WARTIME SPECIALIZATION EVALUATED

The war provided a kind of medical experience that was unprecedented in the United States, and the many unique and unfamiliar conditions were not readily available in Europe or Britain. The investigations related to

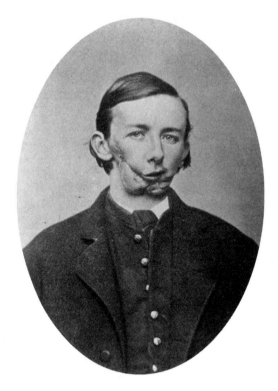

Elbert Hewitt, private, Company C, 6th Vermont Volunteers, age twenty-one years, was admitted into the Frederick General Hospital after being wounded at Winchester, Virginia, September 19, 1864, by a fragment of shell, which carried away a large portion of the superior and inferior maxilla. Three operations were performed by Gurdon Buck. This photograph shows the result of the series of operations. The mouth is symmetrical to the lips, but much drawn to the right side. (Photograph courtesy of the National Museum of Health and Medicine, Washington, D.C.)

the various specializations were by no means complete by the end of the war, and in many cases the methodologies employed were more important than the results. However, the specialists referenced herein commented frequently that they hoped that their investigations would be elaborated through the further research of other physicians. There was an epistemological uncertainty about these new specialties, questions, limitations in knowledge, and a determination to answer these difficult questions.

The publications and case histories of the emerging specialist differ in an important way from the medical and case reports submitted by the general practitioner; namely, they outlined the techniques and ideas about the specific specialty in which they were engaged. Da Costa, Mitchell, Keen, and Buck revealed through their research with Civil War soldiers how to understand, recognize, diagnose, treat, and investigate the various disorders they studied. They problematized the issues that they themselves did not fully understand and posed further research questions to be pursued, inviting other physicians into the specialized areas carved out during the war. These men were actors in the process of medical specialization, and through their work they effectively illustrated the potential of specialism in medicine. Indeed, there were highly significant patterns established during the war, which suggests that these years were important for the development of medical specialties in American medicine.

First, the conditions of the war itself helped determine which specialties would emerge, and the ongoing challenges of the war shaped and directed the practice of these specialties. Second, the institutional landscape of the United States was transformed by the war. Specialty hospitals were designated for the study of specific diseases and disorders, allowing and encouraging physicians to have an opportunity for the rapid accumulation of specialized knowledge; and these specialists, because their service supported the war effort, were paid by the government. Moreover, physicians profited professionally from the institutional support of the Army Medical Museum: they published the results of their experiments and advancements in the field and sent casts and photographs to the museum (for which they were duly credited), and in doing so established identities as specialists. Third, through the Surgeon General's Office, physicians published in detail their methodologies, which were illustrated by Civil War case histories and created a hierarchy of knowledge with themselves at the top. Finally, and perhaps most importantly, the physicians discussed here maintained continuing associations with their Civil War patients, which added layered dimensions to their research. Now they could study the cases produced by the war and the manifestations of the operations performed or injuries sustained for years afterward, giving the Civil War physicians a very enviable and unique perspective within these emerging specialties. Moreover, these findings were internationally recognized.

By the late 1860s the AMA supported the inclusion of specialties in medical schools, and elite physicians continued to advocate for specialist expertise in medical practice. Some of the rank and file remained opposed to specialists, especially at the local level, for fear of losing patients, and the AMA was forced to mediate between the emerging specialists and the rank and file for the remainder of the century. However, this tension was no longer about the efficacy of specialization in medicine, but rather arose because the relationships and boundaries of specialization, and of GPs and specialists, needed to be defined and mediated by the AMA. Significantly, the war specialists were able to achieve a type of dominance through their publications and war record, and this set the subsequent tone for the relationship that would develop between specialists and the AMA in the next decades; specialists were powerful and respected men, and the AMA would have to work with them, not in opposition to them.

The four years of war allowed for exceptional developments in a physician's career, but larger medical and professional reforms in the form of licensing agencies, professional associations, and research universities had to follow. But compared to Britain, as one example, where doctors formed collective opposition to specialization for the remainder of the century, resistance to medical specialization in the United States was resolved quite quickly after the war.[211] One reason was the demonstrated efficacy of medical specialization in practice; another was the drive among elite physicians to reform medical education along more scientific guidelines. The efficacy of the wartime medical model revealed that the time was ripe for change in American medicine. And while American medicine did not reach professional maturity during the war, American physicians did come together in a way that could have scarcely been anticipated in 1860. As more physicians saw the potential of medical science and the importance of institutional bodies such as the Army Medical Museum, the Surgeon General's Library, and specialty hospitals, some of the war physicians also became advocates for better educational models, the regulation of the medical marketplace, and well-defined and enforced standards for medical practitioners.

But there is another, equally, transformative part of this story. In late 1862, Walt Whitman stated, somewhat prophetically, that he saw some soldiers casually digging graves for men of the 51st New York and the 11th New Hampshire. He was struck that "death is nothing here."[212] There were dramatic changes in the way Americans managed death during the war. For some Americans, Civil War death was imbued with religious significance; for others, it was representative of heroism or courage; for others still, it was political or violent; but for a growing many, death and Civil War bodies were increasingly associated with science. And it was these changing attitudes about death that enabled the medical profession to achieve a new supremacy in American medicine.

CHAPTER FIVE

Whose Bodies?

Military Bodies and Control during the American Civil War

T he relationship between the physician and the "dead body" was contested in nineteenth-century America. Although most states allowed criminals to be dissected, not enough people were executed to meet the increasing demands of the medical profession.[1] Medical training, of which anatomy was the cornerstone at the time, was consequently severely hindered, forcing medical students to go abroad for their training or to resort to grave robbing, which was both illegal and socially unacceptable. Indeed, the public feared dissection, which was manifested in at least seventeen anatomy riots in America between the years 1785 and 1855.[2] Although states increasingly passed anatomy acts to control the availability of bodies, the public rejected them and the dissector, who was, as one historian suggests, viewed as a "butcher who reduced the human body to the status of thing, to the condition of meat."[3] Of five anatomy acts enacted in the United States before the 1860s, three were repealed, leaving only two states with such legislation on the eve of the Civil War.[4]

The contests over dissections in the nineteenth century have been well documented—but what about during the war years?[5] Most narratives of the period have instead focused on the procurement of the poor, the homeless, the powerless, the unclaimed, and the black bodies that were "exploited" by the medical profession in the name of scientific advancement. In the war, however, it was the bodies of Union soldiers that were dissected and studied. And yet there were no anatomy riots. It was quite the opposite. American physicians built a large, pathological cabinet from the bodies of American soldiers, which was open to the public, frequently written about, and widely publicized. There was an important, unprecedented, and perhaps acceptable dimension to the wartime dissection of bodies, which was reiterated often: by expanding medical knowledge through dissection, those still living and fighting had a greater chance of being saved.

To understand how the Army Medical Museum amassed such a large repository of body parts, with the public fully aware of the collection of wartime bodies, one must comprehend the changing nature of death that happened with the war. Tales from the front as revealed in letters, diaries, photographs, and newspapers destabilized ideas about the sanctity of the body, and death became more abstract. The medical department tried to control the changing conceptions of death and the body, which for many physicians was almost completely associated with medicine and science. Bodies enabled doctors to search for more effective treatments and to develop their skills through research and experimental medicine, which created a foundation for the medical sciences. The wartime ownership of bodies thus politicized the body by laying the basis for the study of medicine that would grow into demands for anatomy legislation after the war. There was now a written record of experience, including unpublished case records, the six volumes of the *Medical and Surgical History*, and countless journal articles illustrating the need for bodies to better understand disease and medicine.

What most Civil War physicians wanted from medical study in the war was an opportunity to establish their own identities as producers of medical knowledge; but they had to work within the structure of the military medical department. A close relationship between an individual physician and the medical department allowed significant developments in a physician's professional career. But it was a complex process of professionalization, with the competing priorities of doctoring to save the lives of soldiers and attempting to complete anatomical training being intertwined. In contrast to the heated debates between body snatchers and the public before the war, the chief conflicts during the war were between individual physicians and the staff of the Surgeon General's Office over the ownership of bodies. The dissection of wartime bodies was also sometimes contradictory. For example, physicians justified the "exploitation" of the individual body because it would ultimately benefit American medicine as physicians advanced their own research objectives.

For the larger public, the enormous death toll was a cost that almost seems incomprehensible. It has long been accepted that 620,000 men died as a result of the conflict, but new estimates suggest that far more men died as a direct or indirect result of the war—perhaps as many as 750,000 men.[6] Indeed, these estimates, based on the examination of new census records, suggest that 1 in 10 white soldiers died, leaving 200,000 war widows.[7] When searching for the larger meanings of the war, are these found in ideas about honor, courage, emancipation, or the "Lost Cause"? Yes of course, on the one hand. But for many Americans the war was completely associated with death—and Americans have long searched for meaning in that loss. Death, in fact, was everywhere and was visible in a way that it had not been before the war. In the process, Americans were forced to reconfigure ideas about death and the Civil War body.

DEATH IN NINETEENTH-CENTURY AMERICA

Walt Whitman constantly wrote to his mother about his hospital visits and recorded his experiences, in which he detailed the courage and sacrifice of the young men he met.[8] His diaries and letters provide an excellent insight into how death was perceived during the war as he commented on it frequently and reflectively: "Somehow I got thinking today of young men's death—not at all sadly or sentimentally, but gravely, realistically, perhaps a little artistically."[9] He found reminiscing about death not gloomy or depressing but rather "soothing, bracing, tonic."[10] He was not shocked by the death he saw but rather admired the bravery exhibited by the men as death approached: "One night in the gloomiest period of the war, in the Patent Office Hospital in Washington City, as I stood by the bedside of a Pennsylvania soldier who lay, conscious of quick approaching death, yet perfectly calm with noble, spiritual manner, the veteran surgeon, turning aside, said to me that though he had witnessed many, many deaths of soldiers and had been a worker at Bull Run, Antietam, Fredericksburg etc., he had not seen yet the first case of a man or boy that met the approach of dissolution with cowardly qualms or terror. My own observation fully bears out these remarks."[11] Soldiers were expected to demonstrate manly character and courage, but many Civil War soldiers also saw death or mutilation as an inevitable outcome of their suffering. As one soldier observed in a letter home after seeing a bushel of arms and legs being carried out of the hospital by a surgeon, "one gets used to such seens [sic] quicker than you would think it possible."[12]

Indeed, death was so commonplace that there was a detachment about it, as Whitman observed of a patient in Armory Square Hospital after the Battle of Gettysburg: "Notice the water-pail by the side of the bed, with a quantity of blood and bloody pieces of muslin, nearly full; that tells the story. The poor young man is struggling painfully for breath, his great dark eyes with a glaze already upon them, and the choking faint but audible in his throat. An attendant sits by him, and will not leave him till the last; yet little or nothing can be done. He will die here in an hour or two, without the presence of kith or kin. Meantime the ordinary chat and business of the ward a little way off goes on indifferently."[13] Some Americans faced death with a "calm resignation" because they believed "a transcendent beauty awaited them beyond the grave" and that "heroic achievements would be cherished forever by posterity."[14] Indeed, "religious faith offered meaning to life and preparation for death."[15] Perhaps a belief in eternal life made it "easier to kill and be killed" during the Civil War.[16] But it was death without "kin" present that was so different from prewar America, where people usually died at home with elaborate death rituals including bathing, grooming, posing, and photographing the corpse.[17]

While some families were forced to come to terms with losing a loved one and never seeing the body again, some families still tried to have the body of a loved one sent home. But it was not an easy process. Abigail L. Johnson lost her son to disease in December 1862 and attempted to have his body returned for burial: "Soon after [the death of my son Henry], I saw the death of my other son Frank, in the daily papers. I made arrangements for his burial in my other son's grave and was going to have them both in one grave when to our sad disappointment it proved to be the body of a stranger. . . . My son's name was on the bosom of this man's shirt. . . . The circumstance of his death seems to be enveloped in darkness. Oh when will war and bloodshed cease from our lands? When will fathers and mothers have their sons at home to die with them and have the mournful comfort of preparing their bodies for the grave? This is from a mother in affliction."[18]

Handling bodies during the war was often very difficult, and the preceding case in particular led to demands for the greater care of diseased bodies.[19] The Quartermaster Department, which was charged with the burial of soldiers, was notified that friends and family had to be able to establish the identity of the body to be exhumed. Thus, in addition to the death record, surgeons of the general hospitals began the practice of pinning a card on the breast of the deceased containing his name and description, which was to be buried with the body. The object was to remedy the mistake of exhuming the wrong body from going beyond the cemetery. Indeed, the quartermaster was puzzled by the number of cases of negligence of "parties at the hospitals tending to confuse burial records" in his attempts to "procure for the friends of the deceased officers and soldiers the melancholy pleasure of having them rest near the graves of their kindreds."[20]

Some families wanted the return of the corpse, if only to see it one last time in a semi-lifelike state, and thus turned to embalmers. Before the war, embalming was used by medical schools to preserve corpses for dissection, but the practice had not been followed in burial for regular citizens; most who wanted to preserve the corpse resorted to coffins on ice.[21] The Civil War, on the other hand, led to an unprecedented demand for embalming. This consisted of a chemical injection[22] (usually through a femoral artery) after which the embalmer would ship the body home. It cost $50 to embalm and send home an officer and $25 for an enlisted man.[23] Embalming was used primarily by families with money, a fact not lost on the physician Oliver Wendell Holmes, who observed after Antietam that "the slain of higher condition, 'embalmed' and iron-cased, were sliding off on the railways to their far homes; the dead of the rank and file were being gathered up and committed hastily to the earth."[24]

The relationship between embalmers and the regular medical profession was not always smooth; in fact, the medical department viewed embalmers as an "unmitigated nuisance" since they were competing for bodies.[25] Drs. Brown and Alexander, the owners and operators of Embalmers of the Dead[26] in Washington, enterprisingly contacted Hammond shortly after Circular No. 2 was issued to offer their services: "As we understand you propose to establish in this city a national cabinet of surgical anatomy to be made up by contributions from the casualties of the war, and as we believe that we could under your efficient service help in preparing your specimens so as to effectively preserve them from decay, and also by copying them in wax. While still fresh, to a life like perfection, thus producing one of the greatest combined cabinets the world ever saw. We alone use by right of purchase the system of Professor Suquet of Paris for embalming and putrefying the dead either in the whole or parts of the bodies. We should be happy to be allowed to take charge of the entire cabinet, and preserve and arrange the specimens as they may be presented."[27] Hammond rejected this proposal, but it illustrates the contest over bodies.

There was in fact an almost unimaginable scale of bodies to contend with during the war. And these war bodies were not hidden; rather, they were very visible through the new medium of photography. "It seemed that the camera never stopped. Wherever armies went, the Cyclops eye followed. To the battlefield, to the home front, at sea, on the march photographers turned their instruments toward whatever caught their interest."[28] These images were shocking, dramatic, and tragic and shaped the image of the Civil War dead for the American public. Photography was a novel technology in 1861. Americans were fascinated with the idea of shadowed images on glass, paper, and metal and the scenes of war that photographs provided. Indeed, during and after the war "there was a steady demand in the North for war views."[29]

Alexander Gardner's photographs were of particular interest because he focused not merely on the surrounding field or site of battle but rather directly on the dead body. He favored close views, bloated corpses trying to "objectively" demonstrate the destruction caused by the war.[30] Indeed, of the almost sixty negatives that Gardner and his assistants took after the Battle of Gettysburg, three-quarters of the images focused on the dead bodies, dead animals, and mass graves. While it may be argued that Gardner himself was fascinated with death, this was only part of the story. He was in fact was responding to the public's desire for these images. His photographic scenes of death after the Battle of Antietam in September 1862 engendered a great response from the public. Most members of the public had never seen pictures showing the aftermath of battle or such graphic depictions of dead soldiers and bodies, and there was thus a huge demand for more of these types of images.[31]

The images that Gardner and his team produced simply and provocatively showed the thousands of dead "lying singly" and "heaped in piles" as the casualties were literally "falling in rows."[32] Images like his "Harvest of Death" after Gettysburg, the scene of Lee's defeat in 1863, described by Gardner simply as "devilish!," graphically revealed the dead strewn on the field with shoes removed (for the survivors) and pockets turned inside out, waiting to be buried or claimed by the medical department.[33] Of such scenes Walt Whitman would recall: "The dead in this war—there they lie, strewing the fields and woods and valleys and battlefields of the south—Virginia, the Peninsula—Malvern Hill and Fair Oaks—the banks of the Chickahominy—the terraces of Fredericksburg—Antietam Bridge—the grisly ravines of Manassas—the bloody promenade of the War department."[34]

Whitman also commented on "the varieties of the *strayed* dead," the "national soldiers kill'd in battle and never buried at all, 5,000 drown'd—15,000 inhumed by strangers, or on the march in haste," in graves that were merely covered by "sand and mud."[35] He spoke of the ravages of disease or the "mighty reaper," including the deathly effects of dysentery, inflammation, and typhoid. Men were sometimes forced to die alone "in bushes, low gullies, or on the sides of hills" where the only reminder might be a "skeleton, bleach'd bones, tufts of hair or fragments of clothing."[36] Whitman lamented the indignity to corpses, which sometimes "floated down the rivers" or "lie at the bottom of the sea"; but perhaps the greatest indignity of all was "on monuments and gravestones, singly or in masses, to thousands or tens of thousands, the significant word *Unknown*."[37]

Contemporaries were thus overwhelmed with "the work of death."[38] Members of the public now had to understand or come to terms with the new context of death—indignities to the body, vicious wounds and diseases, and often no funeral or burial for the family to attend so they could say goodbye and come to terms with their loss.[39] But it was simply not possible to honor all corpses or engage in traditional funerary rites; there was, then, a "reconceptualization of the meaning of the corpse and of death in general."[40]

CHANGING THE PUBLIC PERCEPTION OF DISSECTION

The medical profession was able to capitalize on the changing attitudes about death and the body. As noted earlier, part of the attraction for American physicians doctoring in the war was simply the availability of bodies and the access to these bodies.[41] Cutting open the body was not mere morbid curiosity; rather, the process, it was argued, might reveal the mysteries of disease and improve the health of the nation. Physicians commented often in case histories and letters of the new relationship between disease and the body that developed with the war. But there was more to the story. Physicians were ultimately working to save Union soldiers. Treating the sick and wounded after battles was a unique but vitally important medical experience. And, as physicians performed their first few autopsies, the "mystery" of the internal body was to some extent revealed, and it became less a fascination with dissection and more a matter of mastering the diseases that ravaged the soldiers. There was also autonomy about the war experience that differed in an important way from other educational interventions in the nineteenth century, such as the Paris Clinical School. Together, American physicians were dictating the way in which medicine was structured and practiced. This was different from the individualized training that many physicians sought from study in Europe and was important in supporting a new type of epistemological authority.[42]

Death became almost completely associated with scientific medicine, and this interest was fostered through the Army Medical Museum.[43] And in building the museum's collection, the deep divide between the rank and file and the elite that existed before the war shrank significantly. Indeed, the museum demonstrated, among many other things, the professional solidarity of American physicians. "There has been a cordial collaboration on the part of surgeons in charge of hospitals, and an entire harmony and concert of action between the medical and surgical departments of the museum. The museum already occupies no mean place among scientific collections, and may be regarded as an object of just pride to the medical staff of the army."[44] Physicians wanting to improve medical knowledge and contribute to the advancement of medical science were optimistic that the bodies and specimens produced by the war would lead the way to developments in medicine—but this was also a way to introduce the project to the larger public.[45]

Framing the specimens as important national contributions, not merely trophies of war, was a theme that resonated powerfully with the public, which flocked to the museum. Otis remarked shortly after the war that "visitors to the museum are so numerous" that he was compelled to extend the hours of opening.[46] By the end of 1867, more than 6,000 people visited the museum, and four years later that number had tripled.[47] Brinton also observed that the "the public came to see the bones, attracted by a new sensation."[48] Indeed, the public interest was shaped by the desire to see the objects produced by the war, to gawk, study, or satisfy a morbid curiosity, but the professionals at the museum attempted to control the response.

In describing the content of the museum, Woodward published accounts in many places, one of which was the popular *Lippincott's Magazine*: "To give any detailed description of such a collection is of course out the question; yet it may be of interest to state there are upon the shelves 2211 specimens of fracture of the cranium including 46 cases of trephining; 10 of depressed fracture of the inner table, without injury of the outer, a rare and interesting condition on which it would be out of place to comment here; 22 specimens of wounds by sabers and other cutting weapons."[49] He went on to review the other divisions of the museum—but these were merely general descriptions accessible to the layperson to draw him to the museum. The public did not understand details because the scientific medicine being produced at the museum was too complicated for anyone but trained medical professionals, a subtle message that was reiterated often.

When people visited the medical museum, they saw six departments: surgical, medical, anatomy, comparative or animal anatomy, microscopy, and miscellaneous articles, each filled with the preparations obtained from military bodies, which had been diagnosed, prepared, and dissected by American physicians. People saw the long rows of glass cases that held

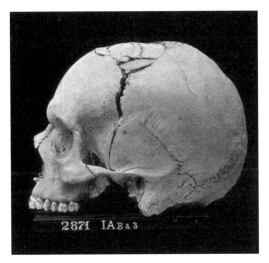

A Confederate soldier was wounded in the demonstration on Washington, D.C., July 12, 1864, when a shell extensively fractured the cranium. He was admitted to Lincoln Hospital and treated by Assistant Surgeon Henry M. Denn. The patient died two hours after admission to the hospital. The autopsy report commented on the number of depressed fractures of the vault of the cranium. (Photograph courtesy of the National Museum of Health and Medicine, Washington, D.C.)

prepared specimens and were "aware of the nature of the collection by the strong smell of carbolic acid."[50] Visitors examined "interesting cases" such as John Wilkes Booth's spinal cord from the cervical region (which was torn and discolored by blood), "transversely perforated from right to left by a carbine bullet, which fractured the laminae of the fourth and fifth vertebrae."[51] People could examine never-before-seen conditions such as the skulls displaying gunshot wounds, gunshot wounds to every part of the body, wounds caused by arrowheads and bayonets, specimens of disease illustrating morbid processes of every kind and samples of diseased organs, parasites, concretions, and calculi. Visitors were also allowed into the museum's microscopial collection, perhaps the most scientific division of the museum, which was described as "one which was not surpassed anywhere not even in the medical school in Paris."[52] Finally, visitors saw photomicrographs and read the extensive and brief medical case histories of the Civil War soldiers.

The testimonials from foreign doctors about the new "supremacy" of American medicine were also widely displayed. One London publication noted that "the Americans are a wonderful people. There are few other nations which would have been capable of utilizing the results of protracted internecine war as to make them available in after years toward the advancement of medical science and the alleviation of human pain."[53] Perhaps more interestingly, Woodward observed that foreign visitors not only were impressed with the originality and nature of the collection but were "struck with the free access given to the general public and to private

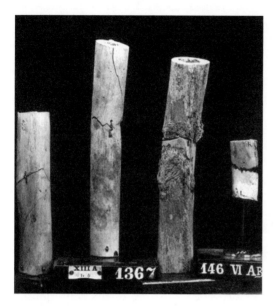

Of these gunshot fractures of the long bones, specimen 146 is a portion of a right humerus at the junction of the upper third, showing a transverse fracture by an unknown missile, and is the result of an excision. The other three specimens demonstrate fractures of the femur from gunshot wounds. The specimens were contributed by Surgeon W. H. Leonard, United States Volunteers (Photograph courtesy of the National Museum of Health and Medicine, Washington, D.C.)

soldiers, who in less enlightened communities would be excluded from such an institution."[54]

Throughout the late eighteenth century and the nineteenth, the public could, and did, pay money to view certain anatomical collections, attend anatomy and physiology lectures, and purchase popular anatomy journals and magazines. There was a morbid, political, or scientific curiosity in being able to see, smell, and even examine the prepared and fragmented bodies; to compare the ideal body in health and the diseased body in sickness.[55] By the third quarter of the nineteenth century, however, the pathological contents of many medical museums and schools were increasingly hidden from public view. As medicine itself became more scientific, more medical professionals and curators consciously emphasized to popular audiences that these collections were strictly about science, not "freak shows" or "cabinets of curiosities," and thus were beyond the realm of understanding for the non–medical professional.

The Army Medical Museum, however, widely advertised and opened its doors to the public, and there were two key reasons why this was so. First, the museum was funded by the federal government, and in the immediate wake of the war the museum was to be a common possession, a memorial of shared sacrifice, for all Americans. "Those of the combatants who survive are now better friends than ever," as John Shaw Billings wrote, "and the museum specimens coming as they do from the sick and wounded of both

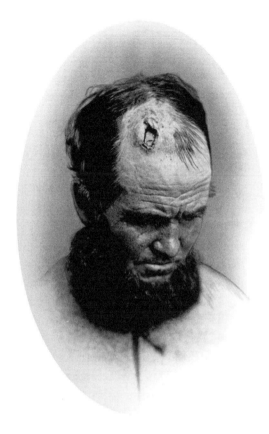

John Parkhurst, private, Company E, 2nd New York Artillery, suffered a gunshot fracture of the frontal lobe on April 7, 1865, at the Battle of Farmville, Virginia. The ball fractured the upper portion of the frontal bone. This patient was photographed at Harewood General Hospital by R. B. Bontecou. (Photograph courtesy of the National Library of Medicine, Washington D.C.)

armies, and contributed by both Union and Confederate surgeons, enforce the lesson of the profession and of its interests, as well as that of our country."[56] Indeed, John Brinton remembered that soldiers and officers who had a limb in the museum "would often come to look up its resting place." By 1867 the museum was one of the "sights" that could not be missed when visiting Washington, and during President Grant's inauguration in 1869 the hours of the museum had to be extended to accommodate the many visitors.[57]

The second related reason the museum was opened to the public was so that laypeople could see not only the importance of the institution for war medicine but also the scientific authority and social prominence of the orthodox physician. As noted earlier, before the war most states repealed anatomy acts, and doctors were looked upon merely as opportunistic dissectors. By 1865 the public came to expect more from physicians and the promise of scientific medicine. Thus, in opening up the museum's collection the war physicians could demonstrate their deeper knowledge of the body and new avenues of medical research that developed through the war.

In the process, orthodox physicians became the leading and often sole authority when it came to the body, which helped cement their ascendancy over competing sects in the postwar period.[58] They decided which cases were interesting, which specimens were worthy of being displayed in the museum, and even which bodies should be autopsied. In other words, physicians determined which bodies were useful; and these "chosen" bodies became the most important part of their war narrative. The wartime activities, however, also revealed the potential of the Army Medical Museum for the larger development of American scientific medicine.

The museum was the first major national center of medical research to be supported by the government. But without the immediate objective of war and thus the larger goal of improving military medicine, civilian and military physicians had to convince Congress to continue funding the museum in the postwar period.[59] Samuel Gross, Austin Flint, and Oliver Wendell Holmes, as an example, discussed the importance of the national museum just after the war in a letter addressed to members of the American Medical Association (AMA). After describing the extensive and impressive collection of specimens, they observed that it was a "great center of attraction for physicians and surgeons from every part of the country," indeed "from all civilized regions of the earth." And this, as Holmes, Flint, and Gross argued, was important for both the continued development of professional medicine in America and, by extension, health care, for "an educated and enlightened medical profession means a great diminution of human suffering" and would meet "the needs of the nation."[60]

This galvanized some members of the AMA into action. In response to their plea, members of local and state medical societies from nineteen states also appealed to Congress for continued funding for the museum. They lauded the museum's rich collection but emphasized above all that the museum would produce medical knowledge for the general good, indeed, for all those whose "welfare and lives depend on medical skill."[61] The government recognized the value of the museum with an appropriation of $200,000, which was approved by the House of Representatives on March 2, 1885.[62]

In the years following the war, John Shaw Billings became the authoritative voice for the medical museum. While the librarian for the Surgeon General's Library, he was also appointed curator of the museum in 1883, and the museum and library were incorporated into one division of the Surgeon General's Office. Plans were also made to develop an Army Medical School, which would operate in conjunction with the museum and library. The purpose remained the same as during the war: to "advance knowledge." And reflecting the tide of medical science, the goal was to have "half a dozen or more of specially trained men busy in the laboratories and work-rooms of the museum, each engaged on his own problems, and the whole for the common good."[63] The museum, as Hammond and the many war physicians envisaged, moved scientific research to center stage. But how did the collection come to assume this prominence? And was the building of this collection controversial?

PROFESSIONALIZATION AND THE CIVIL WAR BODY

We have so far examined the various attempts of the war physicians to study and learn from the Civil War body. But given the contentious nature of dissection and the lack of experience in pathological anatomy among some American physicians before the war, it was at first, as Brinton observed, "no easy matter to popularize the surrender to the Surgeon General's Office of human specimens"; only when "medical officers in the field and hospital felt that the medical department was really in earnest, that a great work was in progress, the objects of the highest interest to military surgery and the wounded of future wars were in contemplation, was the work of preservation efficiently carried on."[64]

John Shaw Billings similarly observed that the Army Medical Museum was specifically created to "preserve specimens illustrative of the wounds and diseases which cause death and disability in war, and thereby facilitate the study of methods to diminish mortality and suffering among soldiers."[65] This central objective was articulated often and helped garner support for the developing research goals and medical practice during the war. Both during and after the war the Army Medical Museum was often referred to as a research center of "national importance" for the "systematic study of the diseases and injuries of soldiers," which were represented there by "catalogues, specimens, photographs and a full set of publications on medical and surgical subjects."[66]

The overall project was for the benefit of soldiers; but in the general descriptions of the museum, the identities of individual soldiers and perhaps even the rights of individual soldiers were subordinated to the greater good. It was often observed that "the collection of books, specimens, records constituting the Army Medical Museum and library are of national importance . . . the contents of the Army Medical Museum and library are unique in completeness with which both military surgeries and the diseases of armies are illustrated."[67] Bodies were not lost in vain if their contribution could be perceived as valuable. After the war the *Medical Record of New York* observed that, through the unprecedented cooperation between military and civil physicians, the museum contained "a collection of scientific treasures that promises speedily to become, if not indeed already, more interesting and valuable than any of its kind in the world."[68] Even one body, then, allowed for the development of scientific medicine in America.

Framing the individual body as useful for the entire army or even country was not without precedence during the war. The court-martial system is one example.[69] Minor offenders were ordered to pay a fine or ride the wooden horse or were given some other degrading punishments, or were sentenced to hard labor in the heavy stockades.[70] The worst cases went before a judge and often received a death sentence. There were 275 Union soldiers listed as executed during the war; those found guilty of a crime against military or civilian authority were often sentenced to death by a firing squad or hanging.[71] Most of the executions were the result of desertion. Although the desertion total has been listed at more than 200,000 soldiers, 80,000 of whom were caught, only 0.19 percent of those apprehended were executed for desertion.[72]

Wartime executions were used effectively to set an example or act as a deterrent for the rest of the soldiers.[73] Troops were ordered to witness the hanging and also the grave, which was usually dug beforehand and situated directly beside the gallows.[74] In the military, it was perceived as necessary to subordinate individual rights to the collective good. For example, Special Order No. 106, Department of the Gulf, issued on May 2, 1863, stated: "It has become necessary to prevent demoralization that the fate of this wretched man should be measured out to all who follow his example."[75] The soldier in question was Private Henry Hamill of the New York Infantry, who had confessed to "plundering and pillaging" and was shot to death in front of his unit on April 26, 1863.[76]

In a similar fashion, as doctors began building the national cabinet, soldiers were compelled to contribute their bones and specimens for the "good of the country." Brinton recalled a story in which he had to convince a group of soldiers: "I was informed of a remarkable injury of a lower extremity. The man had died with the limb on and had been carefully buried by his comrades. For some reason or other that specimen was worth having, but his comrades had announced their determination to prevent the doctors from having it." Brinton, however, persevered: "I visited his mess mates, explained my object, dwelt upon the glory of a patriot giving *part* of his body at least under the special guard of his country, spoke of the desire of the Surgeon General to have that bone. My arguments were conclusive; the comrades of the dead soldier solemnly decided that I should have the bone for the good of the country, and in a body they marched out and dug up the body."[77]

Brinton, like many of his contemporaries, was fascinated by the different ways the body could be used to study medicine and disease.[78] He had begun a private collection of bone specimens accumulated in the West that he added to his personal collection of gunshot wounds of bone, but he was thrilled with the prospect of helping to build a national cabinet.[79] "My whole heart was in the Museum," he wrote, "and I felt that if the medical officers in the field, and those in charge of hospitals, could only be fairly interested, its growth would be rapid, and the future good of such a Grand National Cabinet would be immense. By it the results of the surgery in this war would be preserved for all time, and the education of future generations of military surgeons would be greatly assisted."[80]

Arrangements were also made to "inaugurate a system of exchanges" with the museum of the Royal College of Surgeons in London, the Society for Medical Improvement in Boston, the pathological societies of San Francisco, Philadelphia, New York, and the Smithsonian Institution, and various repositories in Vienna, Berlin, and Paris.[81] Physicians in the nineteenth century often judged the scientific value of medical institutions by the medical museums attached to them. With the wartime acquisition of bodies and specimens, American physicians were able to build a museum that was of considerable interest around the globe, while also demonstrating new forms of professional competence through the physical and intellectual mastery of the Civil War body.

When George Otis wrote Professor Flowers, curator of the Museum of the Royal College of Surgeons in London, in reference to an exchange between the two repositories, he assumed a new professional authority grounded in his wartime acquisition of anatomical specimens. He listed the 3,500 specimens in the surgical series, the 500 in the medical series, the 150 plaster casts and models, the 100 drawings and paintings, and finally the 1,100 microscopial preparations. He also described the illustrations, photographs, and photomicrographs, especially of the series of intestinal lesions of camp fever and dysentery, which he noted were of "exceeding interest." Otis was enthusiastic about the work: "Duplicates of many of these specimens have been prepared, and we are now engaged in photographing the choicest of them." He also promised to send Flowers a series of the museum's photographs, along with a series of "illustrations of gunshot injuries, one for each important region, and preparations of lesions of the intestinal canal in fever and dysentery together with microscopial slides of the same lesions," in exchange "for duplicates from your collection."[82]

By listing the sheer numbers of specimens, and especially by commenting on the unique nature of some of the acquisitions, he was using the bodies produced by the war to help professionalize the work of American physicians. Flowers responded to Otis that the council of his college would be "pleased to donate all of the catalogues of their collection—25 printed volumes in total" in return for "all of the works published by the medical museum, future publications, duplicate specimens (especially if accompanied by a case history)."[83] In the interim he asked for photographs of the specimens.

Two things were clear from the inception of the project. First, building and contributing to the cabinet were viewed and presented as a special mission and a crucial chance to develop American medical education—an opportunity that could not be missed. Second, the medical department framed its research and projects around military bodies and body parts, thereby linking Civil War bodies with the development of scientific medicine. In other words, the dead soldiers could save the living through the medical department's access to the body. The relationship between the quick and the dead was an important one during the war. Indeed, "when death became the concrete a priori of medical experience . . . it could detach itself from counter-nature and become *embodied* in the *living bodies* of individuals."[84] The project could develop, then, only with the medical department's ownership of the Civil War body. But the modern body often operates as the site of political contestation.[85]

WARTIME SPECIMENS AND THE POLITICS OF OWNERSHIP

Brinton initially worked with the hospital steward Frederick Schafhert, who had a long history preparing specimens for Joseph Leidy at the University of Pennsylvania and was "adept in preparing and mounting specimens for a museum."[86] The first preparations were less about scientific medicine than establishing ownership of all military bodies. Brinton recalled the story of a soldier who visited the museum to demand the return of his limb and was immediately informed that "the member in question could not be given up," to which the solider replied, "but it is mine, part of myself," "earnestly enforcing his claim, which to the lay mind seemed reasonable."[87] "Yet,"

Brinton continued, "to surrender a specimen was very much like yielding a principle."[88] Indeed, when Hammond gave Brinton his official orders regarding the museum, he was explicit that, "should any medical officer of the Army decline or neglect to furnish such preparations for the Museum, you will report the name of such officer to this office."[89]

The state and the medical department claimed ownership of military bodies and used this claim to justify dissections that had been considered unacceptable in antebellum America. Brinton's wording regarding ownership is revealing: "A soldier, a private, came, examined the Museum, and with the help of the Assistant Curator, found his amputated limb. It seemed to him his own property and he demanded it noisily and pertinaciously. He was deaf to reason, and was only silenced by the question of the Curator, 'For how long did you enlist, for three years of the war? . . . The United States Government is entitled to all of you, until the expiration of the specified time. I dare not give a part of you up before." Brinton continued, "In the meantime one detachment of you is stationed at the museum on government duty, the other wherever you may be ordered. Such is the opinion of the attorney general.'"[90]

Specimens were collected in two ways. The first, as described earlier, was through Circular No. 2, which required physicians to prepare and submit medical and surgical specimens of interest. Almost immediately the greatest interest had been "exhibited by the medical staff in the undertaking and pathological specimens have been continuously forwarded to the museum from every quarter."[91] Doctors were authorized to buy fluids and chemicals to prepare specimens and were further authorized to make requisitions to the medical purveyors for such articles.[92]

The second way that bodies were amassed was by assigning specific medical officers the task of collecting, preparing, and sending specimens to the museum from the cities in which they were stationed.[93] By order of Hammond, Brinton retained the services of the physician W. W. Keen in the fall of 1862 to "take charge of all such specimens as may be sent to you by the surgeons in charge of the US military hospitals"; he further instructed that "as these specimens accumulate you will forward them in securely fastened barrels to the offices of the Surgeon General at Washington D.C."[94] He similarly wrote to Surgeon William Moss,[95] who was ordered to proceed to Nashville and consult with Surgeon F. L. Town to "make suitable arrangements for the preservation and forwarding of pathological specimens."[96] He was then ordered to make arrangements to procure all specimens from Murfreesboro, Louisville, and Cincinnati to "make suitable provision for the interests of the museum."[97] Moss was given full authority to order whiskey and barrels and anything else he required for the preservation of medical and surgical specimens.

After being assigned this project, Brinton was almost draconian in his method; but the wartime acquisition of bodies was no longer about pillaging graves in the dead of night; rather, there was a remarkable openness to the project. Brinton and his assistants searched for specimens, which had accumulated after each battle in each division.[98] He also issued official letters to all heads of the hospitals requesting that any specimens retained since the outset of the war be forwarded "at once" to the museum.[99] Surgeons received instructions on how to prepare specimens: "In every case of amputation, resection in surgical operations occurring in hospitals affording such specimens [should] have the soft parts roughly removed from the preparation. You will then send an orderly to the dead house at the barracks hospital directed to the care of surgeon Keen who will take the proper steps to ensure its preservation. Each preparation should be marked by one or two strings, a strap of leather so that it can be compared with the history furnished by you in your report."[100]

There was some urgency in the quest. Even prestigious volunteer physicians such as Drs. Hodgen, Perrin, Bartholow, Hartshorne, Gross, and Leidy of Philadelphia, among many others, received orders demanding submission of their specimens.[101] Other eminent physicians such as Drs. Letterman, Armory, Simons, Sumner, Lackey, Culpepper, Franklin, and Mott were asked to cooperate to help ensure that others would follow suit.[102] When specimens were received at the museum, they were carefully compared with official hospital records to ensure that all of the "interesting" ones had been sent. Brinton wrote on one occasion, "I have the honor to acknowledge the receipt of the pathological specimens forwarded by you from St. Louis to the Army Medical Museum. I did not notice among the preparations already sent a gunshot wound of the ear which occurred at Fort Donelson, and was treated in the hospital under your charge. The Surgeon General has directed me to request that it be forwarded and also the round ball which inflicted the injury should it be in your possession."[103]

In his quest for specimens, Brinton also monitored hospitals after major battles. For example, he wrote to Surgeon D. P. Smith at the Fairfax Seminary Hospital in Alexandria, Virginia, regarding the large number of wounded men after the Battle of Fredericksburg. He reminded the doctor of his responsibility to comply with the provisions of Circular No. 2 and directed that "all cases of amputation, resection etc. be preserved for the museum." He further reminded Smith that the first catalog was to be published January 1, 1863, and that he "had better send us all specimens collected by the 28th of this month."[104] Sometimes those collecting the specimens and bodies were welcomed to the battle site. After the Battle of Chancellorsville, the site of what was perhaps General Lee's greatest victory, Surgeon L. Guild was dispatched to collect Union bodies. Nearly 1,000 had died, and more than 1,500 were injured; permission was granted for a pontoon to cross the United States ford to the Confederate's ambulance train for the internment and removal of the bodies. Guild remarked, "General Lee cheerfully gave his permission for the removal of the dead bodies; remarking that he 'did not want a single Yankee to remain on our soil, dead or alive.'"[105]

Brinton himself collected numerous specimens. He first visited the Washington hospitals and procured "amputated arms and legs," then traveled in the vicinity of the hospital and obtained what he could.[106] These first specimens were cleaned, prepared, mounted, and placed throughout the Surgeon General's Office.[107] Eventually the project grew, and Brinton moved what he referred to as his "museum possessions" to the museum's first substantial location, Mr. Corcoran's art building, which had been turned over to the medical department for the Army Medical Museum.[108]

As the project developed, Brinton aimed to fill the holes in the rapidly developing collection. In what would become a pattern of his correspondence, he wrote Assistant Surgeon January in charge of the General Hospital in Newark late in 1862 requesting "brains after postmortems."[109] A month later he wrote Surgeon Dewitt C. Peters requesting specimens of "the heads, lungs, livers and bladders."[110] Assistant Surgeon Alfred Miller, who was stationed at Fort Ridgely, Minnesota, often submitted arrows and Indian bows to the museum. Brinton wrote Miller to inquire as to whether it would be possible for him to "obtain a specimen or so of scalps."[111] The physician J. T. Calhoun suggested to Brinton that it might be prudent to provide each medicine wagon with "a metal can, with a wide mouth and a screw top to hold a gallon each and to contain spirits when furnished." He observed that "this would give every medical officer an opportunity to preserve his specimens. . . . I call to your attention this suggestion as I am convinced if adopted it would secure the museum hundreds of specimens. There could have been hundreds more from Wapping and Gettysburg if these cans were furnished."[112]

Occasionally, to Brinton's chagrin, he would receive specimens without proper records. For example, Dr. John Liddell, assistant surgeon, Stanton

General Hospital, submitted "an interesting specimen of gangrene of the marrow of the femur," which was obtained at the autopsy of a patient named George Curtis who suffered an amputation of the thigh on June 5, 1864. Liddell asked Brinton to "have it figured out" since "at present we have so much to do with the living we cannot pay much attention to the pathological anatomy as we wish to."[113] Woodward too struggled with incomplete case histories: "There is in the museum a very interesting specimen of carcinoma of the pyloric orifice of the stomach without any history, not even the name. This specimen came from Campbell hospital while you were in charge. Do you remember it, and if so, can you not get a history for us out of the Ward Surgeon?"[114]

In a similar case, the physician H. K. Neff wrote Brinton from the Post Hospital, Morris Island, South Carolina, in September 1863 that he was thrilled to be "assisting Dr. Gross in his amputations" and offered to "furnish any number of recent ones; both flesh and bones," but went on to suggest that "this is a god forsaken place to get anything prepared and the specimens are useless unless attended to at once, they become so offensive that we have to dispose of them."[115]

But physicians were reprimanded and even accused of hindering the development of the profession or even medical knowledge by not sending their specimens. As one physician was told:

The Surgeon General directs me to inform you that it has been reported to this office that you refused to save a specimen of a wounded leg of a soldier under your care. . . . The Surgeon General further directs me to say that it is his intention to avail himself of the sad opportunity presented by this war to establish a military pathological cabinet of specimens collected from every military hospital, and to carry out his intention, he has directed that all medical officers in charge of military hospitals of soldiers sick and wounded, shall preserve all pathological specimens which in their opinion might serve to enrich such a collection. He hears with regret that any member of our liberal profession should neglect or refuse to cooperate in so laudable an endeavor to promote scientific knowledge. . . . He should deem it to be his duty to close any official connection that might exist between yourself and the United States.[116]

Other difficulties in building the national cabinet included occasional contests over specimens as the government asserted ownership of all military bodies. S. W. Gross of Davids Island General Hospital became involved in a controversy when the man who had charge of his dead house "stole the specimens and sold them to Dr. James R. Wood of New York."[117] The man in question had "prepared himself after learning at military hospitals in Washington and then on Davids Island" and was "intelligent and had a keen interest in the preparation of pathological specimens."[118] Medical Director Charles McDougall was requested to procure Wood's specimens for "transmission to the Army Medical Museum for which they were originally intended." The museum was intended to appeal to the medical profession's desire for improvement and respectability. McDougall warned Wood that it was the "wish and intention of the Surgeon General to preserve for this Museum every object which contributes hereafter to throw light on medical science."[119] On February 24 McDougall wrote to tell Brinton that the stolen specimens from Davids Island had been recovered and would be forwarded "with as little delay as possible."[120]

While this conflict was easily resolved, some were not. The physician Reed Bontecou and the Surgeon General's Office were involved in a prolonged struggle over bodies. In early 1863, Hammond wrote Bontecou in regard to "two to three hundred pathological specimens" which Bontecou had obtained while in charge of the Hygeia Hospital. He was asked to answer the charge that he had stolen the specimens. Bontecou immediately denied it but protested that he had, during the months of April, May, June, and July 1862, collected "bone specimens to the number of 70 to 80 and wet preparations to the number of 30, which I presumed belonged to whoever collected them, at that time not having heard or seen any order to the contrary."[121] He then claimed that the wet preparations were "accidentally destroyed by the negroes who cleared the dead house."[122] The bone specimens he gave to Professor Thomas Markoe of New York, who worked as a volunteer in the hospital. And the "interesting specimen" that Hammond requested (a femur) had been given to R. H. Gilbert, the surgeon in charge of the Post Hospital at Fort Monroe, who had "ably assisted" Bontecou for a few days.

Bontecou promised to comply with the mandates of Circular No. 2 thereafter and said that he would soon submit the "good collection" he already had.[123] Apparently this was not sufficient for Brinton and Hammond, who continued searching for the missing specimens. Brinton submitted a report to Hammond in June 1863 and was clearly irritated that Bontecou had given away specimens that "did not belong to him, but were then the property of the medical department." Brinton further suspected Bontecou was still collecting specimens after Circular No. 2 had been issued and suggested that Hammond insist on them for the museum, "as they were its property," particularly since Bontecou seems to have been "directly violating the Surgeon General's orders."[124] The following week Brinton wrote Markoe, "I am directed by the Surgeon General to make to you relative to certain specimens of morbid anatomy collected by Surgeon R. Bontecou, and which *properly belong* to the Army Medical Museum. Surgeon Bontecou states that when on duty in the Peninsula, he had collected numerous pathological specimens and that in his ignorance of the requirements of the service, he had given between seventy and eighty of these preparations to you. By the regulations of the department all specimens collected by medical officers *belong to the national museum; no other disposition of these objects is permitted.*"[125]

Markoe was ordered to return to Medical Director Charles McDougall all of the specimens that had been transferred to him by Bontecou "under the mistaken impression that he possessed the right to part with them."[126] The language of these letters reveals the government's determination to have all specimens and the doctors' compliance. Markoe responded that he would "of course give up the specimens," which he was satisfied were government property.[127] He did, however, suggest that he had some "doubt of the fact" that the specimens prior to Circular No. 2 belonged to the Surgeon General. He therefore requested to be allowed to keep "several whole heads not exhibiting gunshot wounds," about which he wanted to write a paper for the *Medical and Surgical History*.[128]

While perhaps slightly morbid, this was not uncommon. Physicians often attempted to hold onto the specimens they had collected prior to Circular No. 2. Dr. James Armsby, for example, had in his private collection photographs of a few interesting cases, which he was accused of not submitting to the museum. He made a sworn statement to Brinton that the photographs in question "were taken while in private practice before entry into the service" and that he had "transmitted every specimen to the Army Medical Museum that he had obtained in the Ira Harris Hospital."[129] Brinton wrote to the physician J. W. Mintzer that "it was reported to this office recently that there was in your possession a half barrel containing a large number of pathological specimens for the AMM. They must be forwarded to this office immediately."[130]

Physicians clearly coveted this unprecedented access to bodies. Dr. Alexander Hoff volunteered to serve in the spring of 1861 and was soon appointed surgeon of the 3rd New York Volunteers. He often wrote his mentor Alden March from his post aboard the United States Hospital Steamer, the *DA January*, about his experiences. He noted early in the war that he was "expecting another load of sick and wounded and should I have any interesting cases I will send you drawings and as much information as I can get."[131] Hoff took advantage of the bodies that the war produced, telling March, "I am gathering for you some specimens of missiles, and will send to you by express some six balls with description when an opportunity presents. I will forward a shell, conoidal cannon ball and also some specimens caused by some of them as soon as I can collect them. The Surgeon General demands everything in that line, but I have made up my mind to put aside a few for the very next opportunity."[132]

Dr. J. E. Ebersole of the 19th Indiana Volunteers similarly appropriated a number of pathological specimens after Gettysburg for his private collection. He too was sent a letter by Hammond reminding him that "all specimens occurring in the Army Hospitals are the property of the Army Medical Museum and must be forwarded by the Adams Express Company to the museum immediately."[133] The physician George B. Cogwell likewise received a letter on June 5, 1863, in which Brinton stated, "It has been reported to this office that there is in your possession an exceedingly valuable pathological preparation which was obtained at the hospital in the barn of Philip Ray near Keedysville after the Battle of Antietam. The specimen alluded to is one of a gunshot fracture of the jaw and humerus, one of the molar teeth having been driven into the head of the latter bone. You had better forward the specimen to this office immediately."[134]

Sometimes physicians claimed that specimens had been stolen and they could not be recovered. The physician H. K. Neff sent a large number of specimens to Washington from Port Royal but left a number that were still in need of preparation at his hotel, "in the care of the proprietor"; when he returned they were gone.[135] Stolen specimens were a recurring problem. Dr. J. W. Mintzer wrote to Brinton in June 1863 informing him that he had recently submitted a "small box of pathological specimens"; he apologized that they were in such bad condition since his assistant had inexplicably "broke open the barrel containing the specimens and its contents were buried."[136] His assistant, Mr. Dowling, was charged with "exhuming the buried specimens," and a further search was instituted. Minzter did, however, assure Brinton that he was busy preparing more specimens in his leisure and would be "happy to deliver them in person."[137]

Indeed, the medical profession's enthusiasm for anatomy was not without its critics. In one revealing case, while surgeons performed an amputation in the woods after the Battle of Chancellorsville, Captain William Corby of the Irish Brigade lamented, "God wished to punish us for past sins and disregard of His benefits, and a certain number had to die."[138] In other cases, friends would wait by the side of the patient so they could immediately take the body home. For example, Martin Karr, a private from Company H, 1st New York Volunteers, had been wounded by a shell in the right knee joint and had an amputation by double flaps in the field.[139] He was later admitted to Douglas Hospital and treated by Dr. William Thomson. His case file noted that during transport to the hospital his wound had become infected with what was likely pyemia. While Thomson was sure, based on the patient's symptoms, that this was what he was suffering from, "the body was not autopsied owing to the desire of his friends to remove him without delay."[140]

In what became increasingly common, the friends did, however, allow Thomson to remove the femur from the stump, and he was thus able to "saw the leg longitudinally," which exposed the "decomposed condition of the medulla" as "constantly observed in this disease."[141] Though most of this soldier's remains were claimed by the family, the femur was submitted to the medical museum, illustrating both the cooperation and sometimes tension between physicians and the public. Some case reports simply give a report up to the moment of death and then stated "autopsy not permitted."[142] In the case of Phineas Brown, who died of tetanus in August 1864 at the Albany State Hospital, the attending physician Mason F. Cogswell remarked in the report that "as his friends were momentarily expected, the patient's residence being only seven miles from this city, no general postmortem was made."[143] Similarly, Assistant Surgeon H. Stone remarked after treating a patient who succumbed to pyemia after the Battle of Antietam that "no specimen was sent because an autopsy could not be made as the body of the patient was taken home by his friends."[144] That they do not go into detail suggests that it was understood that members of the family had prior claim to the body and could take it away. In comparison to the number of autopsies, however, family claims to the body were fairly rare.

If the specimen could be used, perhaps it gave meaning to the soldier's life. Contribution of a body or body part to the development of the national cabinet was portrayed as a final sacrifice showcasing the commitment to the country. Assistant Surgeon J. T. Calhoun sent a number of specimens from the Battle of Wapping Heights, July 23, 1863, and observed that he had "collected them off the field more due to the gallant action of Wapping Heights to be represented at the AMM then their value as pathological specimens."[145] Indeed, Brinton observed that while at first there was some "natural aversion on the part of the wounded soldiers and their friends" and that the "topic was a ghastly one," soldiers did often comply with the request for their specimens: "I recollect one instance of a very rare and carefully studied case of a leg injury. The patient died and was buried in soldier fashion. His bosom friends sat up and watched as the nefarious collector came. So great was his earnestness, so deep his sympathy, so moving his eloquence, so unanswerable his argument that patriotic bones rest better in government cases than in a Virginia trench, that the stony hearts of the watchers were softened. Slowly and mournfully the former comrades marched to the burial spot. The leg was exhumed, the bone taken out and carefully inspected by the mourners, the chief of whom remarked that 'after all John would rather be of some use to the very end.'"[146]

The idea of useful limbs sometimes appealed to a soldier, who would on occasion request to see his contribution to the making of the national cabinet. These men were surprisingly deferential to the staff at the museum. Former Union soldier Lorin Leray, for example, wrote the museum on December 29, 1883, inquiring after his limb: "Dear Sir: Nineteen years ago, Surgeon A. J. Bartlett 33rd Minn., now of Illinois, removed the head of the humerus from my left arm. He writes me that he sent the bone with a minie ball sticking in it to the Army Medical Museum at Washington—it is numbered 6599 in the surgical section. I have never seen the piece removed. Will you kindly have the bone with the ball in it photographed and sent to me? I will be glad to incur all the necessary expense. I hope you will do this as it will be a valuable war relic to me."[147]

There seemed to be pride associated with having a specimen preserved and displayed in the national museum since letters like Lorin Leray's were quite common. Soldiers often wrote not asking for the actual specimen but rather photographs of it.[148] One visitor to the museum observed, "The fact of having a portion of one's body put on exhibition here before the wondering gaze of casual visitors and critical scrutiny of medical students, seems however, not to affect some of the 'subjects' who have contributed the 'bone of their bone and the flesh of their flesh' to the museum. One of the orderlies attached to the museum is *minus* the bone of the right arm, from the shoulder blade to the elbow; but he has the satisfaction—if satisfaction it is—to be able to go and take a look at it every day."[149]

Acceptance of this project was perhaps exemplified best by Major General Daniel Sickles, who had received an amputation in the lowest third of the thigh on the field at Gettysburg on July 2, 1863.[150] Surgeon T. Sim,

United States Volunteers, mailed the amputated leg to the museum in a small coffin with his calling card saying, "from the compliments of General Sickles." Woodward later suggested that after Sickles recovered from the shock of the operation his first thought was "of the museum at Washington, to which he ordered the broken bone sent, in the hope that his misfortune might prove the gain of fellow soldiers in the future."[151]

Woodward was perhaps overestimating the colorful general's love of the project, but the important point is that Woodward spoke widely and publicly about the museum's developing collection. It is revealing of the public's general acceptance of the new AMM that Woodward so freely wrote about the entire museum's collection (medical, surgical, anatomical, and microscopial) in popular magazines as well as in medical journals. After all, this was a collection built from the body parts of American soldiers. But in what was now standard rhetoric, he cleverly linked the bodies, the ongoing work, and the anatomical displays with the advancement of medical science—which appealed to the public's desire for progress in the final third of the century. As Woodward noted, "Under these circumstances it may fairly be regarded as one of the large compensations of human history that the periods of pestilence and war with which our race is scourged from time to time, serve generally to give a fresh impulse to the genius of those who have devoted themselves to medical pursuits, enabling them to make new discoveries, and to accumulate stores of knowledge which serve to increase their usefulness in ordinary times."[152] Although the work of collecting the material of soldiers was "ghoul-like," as Brinton himself conceded, the medical department needed the bodies to develop scientific medicine, which had become a central and very public objective over the course of the war.[153]

BODY OF KNOWLEDGE

"There can be no doubt the [Civil War] has given great impetus to medical study in America, and this not merely the directive of operative surgery and public hygiene, on which its effect has been perhaps most obvious, but in many collateral branches also on some of which a favorable influence from this source could scarcely have been anticipated."[154] So noted Woodward as the objectives of the medical museum developed over the course of the war and after.

The most significant pattern that emerges from the many case reports is the free access to knowledge and experience that wartime medicine provided. The first museum catalog, published in early January 1863, was quite small, showing only 1,349 objects in total, of which, as Brinton observed, 988 were surgical, 106 medical, and 133 extracted projectiles.[155] Through examining the catalog, the staff at the Surgeon General's Office could compare incoming case studies, narratives of service, hospital registers, and autopsy reports to determine what specific diseases they subsequently wanted to study and illustrate in the national cabinet. All of the diseases that pervaded during the war—that defied understanding—could be studied individually or in the form of large research projects. The scope of this project, then, is what distinguishes it from any other educational intervention found in the nineteenth century—whether in France, Germany, or Britain. Civil War medicine, disease, and science offered a powerful, intensive, and, above all, unique medical experience. There was, however, an interesting relation between intent and realization of objectives. The most pronounced effect of the mandate to collect specimens was that physicians were encouraged to see beyond the patient with a view to the knowledge that could be derived from the body, changing basic assumptions about how to study medicine and disease.

As the war progressed, Woodward, Brinton, and Hammond (in conjunction with recommendations from other physicians) let the varied specimens accumulate and then decided which were needed to enhance the collection or to train American physicians. After examining the museum's collection immediately after the first catalog was published, Woodward requested that physicians submit "all abnormalities or irregularities which will make good wet specimens, all pathological conditions (not surgical strictly) which will do the same, and calculi, parasites etc."[156] He further requested "a good series of specimens illustrating disease of the brain and nervous system, a series on valvular disease of the heart, a series of tubercles off the lungs, showing different stages, cavities etc., cancers and tumors of internal organs and specimens illustrating enteric fever and chronic diarrhea."[157]

The staff at the Army Medical Museum always strove to ensure that physicians engaged with Civil War bodies understood that they must collect specimens in a way that would make them of use for the purposes of science. And these objectives were continually published in both military and nonmilitary journals to induce physicians to contribute to the project.[158] In May 1863, the *American Medical Times* encouraged "every physician connected with the army or with its hospitals" to "carefully preserve all pathological specimens, and forward them with accurate histories to the Curator. The name of each contributor appears in the catalogue in connection with the specimens."[159] Brinton too encouraged, even demanded, diligence, noting that because "the value of all pathological specimens depends to a great extent upon the completeness of their history, strenuous efforts have been made to procure an accurate surgical and medical account of every case from which a specimen has been taken."[160] Physicians, after all, had a duty to both Union soldiers and the large wartime community of American physicians, so "it should be reasonably expected of every medical officer of the army that he will have sufficient *professional interest and pride* to keep a correct record of his medical and surgical cases."[161]

The specimens submitted to the museum, particularly immediately after Circular No. 2 was issued, were usually the direct result of battle wounds. J. Dalton, a private from Pennsylvania, had been shot at Gettysburg, the ball entering the right side one inch above the crest of the ileum and remaining in the wound. Shortly afterward he died of his wound. The autopsy documented that "the ball entered the spinal column of the right side at the articulation of the 4th or 5th lumbar vertebrae just in front of their transverse processes destroying the continuity of the spinal canal and facing obliquely upwards through the body of the 4th lodged in that of the 3rd on the left side."[162] The spine was sent to the museum, along with the ball.[163]

Dr. William Thomson submitted the case history of Coleman Boyer, Company L, 112th Pennsylvania Volunteers, who had been struck by a round ball, which entered the right arm above the elbow joint, escaped at the middle of the arm anteriorly, and inflicted another wound in the thumb.[164] Boyer was also inflicted with a back shot in the right opposite side of the ninth dorsal vertebrae and one inch outside the spinous processes, which penetrated the thoracic cavity and then passed through the lower lobe. He soon died of shock, and the entire arm was submitted to the museum. Thomson pointed out that "the specimen indicates the amount of injury possible from a round ball when passing through the elbow joint."[165] Cases such as these represent the original function of the museum, which was to learn from the specimens and effectively illustrate the effect of wound trauma and diseases.

Some cases, however, demanded more comprehensive study and led to the development of new ideas. Frank Vogle, private, Company G, 74th Regiment, Pennsylvania Volunteers, was wounded at Gettysburg by a minié ball, which entered on the front of the right leg, six inches below the knee joint, passed around the fibula, and exited behind the calf of the leg.[166] The case report, submitted by Assistant Surgeon I. Eagleton, is more than twelve pages long, because despite treating the wound prophylactically with carbolic acid, followed by a fermented poultice, tonic, and extra diet, it developed great complications from gangrene, which quickly spread.[167] The doctors after consultation decided to amputate below the knee joint, despite the patient's severely weakened state.

The patient fared well during and immediately after the operation, which was performed by Assistant Surgeon A. Hewson, who was also in residence at the hospital. Within a few days the patient inexplicably suffered "an attack of hemorrhage from the stump." The physicians went to great lengths to try to save Vogle, but he eventually died, and a postmortem was made within a few hours of his death. Rather than merely focusing on the wound, the postmortem was aimed at tracing the cause of the hemorrhage. After the rather lengthy investigation, the physicians determined that a blood "clot had formed before the last ligature was applied, thereby filling the opening." They submitted both medical specimens and the original amputated leg to the museum.

Given that it was in fact wartime, some of the cases and the operations performed were truly remarkable. Assistant Surgeon J. T. Calhoun, medical director of the 3rd Army Corps, performed a very complicated facial reconstruction in the field hospital immediately following the Battle of Gettysburg. Private John Hall, Company 8, 11th New York Volunteers, had been shot, and the shell had torn his cheek, producing a "horrible compound comminuted fracture of the inferior maxillary."[168] The patient was placed under chloroform, and Calhoun, along with assistant surgeons Jameson and Hays, also of Company 8, removed "piece after piece of bone" with a pair of duck billed forceps "suppurating the muscles from the bone." Little hemorrhaging took place, and the operation continued. The bone at the chin had been shattered, and the "soft parts had to be held in place." During the operation, the tongue was carefully kept in sight, and a ligature was passed through its tip and held by Surgeon Hays. After carefully "securing all bleeding vessels and getting rid of all burnt or destroyed tissue, the excessively ragged wound was brought together in accurate opposition by the introduction of silver pins, with a wire figure of 8 suture."[169] The dressings were treated with charpie and water, and the patient recovered "nicely." Calhoun submitted the superior maxillary bone for display at the AMM along with the case history of the operation.[170]

The staff at the museum also used the incoming specimens to identify research projects. Woodward wrote J. T. Cantwell, assistant surgeon with the 82nd Regiment, Ohio Volunteers, from Mansfield on March 12, 1864, to thank him for sending the "specimens of gallstone" but recommended reading Thudichum's *Treatise on Gall-stones* (London), "an excellent work full of instruction," which Woodward believed would help Cantwell's understanding.[171] Some cases helped to elucidate the function of specific diseases that had previously been unknown or little understood. As Woodward wrote on one occasion, "In your letter to the Surgeon General's Office of Oct. 17th you make an observation with regard to the proliferation of the connective tissue of the medulla oblongata and cerebellum in a case of tetanus, which if correct is of such importance that I cannot refrain from expressing the hope that you have preserved microscopial specimens to demonstrate the condition in question, or at least that you have preserved a portion of the tissue involved from which of course such preparation could still be readily obtained."[172]

Woodward had long been interested in tetanus, particularly because most physicians had trouble managing it.[173] Of 509 cases of tetanus recorded in the Union army, 89 percent proved fatal.[174] Also troubling was the sheer pain of this disease. Tetanus can cause painful muscle spasms, or "lockjaw," and back and abdominal muscle seizures; the patient can no longer swallow or breathe at this point and quickly succumbs to death. There was no effective treatment for tetanus. Physicians used chloroform during the "paroxysms of spasmodic contraction" and opium to try to minimize the pain, but without a way to treat tetanus, the goal was to better understand its pathology in the hopes of finding a treatment or preventative. Physicians frequently commented on "great congestion of the brain and spinal cord," which was attributed to lesions found on the connective tissue. But investigations into this disease resulted in few answers. Woodward thus asked Surgeon McGill, who had also been conducting independent experiments on tetanus, to "contribute to the microscopial department of the museum, one or more specimens which may serve to show the nature of this condition," which would then be studied.[175]

In seeking to develop American medicine, each physician had a chance to make his mark or weigh in on current medical or surgical debates. One such forum for debate took place between advocates for conservative surgery, primary or secondary amputation, or resection. Above all else, wartime medicine was a process of learning and experience. Because many physicians had never seen the type of tissue damage and infection caused by the minié ball—pyemia, gangrene, or osteomyelitis (bone infections) in particular—they were often faced with tough choices.

When deciding how to treat war wounds and injuries, physicians, in consultation, usually began their course of treatment with such questions

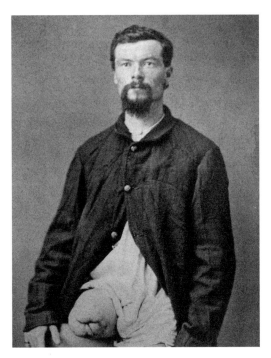

William Cotter, private, Company E, 9th New Hampshire, underwent primary amputation of the lower third of the femur at Petersburg, July 30, 1864. He was admitted to Douglas Hospital and treated by Assistant Surgeon William Thomson. The stump remained irritable, and abscesses continued to bother the patient. Two years after the initial operation, Thomson resected six inches of new bone. The patient was discharged June 6, 1866, but continued to be bothered by abscesses in and about the cicatrix, and in 1871 Dr. N. S. Lincoln removed the head of bone. The patient died in January 1874. (Photograph courtesy of the National Museum of Health and Medicine, Washington, D.C.)

as whether to amputate or to put the limb up in splints. Civil War surgeons had a few options. A primary amputation was performed within twenty-four to forty-eight hours of receiving a wound, and when done correctly, could save a soldier's life. A secondary amputation was performed three or more days following the injury but could be dangerous because infection had time to both develop and spread. Once infection had time to set, an amputation was essentially performed through infected tissues, which would then aid the further spread of infection, causing deadly diseases such as pyemia. Resection meant removing a portion of the damaged bone, with the hopes that the limb would be of use after the healing process had taken place. Finally, there was conservation. Saving the limb involved cleaning, dressing, and treating the wound while trying to strengthen the patient's constitution through proper diet and stimulants.

Physicians had to learn how to judge the severity of the wound, recognize the potential for serious infection, and decide on the best course of treatment. The case histories submitted to the medical museum were meant to teach. William Thomson, for example, championed in some specific cases conservative surgery. His report to Hammond was in part a response to the enormous number of amputations performed early in the

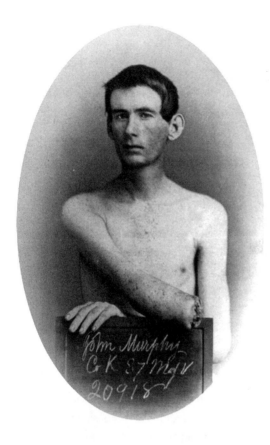

John K. Murphy, Company K, 37th Massachusetts Volunteers, was wounded April 6, 1865, at the Battle of Harper's Farm, Virginia. His right forearm, middle third, was amputated on the field by circular incision. The patient recovered well. This patient was photographed at Harewood General Hospital by R. B. Bontecou. (Photograph courtesy of the National Library of Medicine, Washington, D.C.)

war and a feeling among a few surgeons that some "sawbones" amputated far too readily or conversely that some surgeons waited too long before amputation and infection had time to set in. Thomson, in particular, hoped to shed light on the debate between amputation and conservative surgery.

Thomson was particularly interested in the amputations of the knee joint that affected the popliteal artery, which, he argued, if not done immediately made amputation very unsafe. He made a number of findings in the Civil War hospitals and used as an example the case of G. W. Perkins, Company G, 1st Massachusetts Cavalry, who was struck by a pistol ball in the left leg at Brandy Station.[176] Thomson suggested to Hammond that this particular case was "of great interest" and could be valuable for teaching physicians in the field. On Perkins's admission to Douglas Hospital three days after the injury, it was found that a pistol ball had entered the left knee joint near the outer and inferior margin of the patella, slightly grazed the head of the tibia, and escaped near the head of the fibula. A small portion of spongy bone and cartilage was removed from the wound of exit.

Thomson confirmed that "the joint was swollen and fluctuated distinctly." After etherizing the patient, Thomson flexed the patient's leg strongly during his examination, and a "quantity of dark blood escaped from the wound of exit."

Thomson evaluated the wound cognizant of a number of factors: "The man's youth, his robust appearance, his great unwillingness to submit to an amputation, the very slight injury done to the bones, and a strong desire to discuss some alternatives for the unvarying mutilation considered necessary in such cases. . . . I was fully aware that the knee joint was surely involved."[177] Thomson thus attempted to save the limb. He also pointed out to Hammond that he had much experience of treating this type of injury. Thomson hoped the publication of this case history might teach physicians to be more thoughtful when deciding whether or not to amputate.

Thomson's case history was thus comprehensive. He first explained the process of infection: "From a careful study of a number of cases of gunshot wounds of the knee joint, treated timidly, with simple water dressing I had become convinced that the retention of the products of inflammation in the joint was the prime cause of the enormous abscess in the thigh." He proceeded to explain that, through his experience in the hospital, numerous such cases, when treated without amputation, followed the same pathology. It was important that physicians understand what to look for, so Thomson thus went step by step explaining the pathological process. "The inflammation of the synovial membrane is soon followed by an effusion of serum distending the joint, causing fluctuation and giving rise to tenderness or pressure and pain. There is at that period therefore of swelling and redness. Suddenly this swelling disappears, the outlines of the bones are readily felt, the tension is removed and with it the pain and tenderness."

He had noticed on many occasions that inexperienced surgeons "fancy that the synovitis is yielding to his therapeutics." However, in a few days the "thigh will be found tender and pressure particularly on the inner aspect with slight swelling." This was actually the products of inflammation including pus and serum, which had "generated in the joint" and was now spreading into the tissues of the thigh. This was typically when inflammation occurred, producing abscesses and serious infection, which was signaled by the "great and exhausting discharge." Thus, he pointed out that "an amputation performed after the muscles have been dissected from each other and the soft tissues disorganized have been in all cases that I have seen rapidly fatal."[178]

Thomson decided instead to relieve the pressure and release any serum or pus that might be formed with the joint by making extensive incisions. Prior to the operation, the knee was "irrigated with ice water." Soon, however, the joint became very "tense and swollen" and the patient sick with infection. Thomson treated him with extra diet, tonics, and morphine and attempted to relieve the swelling by incising the wound, after which he placed the leg in a fracture box with straw, dressed it with cold water, and administered a larger dose of morphine. From June 15 to July 1, the patient was monitored almost hourly, and Thomson kept detailed accounts of each visit. But a second hemorrhage took place, which after numerous attempts, could not be arrested by compression on the artery of the groin, and the patient died.

The autopsy was made three hours later by Thomson, who found "a diffused abscess in the popliteal space, following the artery as far as hunting canal but not involving tissues of the thigh." He attributed the hemorrhage to a "very small opening into the anterior tibial about one inch from its origin from an ulceration of the coats of the vessel." He also noted that there were recent adhesions "anteriorly and posteriorly in the left thoracic cavity but no effusion: the left lung was much congested but did not sink in water." The most interesting fact was that the cartilage, of both the femur and the tibia, was almost entirely removed, and the bones looked "vascular and healthy." The cartilage, it was feared, would interfere "greatly with the bony ancylosis upon which the success of the case would depend." The secondary hemorrhage was ruled an accident, possibly the "result of his scorbutic condition which might have followed amputation."

Thomson concluded, "But for this complication it might have been my privilege to report a case of the knee joint treated successfully without amputation. Although the present attempt has failed, I will venture to predict that this method *if employed early* before the joint has been relieved of its morbid contents by a rupture of the synovial membrane will be found worthy of confidence. The most marked benefits followed the incisions in this instance and relieved the wound of all its supposed specific character. The rapid disappearance of the cartilages in twenty days removed one of my greatest anxieties since it renders ancylosis possible before the patient would be prostrated by profuse suppuration."[179] Thomson submitted the knee joint along with the patient's lungs and concluded that the wet specimens and case history would make "valuable preparations" for the museum.

Thomson's case highlights a chief difficulty. Amputations of the lower extremities had a fatality rate of 40.2 percent. On the other hand, treated conservatively, a wound of the lower extremity had the lesser fatality rate of 26.2 percent.[180] A quick amputation could (and did) prevent deadly infections. But it was complicated. The challenge facing the war physicians was knowing and learning when and why to perform an amputation. This learning and teaching process was effectively facilitated through the new medical museum. Indeed, the very purpose of the museum was to help shape and answer these questions and debates among the war physicians.

R. B. Bontecou also contributed to the debate about conservation, amputation, and resection. A particularly difficult class of wounds was compound fractures of the thigh. Bontecou observed in a special report to Hammond, after treating a number of wounded soldiers from Lees Mills, South Mills, Williamsburg, West Point, and Fair Oaks, that "men with gunshot fractures of the thigh were in a pitiable condition" and their limbs were "distended with pus and disorganized blood."[181] He made these cases the subject of resections (removing a portion of the limb containing the shattered bone) rather than removing the entire limb via amputation.[182] This was a poor choice since gunshot fractures of the upper thigh were known to become infected quickly and severely, and it was in fact more efficacious to handle these injuries by primary amputation.

Why then did Bontecou make this call? He believed these men were too sick to survive an amputation. Thus he thought he might have better success by removing the soft parts to "give free outlet to pent up fluids and to relieve obstruction to circulation at the same time moving bone matter and foreign substances."[183] But even so and with meticulous care, "of fourteen cases but one lived to get a firm union of the femur," and the rest died of "pyemic hemorrhage."[184] Amputations of the upper thigh were dangerous, as the femoral artery could be severed, leading to hemorrhage and quick death; however, if physicians did not amputate, soldiers often suffered serious infections. Physicians learned by the record of experience that if they could not amputate early (ideally within the first day), in most cases it was better not to amputate.[185] Thomson and Bontecou, though unsuccessful in the preceding cases, were correct. Making incisions through infected tissues only aided the spread of the infection and often led to pyemia, which had a 92 percent fatality rate.

These debates represent just how challenging Civil War medicine really was but also how physicians worked to develop the knowledge that would aid in surgical efficacy. Elijah Ray of the Palmetto Sharp Shooters sustained a compound fracture of the thigh at the Battle of Fair Oaks, June 1, 1862, and assistant surgeons Dunglison and Hunt agonized over his case. The

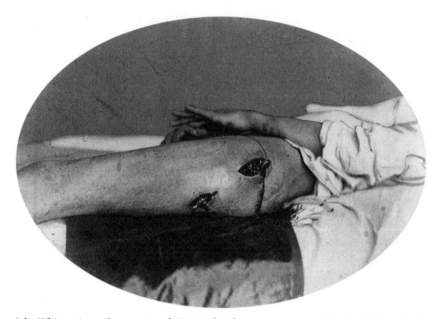

John White, private, Company A, 4th New York Volunteers, was wounded at Fort Fischer, April 2, 1865, by a conoidal ball in the upper third of the left thigh. The ball was extracted by R. B. Bontecou, but White developed pyemic symptoms shortly afterward and died April 27, 1865. (Photograph courtesy of the National Museum of Health and Medicine, Washington, D.C.)

wound was described as a compound fracture of the thigh complicated by the ball still in the wound and great "comminuting from just above the condyles to the middle of the limb."[186] They elevated the limb, and the wound was dressed with cerate and saturated charpie, which was replaced often. Ray was also given tonics, porter, quinine, and a full diet; while he suffered fever at night, he was reported to be comfortable during the day. The doctors continued to monitor the wound and asked in the case file, "Shall we amputate in this case? Our experience in secondary amputation of the thigh is so discouraging that we think our efforts to save the leg are fully justified."[187] After seven weeks of treatment and extensive monitoring, Ray succumbed to pyemic infection. The doctors then dissected the leg, carefully leaving the bullet intact near the great trochanter. They also found huge amounts of liquid matter and pus in the leg, confirming that he had died of pyemia. They submitted the leg, along with the bullet still attached, which was considered a highly valuable contribution.

The very specific challenges of the war created a new context for physicians and invaluable lessons in which to develop the surgical expertise of American physicians. But the experience was also one of unparalleled scope. After the war, Otis noted that, of the great body of case histories that were submitted to the museum, "the value of these materials has been foreshadowed in referring to their nature and extent. It may be emphatically said that they throw much light on some of the great moot points in surgery . . . for example, on the question of the propriety of excising the head of the femur for injury, fuller data than are now extant in the entire range of surgical literature; and that it may be hoped, without temerity, that they include the elements for the solution of many grave surgical problems."[188]

Otis was correct about the importance of these case notes. The histories did, for example, reveal that with a compound comminuted fracture there was little chance infection would not prevail. W. W. Keen, for example, looked back on these larger surgical debates after the war and explained why, in his opinion, amputation if performed early was the best course: "It was my duty to gather and forward all the specimens that I could lay my hands upon. Among them I remember more than a score of knee-joints, every one of which with our then surgical resources should have been amputated. Conservative treatment of joints was an impossibility until antisepsis and asepsis made it not only a possibility, but a duty. The popular opinion that the surgeons did a large amount of unnecessary amputating may have been justified in a few cases, but taking the army as a whole, I have no hesitation in saying that far more lives were lost from refusal to amputate than by amputation."[189]

The intellectual and professional transformation of American medicine encompassed these new surgical perspectives. Civil War physicians, perhaps surprisingly (given the popular depictions in movies like *Gone with the Wind* or *Dances with Wolves*) had a war record of which they could be proud. For the almost 30,000 amputations recorded in the Union army, the mortality rate was 26.3 percent. By contrast, among all the amputations performed in the French military hospitals just a few years later during the Franco-Prussian War, the mortality rate was a staggering 76 percent.[190] The fact that American physicians had rushed to the great French hospitals to study and learn medicine just a few years earlier suggests that during the Civil War these new opportunities for medical education had begun a transformation in American medicine. Indeed, not only was the caliber of American surgery improved, but during the war and after American hospitals boasted much lower mortality rates than their European counterparts, which some physicians attributed to the lessons learned during the war—particularly the use of disinfectants

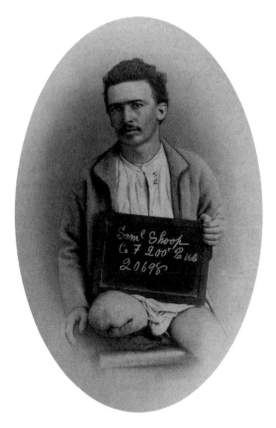

Samuel Shoop, Company 7, 200th Pennsylvania Volunteers, underwent primary amputation of the thigh. (Photograph courtesy of the National Library of Medicine, Washington, D.C.)

locally on wounds or during surgeries, as a prophylactic, and in the hospital environment.

One can also trace a new professional authority among the war physicians that was couched in the developing language of science. As one example, physicians increasingly separated the identity of the soldier from his body, which represented the changing ideas about science and medicine, or rather about the social distance between the doctor and his patient. This helped to establish a common language, an experiential distinction from those who lacked such access to bodies. Dr. John S. Carpenter submitted to the museum a ruptured femoral vein, which was "unique."[191] Other letters simply noted the number of specimens; for example, the physician John Morgan submitted "by the boat that leaves tonight one keg containing 19 specimens and a full report of each case and also a list of all the operations that have been performed."[192] Some physicians, such as W. F. Norris, often sent as many as 40 pathological specimens in one keg.[193]

Many of the case books are simply entitled "specimen histories" and contain hundreds of case reports relating to the specimens, which reduce the soldier to his most useful parts or rather the parts that might move medical knowledge forward:

I have the honor to transmit herewith the following surgical specimens for the Army Medical museum: William Haynes, Priv. Co. F 38th Wisconsin, bones of hand and 2 inches of lower portion radius and ulna; Orson Randolph, Priv. Co. C 67th N. Y. V. Knee-joint; David Hyam Priv. Co. C 5th New Hampshire-two specimens-knee joint and head neck and upper portion of shaft of femur; Wm Johnson, Priv. Co. F. 1st. Head and upper portion shaft of tibia, missile lodged in head of tibia; John Doran, Priv. Co. D. 1st bones of foot and lower third of tibia and fibula; Walter D. Boyce, Priv. Co. D. 124th N. Y. V. seven inches shaft of right ulna forearm; John B. Leshender, Priv. Co. L 4th N.Y. Complicated dislocation of ankle joint-foot and lower tibia and fibula.[194]

Physicians formed an intimate connection with their "specimens." Since their professional identity was now connected to their specimens, many tried to ensure the contributions were useful: "In the photograph album which I had the honor to send to the Army Medical Museum on the 18th of September there is on the 30th page a picture of a plaster cast of a shoulder joint from which the head of the humerus had been removed. In as much as this cast shows but imperfectly the nature of the operation and its result . . . I would respectfully request that the picture of Gallagher's shoulder on page 30 be removed and replaced by the enclosed picture of an excision of the tibia. I make this suggestion with a view to correcting what I consider a fault, and thereby increasing whatever value to the collection it may have."[195]

Physicians also learned and gained experience from specimens obtained from living bodies. The physician J. B. Brown, of the General Hospital at Fourth and George Streets, Philadelphia, submitted the specimen of John Martin, a private, Company G, 4th New York Volunteers, who was wounded in the left leg, below the knee, at Antietam. The case was deemed interesting because of the path the ball took: it entered at the "inner aspect of the left tibia fracturing it and the fibula at about 4 inches above the malleoli, passing down through the medullary canal of the tibia and emerging at the inner border of the astragalotibial articulation extensively comminuting all the bones in its course."[196] The leg was amputated below the knee and healed "kindly" by granular adhesion. The operation was a clear success—it was noted that Private Martin was left with "quite a useful stump."[197]

As physicians visited the museum and read the corresponding case history, they saw the complexity of scientific medicine, which orthodox American physicians who doctored in the war were now uniquely qualified to manage. As the century progressed, the museum's collection reflected the aspiration of American surgeons to continue to contribute to the development of the medical sciences. As John Shaw Billings observed in 1888 of the Army Medical Museum,

> An important feature of our National Medical Museum should be to show methods of research and of instruction for the benefit of the investigators and teachers of the country. . . . For example, as soon as Koch's researches became known in this country, physicians, and especially medical teachers who visited the museum asked if we could show them the apparatus used by Koch and Pasteur in bacteriological work, and eagerly examined the few specimens of cultures in solid media which we were able to exhibit. The anatomist comes to the museum quite as much to see methods of mounting and preservation as to see the specimens themselves; the physiologist does not expect to see function directly exhibited, but he does hope to find information about kymographs and constant temperature apparatus, and he wants to see whether Kuhne's artificial eye is so useful for teaching purposes that he ought to get one to illustrate his lectures.[198]

The themes of death, contests over the body, and scientific medicine intertwined in interesting and important ways in the Civil War. The body and the physician were now inextricably linked as doctors worked to repair the damages of war. Troops were exposed to never-before-seen diseases, which altered the body and paved the way for the medical department's access. Civil War weaponry also destroyed the body, but physicians promised to heal the wounds and thereby earned access to specimens and bodies. At great human cost, the medical profession benefited from the connection between disease, war, and the body. They doctored in the war to preserve the health of the republic, but it was also an important period of training and professionalization for orthodox physicians. The diseases that ravaged soldiers' bodies shaped the projects and directed the specific aspects of scientific medicine; but often the individual soldier had to relinquish ownership and control of his body for this knowledge to be

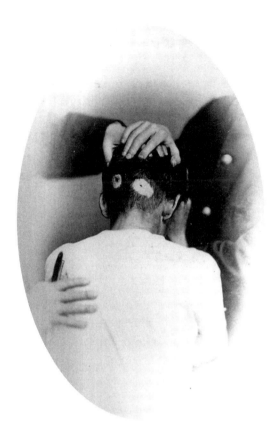

Benjamin F. Chappell, sergeant, Company H, 8th New York Cavalry, suffered a gunshot wound of the skull near Petersburg, April 1, 1865, and was admitted to Harewood General Hospital and treated by R. B. Bontecou. An operation of trephining was performed to remove a circular piece of bone. The patient died shortly afterward, and the autopsy revealed numerous large, pus-filled abscesses in the left lobe of the cerebellum also implicating the medulla oblongata. (Photograph courtesy of the National Library of Medicine, Washington, D.C.)

developed. Soldiers were asked to give up their "bones for the good of the country" and for other soldiers who would benefit from the knowledge generated from the individual body. All this developed in relation to the changing attitudes about death and dissections during the war.

Dissection had been contested before the war, but during the war physicians built a national cabinet that far exceeded any expectations. In an 1864 in a letter to Thomas Longmore, professor of Military Surgery, Army Medical School at Netley, Joseph Barnes elucidated the challenge of wartime medicine and also the medical department's greatest achievement:

> With a system compressing nearly two hundred general hospitals, with eighty-six thousand beds extending from Maine to the Gulf of Mexico and from the Atlantic to the Pacific the evil is unavoidable, but we may claim as near an approach as to perfect accuracy as is possible in a work of so great a magnitude. In this connection the establishment of a "National Cabinet" has proved entirely

successful, the collection of specimens and drawing of casts, illustrations of injuries and their results, has assumed a practical value hardly to be overestimated.[199]

The idea of scientific development appealed to the public in the third quarter of the nineteenth century, and they flocked to see the collection. Indeed, there was a "new elitism based on the organized intellect of a scientific age" from which the orthodox medical profession benefited.[200] The war allowed, even demanded, the acquisition of specimens and bodies and, in doing so, altered perceptions of the body—how disease functioned within it, what diseases looked like, and the different ways the body could be studied to develop knowledge. Physicians collected specimens, dissected bodies, and submitted case notes and their research findings. They published the results of their work in numerous medical journals, contributed to the *Medical and Surgical History*, and even published in popular magazines like *Lippincott's* to ensure that the public was aware of their labors. The history of the wartime bodies, captured in case records and specimen histories, tells many different stories, but the underlying commonality is that physicians formed a professional identity through this access and created superior practical and epistemological standards for American medicine.

CHAPTER SIX

Cholera and the Civil War
Medical Model in the Postwar Period

n 1871 the physician Joseph Woodward observed that the "science of
medicine is essentially progressive: with increasing knowledge comes
more subtle skill, and the advances already made warrant hopeful-
ness as to the future."[1] He was referring to the new ideas and direction for
American medicine that took shape with the Civil War. By 1866 the many
wartime experiences, challenges, innovative research ideas, and management strategies were gradually being adapted in the postwar period to
manage new crises and health threats. Nowhere was the impact of the war
more apparent than on the management, understanding, and investigation of infectious disease. It was perhaps timely, then, that America had to
deal with a serious public health threat just months after the war's end. In
1866 Asiatic cholera appeared in America, and while this devastating and
deadly disease ravaged Americans, regular physicians were called upon to
study and manage cholera. Once again, the techniques, ideas, and literature were institutionalized through the Army Medical Museum and the
Surgeon General's Office, supporting the progression and development of
the methodologies pioneered through the Civil War.

In 1866 Americans had just been through a devastating war in which
almost 750,000 people died, and two-thirds of these deaths were due to
diseases. These staggering statistics demanded that the federal government
take a more active role in managing cholera in 1866. Thus, while it was
an opportunity to produce medical knowledge and further train American physicians, cholera was above all a social problem. The military, along
with local health associations, aimed to minimize any further threat to the
populace. The objective in these investigations, then, was both to better
understand the nature of cholera and to develop a preventative strategy.

There were no easy answers about the etiology of cholera. As in the previous cholera epidemics in America, physicians painstakingly studied and

experimented in the attempts to understand the disease. But there were larger differences in the way the epidemic was managed in 1849 and in 1866, which I would suggest can be traced to the Civil War. First, the federal government sponsored the investigations into cholera. Second, the sharing of knowledge between the military, civilian, and local physicians, including by 1866 northern and southern physicians, was integral in developing larger strategies to manage cholera. Third, the knowledge that American physicians produced regarding cholera mirrored the international response to cholera. Fourth, in the attempt to understand cholera's etiology, some physicians increasingly focused on laboratory-style investigations. Finally, though physicians in 1849 had used sanitary precautions such as cleaning the streets, purifying cesspools, and supplying pure water, the conversation about prevention, particularly how and why disinfectants worked, was shaped within evolving understandings of infectious disease and thus grew more sophisticated. The American medical profession matured through these investigations, further consolidating and extending its professional authority.

CHOLERA: *The Disease*

From 1866 to 1873, the Civil War medical model was vigorously deployed in the management of cholera, including the isolation of the sick, the mandatory reporting of cases of disease to the Surgeon General's Office, disinfection of people and the environment, preventative strategies, epidemiological science, research and investigation, and the dissemination of this knowledge locally, nationally, and internationally. The very nature of cholera added a sense of fear, desperation, and urgency to these investigations. After contracting the disease, "victims would be well in the morning and by nightfall, dying after a few hours of intense vomiting, diarrhea, cramps, clamminess and shrunken features."[2] Most victims were dead within forty-eight hours, and the dramatic dehydration that characterized the disease "gave the skin an ominous bluish tint and the new corpses seemed to decompose more rapidly than normal."[3] One of the worst symptoms, which was commented on frequently in the case reports, was the severe diarrhea, which took the form of "rice water stools" and was often so intense that patients would collapse before physicians could have any effect. Indeed, because of the fear and risk of treating this disease, Joseph Woodward asked that any physician that distinguished "themselves by faithful attendance to cholera patients" be brought to his attention so that they could be properly compensated.[4]

Cholera has a rich history and has sparked a multitude of investigations. On its first appearance in the West in the early nineteenth century, cholera was generally thought to be a nonspecific miasmatic "filth-disease." Anticontagionists believed the disease was caused by some kind of poison or immaterial influence that would infect a susceptible body, and its propagation was tied to the environment—soil or a chemical condition of the earth or atmosphere. Contagionists on the other hand believed the disease was produced in the bodies of sick people, transmitted by exhalations and inhaled or ingested by healthy people, who then became sick (thus traceable to human contact). Others still were contingent contagionists and believed that transmission was dependent on factors such as individual susceptibility, class, habits, filth, race, weather, diet, the virulence of the virus, and local factors.

In 1840 the English physician William Budd contended that cholera was caused by a contagious, living organism that was transmitted by water containing cholera excrement. In 1849 the English physician John Snow argued that cholera was a contagious, specific, waterborne poison that could be communicated via traces of excretions and vomitus most likely found in a water supply. Five years later he confirmed his contention in two separate epidemiological studies into the mode of transmission, confirming that cholera was spread by contaminated water.[5] Anticontagionists were willing to concede that perhaps impure water was a factor in the disease; however, they maintained that predisposition was necessary for the disease to erupt. The most famous contingent contagionist of the period, Bavarian sanitarian Max von Pettenkofer, also published on the dangers of a contaminated water supply; however, for Pettenkofer, as fecal matter left the bodies of cholera sufferers it was harmless, but once it had time to decompose in alkaline fluids, or groundwater, the poison would become infective.[6] Pettenkofer's views represent an overlapping of ideas surrounding cholera. For example, he suggested that a cholera epidemic depended on "a specific germ," the "local and seasonal conditions required to transform it into the actual cause of an epidemic," and finally, "individual predisposition."[7]

The germ theories surrounding cholera were numerous and complicated. However, as in the case of Max von Pettenkofer's ideas, these theories were by no means static.[8] Some physicians, in fact, acknowledged that cholera may or may not have been contagious and were quite open-minded with regard to causation. Anticontagionists generally objected to rigid and repressive quarantine measures, but by 1866 there was a shift from strict "medical policing" (as in the quarantines of 1840) toward new models of public health, which included concepts of prevention, disinfection, and medical inspection, which were variously adapted (for different reasons) by contagionists and anticontagionists.

By the second half of the nineteenth century, American physicians understood that cholera spread in overcrowded and filthy conditions and had been difficult to contain with quarantines.[9] Cholera had always been associated with a "poison" in the atmosphere, or linked to the environment, and was not readily seen as contagious (like smallpox). The major attempt in managing the disease during the 1840s was through preventative measures such as cleanliness and sanitation. In 1849 the bulk of American physicians were reluctant to consider the possibility, let alone accept the idea, that cholera was caused by a microorganism. And yet the idea was "less bizarre" or perhaps even plausible by 1866 (though predisposition remained an important concept in the 1860s).[10] As Charles Rosenberg suggests, the very idea that cholera might be caused by a microorganism was met with a "mixed but promising reception in the United States," which makes an interesting starting point to this discussion. Some physicians who were charged with managing cholera in 1866 and 1867 had not been responsible for it in 1849 or 1855—but they had served in the war and had seen evidence of disease transmission in the hospitals.

Rosenberg argues that "when in the spring of 1866, the United States was again threatened by cholera," the ideas of Snow, Budd, and Pettenkofer "had been current in medical circles for a decade and were widely accepted by American physicians."[11] Other historians have suggested, "At Snow's death in 1858, few people working in public health and sanitation believed his theory of the cause and transmission of cholera."[12] In the American case, there is evidence that Snow's and Pettenkofer's theories were known certainly among elite physicians; the case reports often refer to water supply or soil when discussing transmission, but there is little evidence that these theories were wholly accepted. There was still opposition from some of the profession in 1866. Part of the problem, as noted in many case reports, was that few American physicians in 1866 had their own practical experience with the disease. Thus, while most elite physicians subscribed to these theories or had at least read about the fecal contamination and water carriage theories in European publications, only a select few had actually studied it.

By 1866 a transition related to the investigating physicians themselves was well under way: how they studied and managed disease, the equipment they used to investigate disease, the questions they asked, and the dissemination of this knowledge among practitioners. In roughly the same period, some English physicians, such as John Simon, wanted to conduct chemical and microscopial examinations on the morbid processes of cholera but could not since between 1855 and 1866 "cholera was absent from England, and no material was available for experiment."[13] Thus experiments that could elucidate the etiology of cholera were not resumed until the 1860s in Britain along with Prussia (later united Germany), France, Russia, and America. For American investigators, this did not translate into the discovery of the cholera vibrio, but it did bring American physicians into the international debates surrounding cholera with a new vitality.[14]

By the end of the nineteenth century, cholera's "miasm became a vibrio transmitted in crowded places without adequate excrement disposal."[15] But numerous research projects preceded this development. And cholera was a disease that generated ongoing debates even after the Prussian bacteriologist Robert Koch isolated the cholera germ.[16] Through the war and the cholera outbreak of 1866 and 1867, such traditional measures to manage disease threats such as disinfection and quarantine were still used, but they were no longer merely driven by an understanding of disease linked to "filth"; by this time, more scientific methods influenced many of the measures taken.[17] And by 1866 there was a well-tested infrastructure in place to support further medical ideas and developments.

SURGEON GENERAL'S OFFICE AND AMERICAN MEDICINE: Tracing the Disease and Networks of Knowledge

In 1866 cholera caused more than 1,200 deaths in the army. Cholera ultimately moved as far west as Fort Leavenworth, Kansas, and in the southwest as far as Texas. But because cholera was transmitted between the civilian population and the troops, the cross influences in the management of cholera between civilian and military practitioners and northern and southern physicians were significant, and these influences shaped the larger response to cholera.[18]

With northern generals in command of southern military districts and the Radical Republicans in Congress producing new institutions and social reforms for the freedmen, the control exercised by the Surgeon General's Office during the cholera epidemic was similarly an extension of the scientific authority that the medical profession had established during the war. However, in the eleven unreconstructed states were northern doctors in southern locales managing the threat of cholera. Indeed, in the summer of 1866 cholera raged through the South: from New York to Savannah and

Tybee Island, Georgia, New Orleans to Jackson, and Baton Rouge to Texas. The disease moved with troops from Newport to Nashville, into Memphis, passing up the river to Arkansas. Cholera was reported in remote locales, such as the plantations on the Red River in Shreveport, Louisiana, and also in the city of Shreveport—with the United States military post squarely between the two.

Health ordinances were subsequently passed in these states to help trace the disease. And many of the official case reports that were submitted by the United States surgeons show that, in trying to both manage and trace cholera, it was common practice to consult with local or city physicians while compiling official information.[19] This provided an opportunity for southern physicians to become practically acquainted with the Union medical model, but it was also a chance for American physicians to manage this threat together and share knowledge on a local and national basis.[20] Indeed, Barnes and Woodward utilized both the federal government's expansive resources and networks of knowledge in these investigations. For example, they also ordered army doctors to share findings and compile information from the Freedmen's Bureau doctors then stationed in the South, and this sharing of knowledge ultimately helped stop the spread of the disease.[21] This was not a southern or northern problem but an American problem; the federal government and the Surgeon General's Office led the campaign against cholera, and the subsequent publications, particularly for managing or halting the spread of the disease, were subsequently disseminated to state and local medical societies in the North and South.[22]

The medical department was in a unique position to amass information about cholera because of its record of experience in managing disease, the improving transportation systems after the war, the movement of the military, and the presence of military posts, which made the transmission of the disease more likely but also traceable. In 1866 the military's immediate strategy was to work with various physicians, societies, organizations, and civilian boards to produce knowledge about cholera. This strategy, as demonstrated during the war, was well tested and largely successful.

Within the larger response, there was, then, a continuation of ideology among some of the physicians that had doctored in the war. Many state public health officials in 1866 had been directly involved in the U.S. Sanitary Commission or state sanitary commissions during the war.[23] For example, F. Hamilton, J. H. Cuyler, E. Harris, C. R. Agnew, and C. J. Stillé served on the board of the American Association for the Relief of Misery on the Battlefield (1866) and continued working toward the development of public health reform with members of the regular army.[24] Many of these men had seen the efficacy of sanitary science during the Civil War, and this translated into calls for public health reform, which ultimately led to the creation of the American Public Health Association and the Marine Hospital Service (in the 1870s).

As one example, the Metropolitan Board of Health in New York (created in 1866) was a great stimulus to public health in the United States largely because it "successfully organized itself to conquer an epidemic."[25] But the connection with the Surgeon General's Office was an invaluable resource for members of this body. Elisha Harris, a member of the Council of Hygiene in New York (1864)[26] regularly exchanged letters with Woodward and Barnes for information "regarding Asiatic cholera and diarrheal diseases at the military posts in New York harbor in 1867."[27] Letters were exchanged, and in response Woodward typically discussed the posts in which cholera had occurred, the date of the first recorded case, and its spread, including where the infected person traveled and whether cholera was spread from person to person from this first infected case.[28] The findings of the military and the New York Board of Health, which included information on specific case histories, air, water, and contact theories, the pathology and epidemiology of cholera, common remedies, and successful management strategies such as disinfection, were shared and incorporated into the larger response to cholera.[29]

Other states also enacted legislation establishing and regulating quarantines for the protection of the states (state and national boards of health were years away). But these local associations or city councils were taking shape in the form of small civil boards of health or local sanitary associations, even police departments, and were specifically created to manage cholera. However, there was no tangible authority in these bodies, and thus in 1866 these associations also operated in conjunction with the military,[30] in some cases to prevent cholera from entering the United States:[31]

Well grounded apprehensions of the appearance of Asiatic cholera as an epidemic early in the present fiscal year (which began July 1, 1865) required prompt action for the protection of our troops. A rigid military quarantine was established on the southern Atlantic Coast and sanitary precautions enforced. The adoption of these measures availed to control or eradicate the disease at the recruiting depots and forts where it appeared before it assumed its usual alarming epidemic form; and official recognition has been given to the meritorious services of medical officers' whose fidelity, energy, and skillful administration succeeded in averting or diminishing the horrors of widespread pestilence.[32]

In addition to epidemiology, other interests of the Surgeon General's Office included modes of transmission and the "nature" of cholera. Thus, Woodward issued a circular letter to the surgeons in charge of the general hospitals asking for essays on cholera.[33] The case reports, Woodward noted, "were made with commendable diligence by the medical officers brought in contact with cholera during the year."[34] From these reports, along with the civilian response, Woodward was able to make a credible picture of the epidemic. The first report, *Circular No. 5*, concerned the cholera outbreak during the last six months of 1866. The second report, *Circular No. 1*, concerned cases of cholera and yellow fever in the Army of the United States in 1867. A third report published in 1875 concerned the 1873 cholera outbreak in the United States, which summarized, analyzed, and developed all of these findings.

Joseph Barnes and Woodward sent letters to all regiments asking if the disease "originated among recruits." (In other words, did a person somehow poison the environment thereby creating the conditions in which the disease would pass to vulnerable bodies?) Or was it "transported from other infected points?"[35] (In other words, did the disease move with human carriers?) Or did it seem to have a "spontaneous origin at the post"? In all of the international conferences on cholera in 1866–67, the "evidence of transmission of an infectious cause from place to place" was a key concern—it would help answer questions about transmission and thus help determine preventative strategies.[36]

An example in the American case began when Woodward wrote to J. H. Franz, assistant surgeon, United States Army, in early 1867 to inquire about a recent case of cholera. He asked Franz to pay careful attention to whether the disease "originated on the field" or "was imported."[37] Franz reported that the first case developed with a man who had spent the night in Richmond "in debauchery" and then returned to his regiment, where four more men, who also visited Richmond, were attacked with the disease.[38] Two days later, ten more cases were diagnosed. The cases were all quarantined by the sanitary police. Franz inspected the cooking utensils and found everything to be in good order. He thus reasoned that the men were "exposed to the poison" while in Richmond, but with the goal of "ascertaining the correctness of this supposition," he made inquiries of the local board of health and "learned that the disease did not assume an epidemic form until sometime after the first cases occurred in camp." He noted that during July and August detachments of recruits were received from New York Harbor and Newport barracks and that the Sanitary Superintendent of the Metropolitan Board of Health informed him that cholera prevailed in the former at that time. He determined that cholera must have originated in Richmond or was imported from New York or Newport barracks.

The exercise of tracing the origins of the disease was a valuable one, even though it did not produce conclusive results. For that to happen, the source of the disease would have to be isolated, but it was possible to compile much information about its movement and ideas about the modes of transmission. Franz's objective being to ensure the camp was hygienically sound, he adopted a number of measures, including situating the camp where it was "well ventilated," not "overcrowded, elevated with the grounds well drained," along with the employment of sanitary police.[39] Of 255 cases, 103 were fatal, and the rest subsided. He did not specify exactly what the disease was other than referring to it as a poison—but he gives an interesting theory for how it traveled: "Morbific matter has been conveyed long distances in clothing and excluded with contact from air and that upon unpacking and exposing the disease it has broken out in isolated places. May not the clothing of the recruits packed in their knapsacks have constituted fomites, which being unpacked here emitted material morbi?"[40]

One disease theory at the time suggested that cholera could be transmitted directly via fomites, which could be "nurtured" in infected clothes or linens. Franz was curious as to whether the warmth and secure nature of the backpack somehow nurtured or harbored the "material," suggesting the disease was some sort of "virus," which, when released to the population, became infective. But this was not straightforward either. Was the backpack, for example, comparable to soil and thus somehow nurturing or igniting the "material"? Or rather, was a disease-causing fomite merely being transmitted via the backpack? Reflecting his uncertainty related to germs, he also stated that "the first victims were those whose previous debauching and indiscretions in diet, made them peculiarly susceptible to its noxious influence."[41] He was a contingent contagionist, but Franz supported emerging research, which suggested the existence of some kind of separate entity that was portable and transmissible. More practically, as part of their sanitary regiment, regular physicians were required to either destroy or thoroughly disinfect clothing and bedding from infected regiments.

Joseph Barnes and Woodward continued tracing outbreaks of cholera between locales in the attempt to determine origin and transmission. For example, Bvt. Major R. B. Browne, assistant surgeon at the United States Post Hospital, Galveston, Texas, reported to Barnes, "The cholera introduced among the troops stationed at this post by the arrival of detachment of unassigned recruits from Harts Island New York on the 22nd . . . has apparently died out as no new cases of cholera has exhibited itself among the troops or citizens of Galveston since the 24th. The post of Galveston Texas may be therefore considered at this time as perfectly healthy and entirely free from all infectious or contagious diseases."[42]

The term "infectious" (indirect) or "contagious" (direct) suggests worry about person-to-person transmission but also uncertainty about origins. Barnes and Woodward thus asked physicians to consider how and why cholera was erupting in the first place. Medical Director Jos. R. Smith, 4th Military District in Vicksburg, submitted a report to Barnes on April 19, 1867, detailing the mode of transmission and introduction of cholera to Little Rock and Helena in August and Huntersville in September 1866.[43] Little Rock and Huntersville were separated only by the Arkansas River and were connected by a pontoon bridge stretched between the two banks the greater part of September 1866. In this particular situation, the constant movement of these boats was very problematic: "During the latter part of August scarcely a boat arrived at Little Rock, on which rumor did not affirm cases of cholera to have occurred. Many of these boats I visited in person to see such cases if there. In no instance did I find a case of cholera though on several boats, cases of [cholera] had occurred (followed by death). . . . Careful inquiry has failed to discover the particular case, if any, by which the disease was introduced."[44]

When physicians could not locate the exact source, it was common practice to try to prevent the spread of the disease between human carriers. Joseph Brown, of Fort Columbus, New York, wrote Woodward in June 1866 to discuss his fears related to cholera. He especially advised against any sort of overcrowding, which he suggested was "indisputably a dangerous experiment" and of which "experience has fully shown in frequent instances the most appalling consequences."[45] He advised measures to reduce conditions in which the disease might thrive: "At the present time when cholera may be expected, every contingency should be avoided instead of being overlooked. Recruits are sent to this depot from various recruiting stations in many of the largest cities in this country and the chances are certainly multiplied that if there be any portability in the infection of cholera it may be introduced here. To introduce it to an overcrowded garrison on a limited area would unquestionably be a serious matter."[46]

On July 26, 1866, Brown wrote Woodward again from Fort Columbus about the serious outbreak of cholera that had begun earlier that month (for which he had been prepared). The first case of cholera was reported July 3, 1866. The patient was admitted to the hospital in "profound collapse" and died the following morning. Brown immediately began to trace the movements of the patient. He traced the outbreak to Minneapolis, where the patient had been with his regiment, listed only as "Co. D recruits." The following day another man from Company D was admitted to the hospital with "cramps, rice water discharges, vomiting," and he "commenced collapse almost immediately."[47] Brown could not find a connection between the men in Minneapolis, but more cases began to occur at Fort Columbus. This was complicated by the fact that Fort Columbus was a transfer point for regiments, and there was a continual influx of new recruits and often conditions of overcrowding.

For example, on July 14 there were as many as 1,226 men on the island. Because of the continuous development of new cases on the island, Brown conducted a complete examination of the sanitary condition there. He examined the quality of the water and vacated the prison. He reported that "every precaution is taken to disinfect and properly dispose of the defections of cholera patients who are isolated from the convalescents and these again from the ordinary sick in the hospital. The wards are also regularly disinfected and kept clean and the bedding and bed sack continually changed and renewed."[48] Though he primarily focused on the environment, his report elucidated some interesting points. Brown wrote to Woodward again from Fort Columbus, New York Harbor, on August 1, 1866, and noted that he was concerned with the civilian employees who worked at the post but returned home to Brooklyn at night. He thus requested that an official order be issued which would prevent what he believed "was the certain importation of the epidemic."

The physician T. McParlin similarly wrote to Barnes from Fort Delaware in December 1866. He noticed that during the spring and early summer months "intermittent and other fevers were unusually prevalent" upon the banks of the Delaware River and continued until early in the month of August when an "isolated case of epidemic cholera made its appearance."[49] He was puzzled that the usual cause of the disease in "ascending the banks of the rivers was not observed in the occurrence of this epidemic."[50] Rather, its first appearance was reported in an isolated case that occurred July 22 at New Castle, Delaware, in an "aged resident in town." The disease continued to spread and was reported as an epidemic in Delaware City, a small town at the eastern terminus of the Chesapeake and Delaware Canal ten miles downstream from New Castle. The disease was confined to the "lowest class of the community" and not arrested until about September 20, by which time it had become "epidemic in New Castle the point first visited."[51] He isolated the case immediately and established a quarantine, and all fruit and unripe vegetables were banned from the island. Moreover, to ensure that all "further importation be prevented," he suspended the work of the civilians.[52]

While predisposition remained an important factor for most physicians, others began to adopt strict, almost draconian, measures to prevent possible contagion. For example, U.S. Army surgeon George Taylor, a chief medical officer from the District of Texas, Galveston, advised keeping cholera patients in a "perfect state of rest and to prevent evaporation from the surface of the body by close covering."[53] Thus, instead of only disinfecting the environment, he disinfected the patient. His measures imply that he believed that the bodies of cholera sufferers could indeed emit an infectious virus that would then be transmitted to those who came in contact with the body. He thus advised quarantining and isolating patients from the rest of the command, keeping them warm, and treating them with stimulants such as carbonate of ammonia. He believed these measures together would "prolong life" and ensure that the disease did not spread among the troops.[54]

The themes of water over air and direct contagion versus communicability were factors that were continually considered in these reports. Assistant Surgeon George McGill wrote a special report from Davids Island, New York Harbor, in February 1867.[55] A local miasmatist, McGill from the beginning felt that Hart's Island was ripe for a disease such as cholera. It was used as a rendezvous for troops recruited or to be mustered out and as a prison from the winter of 1863–64 to the spring of 1866. He observed that approximately 5,000 men a day "received their rations and cast their excretions" upon the surface of the island and on the island's "western extremity, where barracks were constructed the soil being comparatively thick, received organic remains and yielded products of their slow decomposition." He further noted that when the "atmosphere on the surface was confined and damp, these products accumulated and recombined" especially under the barracks. He suspected cholera was a living "organic ferment" that became virulent in the soil, gained pathogenicity, and then spread to other people. As one historian has demonstrated in regard to Pettenkofer, this was an important version of a living germ theory of disease.[56]

McGill noted that policing was not given sufficient attention, food was not prepared with proper care, and personal cleanliness was neglected. He then outlined a number of predisposing factors that contributed to the outbreak, such as "feeble vital energy" and "prostrating agencies of diet and filth," in combination with the "debilitating effluvia" at Hart's Island. Though he held a localist interpretation of disease transmission, his experience with this disease proved challenging. He noted that diarrhea came first, and then as the "excrement of cholera fell into the soil it must have generated the so-called specific agency of cholera."[57] Like Pettenkofer, he believed the disease would not become virulent until it was incubated in soil and ingested by a person with predisposing factors. But the experience with cholera complicated ideas about contagion. "Certain persons exposed themselves recklessly and escaped. Friends cast themselves upon the bodies of the dead and remained lying upon them for many minutes having previously experienced the bad circumstances of atmosphere and diet of those who died . . . moreover, men assisting in postmortems and recklessly courting contact with sections of tissue escaped, while others of temperate habits fell speedily."[58]

In trying to determine the mode of transmission, McGill pondered a number of anomalies. What explains "when the operator in a postmortem having cut himself early in his work carries the same to its end exposing naked tissue to tissue organically living and acting morbidly, yet escapes?" He examined this problem more closely. Was it a specific disease attributable to a specific exciting cause? If it was a material, then why did people who received it in excess "whether it arose from the soil or was engendered in the air" often escape? He studied symptoms, living patients, and bodies to reach his conclusion: "My observation has left me with a theory that cholera is a member of the family of diseases in which we have a morbid action of life inducible in men rendered fit by predisposing circumstances and by quality of vitality, perhaps inducible in like manner in all organic cells so its extension, infection etc., at distances varied by the degree of predisposition and transportable in organisms not in material."[59]

He concluded that forces could react with the cholera material (once part of the animal body) to produce the disease in certain susceptible people. His theory suggested that these minute products possessed properties that could be stimulated within certain atmospheric environments. Whether they were living organisms or chemical compounds was still unclear. But

McGill recommended sanitary measures and disinfection above all to manage the disease. He made no mention of quarantine measures but advised eliminating filth from the barracks and island in which the troops were stationed.

There was tremendous fear associated with cholera, which gave heightened urgency to the situation. William Sloan, medical director, Department of the East, arrived at Hart's Island on July 31, 1866, and described the situation as follows: "Dr. Calhoun was dead, Dr. Rowe convalescing but in bed and Dr. Webster worn out. In the hospital were eight patients sick with cholera, well marked and of a malignant type, six deaths having occurred within the previous thirty-six hours. The *personnel* broken down and demoralized, the stewards sick, and the ward-master dead. My first care was to police the wards and to regulate the hospital."[60] It was particularly hard to face the loss of Dr. J. T. Calhoun, who died of cholera within ten hours: "Thus ended the career of a kindhearted, energetic conscientious, and intelligent medical officer, whose services in the field and at the post had endeared him to all with whom he had served. He was stricken down while in the zealous discharge of his duties, and his memory will long be cherished by his old associates and by his former patients."[61]

Sloan proceeded to examine the condition of the camp and found "diarrhea very prevalent and the morale of the men much affected." He was intrigued by the "malignancy of the disease," which suggested that "some epidemic form of the disease must exist." Part of his reasoning was that a "rigid police had been enforced, fumigations and disinfectants most literally used everywhere and still the disease was on the increase."[62] His first objective was to stop any further spread of the disease, and he thus recommended moving all healthy recruits off the island, burning the straw from bed sacks along with blankets and clothing, and disinfecting any baggage or bedding with "active chemical agents." He ordered fumigations of the barracks with sulfuric acid, nitric acid, and chlorine. But despite these measures, the disease raged, attacking in particular the teamsters, "which up until this time employed immunity" to the disease. Though he still attributed the appearance of cholera to local causes, he raised some important points that would support the development of preventative medicine in the bacteriological era.[63]

First, he emphasized the importance of isolating the sick and preventing any further spread so that the cycle of transmission would be stopped. He also suggested that the immunity he thought certain attendants had as a result of their strong constitutions did not exist. He also observed that the number of cases continued to increase, suggesting that it was an "unfamiliar force" or epidemic.[64] Moreover, he spoke of cholera as a *specific* disease with characteristic symptoms: "The disease was undoubtedly Asiatic cholera presenting all the symptoms of a malignant form: diarrhea, vomiting, and purging of rice water, cramps, collapsed surface, shrunken features, anxious expression, sunken eyes dark and hollow, inelasticity of the skin, incessant thirst, sensation of heat of body and extremities, entire suppression of urine, nervous agitation and sometime slight delirium, finally coma from uremia, loss of pulse and death. After death in many cases the elevation of the temperature of the body and the muscular movements were very striking."[65]

There was a transition under way. Most case reports increasingly suggested that the disease was traceable in some way to human contact; medical attendants were believed to be at risk of contracting the disease, and some physicians believed that the disease could be imported from an infected to a healthy locality. The idea that predisposition and poor sanitary conditions would "spark" the disease still prevailed in some medical circles, but this was gradually changing as well. The physician S. Horner, of Post Hospital, Louisville, Kentucky, observed after extensive experience with the disease that the greatest number of cases came from one company and suggested that the disease was somehow connected to the preparation of its food. He also noticed that when the company was ordered to Bowling Green, "it took the disease with it," as six more cases had been reported since its arrival there. He tried in vain to "trace the cause to indiscretions of the men," but the "rapid multiplication of cases compelled me to abandon this idea and to recognize the fact that it existed in its true epidemic form."[66] Similarly, Drs. McGill and Merriman reported that once cholera was introduced at Fort Harker it grew in virulence and was "unfortunately carried thence across the plains." Moreover, in carefully tracing troop movement, it was determined that the 38th Infantry had brought the "germs of the disease with them from Jefferson Barracks."[67]

Physicians of the period debated theories of transmission, specifically importation versus local development. But just how complex was the discussion is well illustrated by the physician William Carroll's official report: "As to the portability of cholera there can be left no doubt; it was brought to the island and all of the residents were attacked by it.... From the fact of some of the nurses having been attacked by diarrhea soon after nursing severe cases, I incline to the belief that a zymotic poison is produced from the patient or his evacuations, which under certain conditions of atmosphere and health, not now understood propagates the disease."[68] Carroll also suggested that while "fear" may have predisposed the patient to the attack, neither "courage" nor "previous good health" nor "medical aid" offered the "slightest effectual resistance."[69]

Joseph Barnes later furnished the military records to public health officials concerning cases of cholera that occurred at the military posts on Governor's Island, Hart's Island, Davids Island, and others in the New York Harbor. The results were then tabulated so that a comparison could be made with the records of the new local boards of health then managing cholera. It was publicly claimed that "the record affords new and convincing evidence of the value of that ceaseless vigilance by medical officers which is seldom perfect excepting under military authority."[70]

Of course, the military medical department had witnessed the effect of many soldiers crowded together in camps and hospitals and had seen epidemic diseases thrive as a result. Cholera would similarly threaten the poor, or rather those that were crowded together in tenements or slums, where unsanitary conditions tended to thrive (the affluent often retreated to the country during disease outbreaks). It might have been difficult for the state to coordinate any effective response to cholera in 1866 without the involvement of the military, which compiled enough case histories and thus fairly convincing evidence that either Snow's or Pettenkofer's theories were correct and that there seemed to be apparent transmission via human carriers to give currency to the idea of contagion. The military medical department invoked the well-tested system of producing knowledge: circulars were issued to collect information about the disease from medical officers in the field, the knowledge was then analyzed, statistics were tabulated, and another circular was sent out "for the information and guidance of all medical officers" but also local health boards, which later translated into public health reform.[71]

By 1867, Joseph Woodward examined the numerous reports and came to an important conclusion regarding quarantines. Although it was politically contentious, he could not discount the overwhelming evidence in favor of quarantine, data that were "too numerous and too important to be overlooked."[72] In tracing the origins of the disease, he determined that there were two chief centers, and through the case reports he compiled an epidemiological picture and demonstrated why quarantines were necessary: "Originating in the overcrowded barracks of Governor's Island, New York Harbor, in the immediate vicinity of an infected city, through which recruits passed with more or less delay before arrival, the infection spread by readily traceable steps to Hart's Island and other posts in the harbor to Tybee island Georgia; to Louisiana, by way of New Orleans; to Texas by way of Galveston; to Louisville, Kentucky; to Richmond, Virginia and to La Virgin, Nicaragua bay. From Richmond it was carried to Norfolk, Virginia; from Louisville to Bowling Green, Kentucky." He concluded that the disease was probably "carried from New Orleans up the Mississippi River to various points on that stream, and west of it, and though the whole chain of evidence is not yet complete, there are a sufficient number of known cases of the transfer of the epidemic from one post to another in this region to put this view of the whole movement beyond a reasonable doubt."[73]

In case quarantine did not prevent the importation, however, he also recommended thorough sanitary measures. Indeed, he observed that once the epidemic appeared it often moved quickly through the rest of the camp, but success with certain hygienic measures prevented it spreading to the general population. For example, Woodward complimented the measures taken by the physician E. McClellan of Fort Delaware, who had established a "quarantine" and saw to it that all "fruit and unripe vegetables were excluded from the island." He also kept a "close watch on the men's sink and anyone found with two or more discharges from his bowels was immediately placed under treatment."[74] McClellan recommended that all posts be placed in the "highest sanitary conditions" and that "rigid quarantines be enforced."[75]

In 1883 Robert Koch was dispatched to Egypt to collect "epidemiological evidence on the question of importation versus local development so that he could advise the German government on quarantines."[76] Although by 1883 researchers were trying to incorporate germ science and laboratory techniques into their work (and in the French and German cases their work centered in the laboratory, whereas this was very new in 1866 America, and of course the researchers were not searching for causative bacteria). Many of the techniques adopted in the two periods, however, were identical: inspecting potential disease carriers, isolation and quarantine, disinfection and sanitation, and government-sponsored investigations into the etiology of the disease.

These investigations revealed new complexities for disease management, but we also see the shaping of public health in the bacteriological era. For example, there was a perceptible shift from "inclusive" concerns (primary concern with the environment) to "exclusive" concerns (focus on disease agents, people, and their interactions).[77] In 1866 the physician's gaze generally centered on the environment, but this was becoming unacceptable as troops moved around the United States and seemed to transmit the disease to previously healthy locales. If cholera was not "a disease of locality," how, then, did it travel? These uncertainties about the etiology of cholera stimulated further investigations. However, in the meantime, people were increasingly targeted as the potential source of contagion. This did not mean that physicians subscribed to the idea that microorganisms were transmitting cholera. Some physicians suggested that "ferments" could travel as well; others maintained that predisposition was a necessary factor; and others still suggested certain atmospheric conditions caused the spread of the disease. Thus, the way in which disease was managed shifted first, and specific understanding of why these measures worked developed as bacteriological models became known and understood.

This shift from "sanitary hygiene" to preventative medicine, in which bacteriological science and the laboratory were linked with specific modes of management, would take a little longer to become diffused, accepted, and practiced in America. But the knowledge produced in the investigations into cholera were used to manage and prevent the disease at its most vulnerable points (e.g., suspected points of passage), which suggested a more sophisticated approach to disease management. Moreover, new preventative measures were developed, such as the purification of drinking water. There was a record of experience and pathological evidence that was developed regarding cholera, and newer ideas about the management of cholera were beginning to gain currency. But even so, the uncertainty regarding the disease proved yet again a powerful stimulus for investigative medicine.[78]

CHOLERA AND THE CULTURE OF CIVIL WAR SCIENCE:
Investigating the Pathology of Cholera

By 1849 the chief method for managing cholera had been through sanitary practices—isolation, quarantine, and cleanliness in particular. Those who subscribed to *de novo* origins and the "diffusion of poison" were content to focus on the environment. Through the war and afterward, more physicians increasingly debated the role of human-to-human transmission, which moved the focus from the environment to people. Circular No. 3, issued on April 20, 1867, asked physicians to communicate the successful methods of treatment and the results of autopsies in hopes of revealing the nature of cholera.[79] However, there was little consensus about a specific pathology of cholera because the many autopsies produced different results.

Therefore, it was the further development of investigative technique that was important in these investigations.

Physicians studied cholera under the following headings: deaths of cholera, cholera morbus, acute diarrhea, chronic diarrhea, acute dysentery, and chronic dysentery.[80] There were a few specific ways that physicians structured their investigations. The most common was through the patient, who was examined with a view to understanding cholera in its various stages (premonitory, inflammatory, or collapse). Second, physicians conducted postmortems in the attempt to understand the specific manifestation and course of the disease. Some physicians focused on the microscopic appearances and chemical makeup of diarrhea, urine, and vomit, looking for clues in the excrement of their cholera patients. Others focused on the applications of various remedies in the hope of finding a way to arrest the disease. Finally, some physicians conducted chemical and microscopial experiments on water supplies. The reports were compared and tabulated in the hopes of determining the etiology of cholera. Collectively, the investigating physicians painted a picture of the disease, and the information was transmitted in the form of circulars to local boards of health, individual physicians, and the Surgeon General's Office. Examination of this research gives a sense of the complexity of scientific medicine in the immediate wake of the Civil War.[81]

One of the most interesting features in these investigations was the incorporation of clinical facts in developing theories about the disease. George McGill's case histories, for example, reveal the increasing importance of laboratory-style experiments in investigations. For example, in the case of Private Richard Withington, 6th Independent Company, 1st Battalion, described as a "native of Massachusetts of intemperate habits," McGill undertook a thorough investigation. The patient suffered very much with symptoms such as "aggravated diarrhea," "nausea," "cramps in the legs and feet," and a "watery discharge."[82] Hours after admission, he began "vomiting profusely" and started to decline. McGill tried to arrest the disease by administering camphor emulsion every two hours, and attendants tried to massage the patient's cramps, which had spread from the feet to the calves, but he could "barely stand to be touched."

The patient was quarantined in the quartermaster's storeroom, in a tent "with a very nice bed." McGill ordered the ground covered with rubber cloths, and the patient was sponged with turpentine to ensure no exhalations would be released from the body, which McGill (not surprisingly) reported as "very clean." With his case report, he submitted a diagram showing the patient's sunken features. He treated the patient with extract of ergot along with emulsion of camphor, to little effect, as the patient promptly vomited, which was recorded as "rice water with a little reddish color." The patient continued to suffer with cramps, "hard breathing and contraction of the muscles"; he was variously hot and cold and "rapidly fading" with profuse diarrhea, before falling into a coma and finally expiring.[83]

McGill proceeded to study the rice water discharge microscopically. He found what he called "bodies" or "oil globules" and shreds of epithelial cells, which he compared to the "numerous very minute cubical crystals so called because they strikingly resembled the blood crystals described by Virchow." He examined things like the "bodies resembling starch granules of a bluish color," which were seen in the dried excrement, and the "brownish red starch like bodies" observed in the vomit and the albumen, which was "detected in the clear supernatant fluid of the rice water evacuation."[84] Indeed, one disease theory at the time suggested that there was a "zyme" in the discharges that came from "epilethium shed from intestinal villi" or a "flux of the mucus membrane of the gut."[85] McGill subscribed to the theory that fecal matter had to go through some process of decomposition before becoming infective.[86] He looked at the discharges and stools, trying to identify abnormalities or "germs," particularly at what stage excrement became infective—as it left the body or after being exposed to certain environmental conditions. And he performed Pettenkofer's test for bile (which was used to determine the level of bile acids in the blood and to see what role these substances played in the disease).[87] He observed that a "red color developed after the formation of a white precipitate on the addition of sulfuric acid," which he found to be a "characteristic reaction with the vomit, with colors pronounced, though not deep."[88]

McGill also examined the colon; the fluid of rice water discharge; the small intestines, which he noted were "hyperanemic generally"; and the bladder, which was contracted and empty." He next examined the ileum, including the "curdy substances, sanious fluid and gases," the intestinal walls, mucous membranes, solitary glands, and the veins. He performed a microscopic examination of the "blood crystals in the epithelium, which were observed in the contents of the diseased segments," along with the "altered blood corpuscles, oil, globules and shreds of foreign tissues." He found that "minute crystals of blood have formed in some of the cells," which he concluded only after "repeated observations." He examined the blood, both the red and the white corpuscles, which he found to be "more numerous than usual" and very viscid. He also examined in detail the "many fields of the red blood corpuscles," which he found "were so densely crowded together as to constitute a plenum."[89]

While most of his observations did not suggest anything abnormal, he found the intestines remarkable. He studied the congestion and the mucous surface, which he observed still had the epithelium (some physicians believed that during an attack of cholera there was a shedding of the epithelium cells). He then passed his "fingers over every line of mucous surface from the stomach to the rectum," trying to gauge the effect of the discharge from the bowels, and he conducted a microscopic examination of the "white substance obtained from the renal pyramids," the "reddish bodies," "ovoids," blood, "oil globules," "epithelium cells," and the "body fluid separating them."[90] Finally, he "cast portions of the intestines into pure glycerin" so that he could make further examinations of the sections. He hoped to find answers about causation, or whether the "specific activity of the disease could be detected in the intestinal liquid of cholera patients, or if somehow the disease was reproducing in the intestinal canal."

The detail of this report was not uncommon among physicians and provides just one example of the autopsies and laboratory-style investigations done with cholera victims.[91] While the autopsies did not reveal the cause of cholera, investigations such as McGill's demonstrated the new possibilities for studying disease and paved the way for acceptance of Koch's cholera vibrio in 1883.

In the course of these investigations, physicians also had the opportunity to test Snow's and Pettenkofer's theories. Physician T. A. McParlin and Assistant Surgeon Hartsuff contributed what Woodward referred to as "important practical experiments" related to the purification of their command's drinking water. McParlin and Hartsuff examined troops who had contracted cholera while stationed in New Orleans and other ports in Louisiana during 1866. They described the various aspects of the disease but were most concerned with tracing its mode of transmission. The camp was situated in an "unfavorable locality," and the preparation of the food and the water supply was deemed "inferior."[92]

McParlin ordered that "pure water be procured and issued to the troops at once," and he distributed either rainwater or distilled water. He was happy to report that as a result of these measures the troops had "enjoyed great immunity from the disease."[93] Importantly, he discovered that when rainwater was scant, some men used river water, and "soon cases of cholera developed." He immediately supplied pure water, and there were "no more cases in that regiment."[94] He suspected the disease was propagated through the water, but rather than conducting controlled experiments on the water supplies, he found it out largely by accident, as was not uncommon in the period. The "popular experiment," as John Simon noted in 1881, was "the experiment that accident does for us."[95]

The 9th Regiment, United States Colored Cavalry, and the 39th United States Infantry, proved McParlin's and Hartsuff's suspicion that water was involved in the transmission of cholera: "They were supplied, but not sufficiently, with distilled water until the cisterns at the Sedgwick were repaired, filled and furnished rain water to them. The men preferred to drink the river water because it was cold and did so against repeated warning, accepting the risks of disease rather than wait for the water to be cooled and aerated. Case after case of choleric diarrhea followed."[96] This suggests that the water carriage theory was not understood or widely accepted in all circles (particularly among laypeople). Hartsuff, however, later reported that "critical inspection failed to develop any other probable cause except the use of river water" and recommended to "remove the regiments away from the river far enough to prevent the men obtaining it." He found once again that after adopting these strict measures "cholera has since ceased in the regiment."[97] On the basis of his experiments, "circumstances have confirmed so strongly the importance of pure water that even troops in transit or remaining a few days, its supply is recommended."

The investigations thus placed a primacy on water supplies. There was also an emphasis on the movement of the troops and on attempts to control disease though inspection stations as they traveled, which suggests the development of very modern thinking about disease transmission. In other words, for some the thinking on the matter had evolved from merely associating disease outbreaks with specific locales and filth to an association with people: "So far as I am informed, it appeared at Galveston July 22; Fort St. Philip Louisiana (in troops from New Orleans returned to their station), August 10; Whites Ranche, on the Rio Grande Texas, August 10, among troops. Dr. Merrill, one hundred and sixteenth United States colored troops, reports that several cases appeared among Mexicans at the station, a mile from camp, many days, perhaps a fortnight, and that the disease was brought by citizens from New Orleans. . . . The recruits who arrived at the Jackson barracks in July were carefully inspected on arrival and placed in camp."[98] This was significant: *all* soldiers were inspected upon arrival, not merely the men showing symptoms, which was an important response to cholera. The military's official response, then, was strict sanitary precautions and medical inspection. But Woodward also incorporated increasingly sophisticated scientific investigations into his strategy.

Woodward agreed, for example, on the importance of the "character of the drinking water used during epidemics of cholera"; the many reports confirmed the danger of contaminated water and also mirrored the findings in Europe and London, which similarly emphasized certain organic impurities of the water furnished.[99] Based on the data collected, Barnes ordered a chemical examination of the drinking water of the troops and sent samples to the laboratory where B. F. Craig, assistant surgeon, U.S. Army, was ordered to complete a report on the water obtained from areas in which the epidemic prevailed. In contrast to Hartsuff, who produced information on the dangers of water supply as part of a "popular experiment," Craig's assignment involved scientific experiments being developed to manage cholera. The pattern was significant. The activities of the troops were monitored, which allowed Hartsuff and McParlin to make observations about the role of water and the development of cholera. This information was then reported to Woodward and Barnes, who ordered a controlled laboratory experiment of the water supplies to confirm and interpret the findings in the field.

CHOLERA AND THE DEVELOPMENT OF
EXPERIMENTAL MEDICINE

The value of experimental knowledge or science-based practice was reinforced in these investigations, particularly because there was an immediate effect on medical practice.[100] The official investigations, and subsequent publications, thus explained how to apply disinfectants in the management of infectious disease. With no clear answers about the etiology of cholera, as Rosenberg has shown, by 1866 it was the practical recommendations of Snow and Pettenkofer—purifying water and disinfecting clothing and bedding, which was of the most interest to physicians. Acting on the orders of the Surgeon General's Office, it was Craig's objective, then, to explain the practice and principles of disinfection and to make this material available for physicians and local boards of health. His report was prolific. He demonstrated first how to disinfect all infective discharges from the body—vomit, urine, and especially diarrheal discharges. Second, he explained the methods used to disinfect or purify water supplies. Finally, he advised which disinfectants to use as preventatives.

Craig began by examining five samples of drinking water from posts in the New York Harbor where cholera had occurred and made a study and comparison of the water samples with a "view to the determination of their organic matter."[101] Craig found enough organic impurities in the water to officially recommend the purification of all water supplies. He argued that while rainwater was acceptable, the best source was distilled water. He performed rather detailed experiments that focused on finding an agent capable of destroying organic matter without harming the water.[102] He proceeded to offer some important practical advice to physicians on exactly how to purify water with a solution of permanganate of potassa, which he suggested worked by exerting an "oxidizing power over the organic matter." Permanganate also, Craig suggested, worked as a treatment for groundwater: "Water as the great final receptacle of all soluble substances is almost always contaminated with organic matter especially in the neighborhood habitations of man, and the investigation made by Pettenkofer and others, point to the upper water bearing a strata of the earth as a great habitat and reservoir of cholera poison."[103]

In light of the evolving understandings of infectious disease, these investigations are revealing. Disinfectants seemed to counter or kill certain infectious-disease-causing matter—but by what process? Much was made about the role of disinfection and prevention. But one could make the argument that the use of disinfectants actually hindered acceptance of the "germ theory" because the success was initially associated with the elimination of "putrid odors," then associated with the miasmatic theory of disease. Before the development of the "germ theory," sanitarians used disinfectants to whitewash and clean bedding and clothing, but they were not targeting anything specific. They were merely eliminating the bad air or putrid smells from the environment. Disinfectants had long been used by anticontagionists or localists; "pestilence and sanitary evils" seemed to coexist, and thus the efficacy of disinfectants seemed to prove miasmatic theories correct. There is, however, a more interesting story. For some physicians of the Civil War era, the use of disinfectants led to questions and investigations about the very *nature* of disease—how a disease seemed to function in the body, who was spreading the disease, and what might counteract a disease process. Indeed, it was the detailed investigations and drives to understand cholera's diffusion that led to more sophisticated experiments about why disinfectants were successful (and why they sometimes were not). These questions first took shape during the investigations into gangrene and erysipelas and were further developed in the cholera investigations.

Craig was, however, quick to point out to Woodward that the "methods in which disinfectants act are not yet understood in all their detail." But he suggested that perhaps the name of "disinfectant may in its narrowest meaning be limited to those bodies which destroy or render inert certain products of decomposition in organic matter, or from morbid action in the living being through the agency of a reaction in which the disinfectant itself undergoes chemical destruction." Craig's focus was on the "antiseptics or bodies which antagonize putrefaction" simply because they had an "important practical application."[104] From the outset Craig recognized that disinfectants were successful because, in addition to prevention, they acted in two possible ways: they altered a chemical process or killed an actual living body.

The German chemist Justus von Liebig explained the disease in chemical terms in the 1840s, discussing the disease process in terms of fermentation, putrefaction, and decay, where "disease was seen as spreading internal rot, that came from external rot, and could be transferred to others."[105] He looked at the chemical changes or breakdown in organic molecules caused by ferments. Liebig's theories held that ferments were not disease entities but rather "catalysts that could, in the right bodily and environmental conditions, initiate disease processes."[106] Craig's theories were also rooted in ideas of decomposition and degeneration: the idea that some kind of chemical miasma reacted with the body, blood, or tissues and that, as organic material decomposed, putrefaction would result. As noted in chapter 3, Joseph Woodward classed disease ferments under the heading "zymotic diseases," which emphasized the chemical link between disease and fermentation. Thus, it was easier for most physicians to reconcile pathological processes with chemical theories of disease, but this would change soon as well. The theories of Louis Pasteur (who later demonstrated that fermentation *required* the action of living microorganisms) also became of interest to Craig and other physicians investigating the properties of cholera.[107]

For countering putrefactive fermentation, Craig advised using what he called "the volatile antiseptics," such as the metallic salts, including chloride of sodium, and many of the more stable forms of organic matter, such as sugar or alcohol and resin: "It has been very clearly observed that the most efficient of the volatile antiseptics possess probably in virtue of their power of imparting stability to matter, a poisonous influence over those organic germs which play so important a role in the propagation of putrefactive fermentation; and in fact over all the lower forms of organic life."

How could volatile antiseptics, then, be applied in the management of cholera? He explained their usefulness in managing cholera. He began with the "big picture" or, rather, the larger diffusion of cholera stuff, "where the virus of a disease is diffused through the air or impregnates buildings." In a very interesting comparison, Craig referenced the management of the cattle plague in England. Historians have examined the significance of animal models in pathological research that helped gain support for bacteriology after the 1870s, but there has been little consideration of this development in the American case.[108] Craig's comparison of the cattle plague in England in the summer of 1865 and the cholera outbreaks in 1866–67 was an interesting one. By 1860 many elite physicians believed epizootics were contagious and were spread between animals through the transmission of some disease-causing matter or germ.[109] It was somehow easier to accept the idea of germs spreading between animals than germs between people, at least initially. But as one historian has suggested, the findings of the Royal Commission on the Cattle Plague published in 1866 "raised the profile of germ theories of disease" and raised the very real probability that "laboratory research could produce information that would change practices for the better."[110] Indeed, this report was "seen as a model of advanced medical research."[111]

Thus, in his investigations, Craig looked to the cattle plague and developed his research within some of the larger questions of the day, particularly those relating to the prevention and management of contagious disease. Craig studied, for example, the role of volatile antiseptics, including carbolic alcohol and fossil oil, and their efficacy in checking decompositions. During the cattle plague, he observed, "The two homologous substances, cool tar alcohols, carbolic and cresylic alcohols have been used separately and conjointly as a means of arresting this spread of the cattle plague in England. . . . The power of even small quantities of these liquids in arresting putrefaction and in destroying the lower forms of animal life is very great. . . . Carbolic alcohol, now on the supply table of the medical department, can be obtained from medical purveyors."[112] And as an extemporaneous means of fumigation he also recommended "the occasional burnings of a few sulphur matches."

He then turned to the treatment of cholera evacuations. Craig mostly thought about the propagation of disease in Pettenkofer's terms: "The theory of the mode of propagation of cholera which is the most widely received and has in its favor the greatest amount of evidence that the virus is not eliminated as such from the bodies of cholera patients, but that it is formed in their discharges by some specific process of decomposition, a process which is supposed to go on only in alkaline fluids." Thus the goal was to "retard putrefaction in the discharges" and, if possible, to keep them in an acid condition. The best disinfectant for this purpose was sulfate of iron or chloride of zinc, to be used either in powder or in saturated solution in vessels in which the discharges of cholera were received, such as privy vaults and boxes, and applied to discharges themselves.[113] Moreover, as an additional precaution, he again advised the occasional use of sulfur fumigation in localities that had been exposed to infection.

Finally, he discussed the use of "destructive disinfectants," such as chlorine or permanganate of potassa, which seemed to work by oxidizing and consuming "whatever organic matter they come into contact with by attacking the more advanced products of putrefaction." He made some important recommendations. The quantity used, as one example, had to be large enough. Physicians were sometimes thrown off by the smell of disinfectants. Chlorine in particular had a powerful odor, and thus physicians often thought that as offensive odors (e.g., discharges) were removed, a disinfection had been successful. However, as Craig warned, it might be the disinfectants that underwent "destruction themselves before they attack the more dangerous organic virus." The proper use for oxidizing disinfectants, he warned, is, rather than dealing with great masses of it, to try to ensure that effluvia was decomposed and that small quantities of organic matter were destroyed. He also explained that permanganate was the best disinfectant for clothes and bedding and that carbolic acid, lime, and charcoal worked well for whitewashing.

Craig's reference to the cattle plague, much like Woodward's reference to Virchow just a couple of years earlier, demonstrates the various ways scientific research and ideas about germs were developed in the third quarter of the nineteenth century. Pasteur's germ theory or Lister's surgical revolution did not overwhelm and transform medicine overnight; it would take a few more years before these ideas were diffused into medical practice, but the conditions created during the war years and after led to increasing acceptance of the idea of "germs" and disease. Indeed, the language throughout Craig's report was revealing of the changing times. In the 1850s and early 1860s, it was common to refer to disease processes purely as chemical, but by 1865, largely as a result of Pasteur's research, some scientists discussed disease as "vital processes," "organic germs," and "lower forms of life" in the disease process.[114] While "germ theorists" were still a small minority in the United States, the publications coming out of the Surgeon General's Office had a wide readership, and these ideas were slowly beginning to gain currency. Whether diseases were the result of chemical or living processes, however, the experiments centered on how antiseptics either could bring about the "final decomposition of infectious and offensive matter" or could "change and prevent decomposition," both of which were countered with disinfection. The most important aspect of his report was the detailed instructions for applying disinfectants. Moreover, Woodward and Barnes ordered that these findings be adopted by the local boards of health then managing cholera. Thus, the research produced in the laboratory at the Army Medical Museum had a concomitant benefit on civilian health.[115]

In 1867, on the heels of his experiments with gangrene and bromine, Roberts Bartholow published a small treatise entitled *The Principles and Practice of Disinfection*, which was based on three papers read before the Cincinnati Academy of Medicine. Bartholow pointed out that, of late, "the practice of disinfection has acquired greatly increased Importance. The alarming ravages of the cattle plague and the present epidemic of cholera" have led to demands for "new and exact methods" of science to combat these "mysterious animal poisons." Disinfections, as demonstrated by various commissions and investigators, were intended to act in two ways. First, they would kill matter developed in the "process of putrefactive decomposition of animal and vegetable matter." Or, second, they would target "that peculiar organic matter," such as "virus, materies morbid, morbific matter, diseased germinal matter etc."[116] His study included the results of his experiments on animals of the toxic effects of the gases developed by the process of putrefaction and the results of his trials on the uses of various disinfectants.

His work was all the more relevant since he had "a large field for practical observation in a number of years devoted to hospital practice."[117] What had Bartholow learned during his years in the Civil War hospitals? Simply that the object of "disinfection is to prevent disease." Craig's first study similarly centered on ways to prevent a "virus of a disease which is diffused through the air or impregnates buildings"—in other words, ways that might kill any airborne germs.[118] But the conversation grew more sophisticated. Disinfectants were used to kill diseases; if not, diseases would grow and multiply. As Bartholow warned, the specific virus "of disease has unquestionably a power of growth and multiplication independent of those external conditions to which we give the name bad hygiene; but it is also true that these conditions favor its growth and decrease its diffusion."[119]

Like Craig, Bartholow began his examinations with two complicated questions: How did disinfectants work? Did they kill living or chemical matter? Bartholow argued that Pasteur, building on the work of Schwann, Mitscherlich, and Schroeder, along with contributions of Angus Smith and

Tilbury Fox of England and others, demonstrated that living organisms "are necessary to the process of putrefactive fermentation."[120] He posited that if the "presence of organized germs is necessary to the putrefactive composition, then the most effectual disinfectants will be those of the antiseptic class, most destructive of these germs." Thus, air or rather "bad air" (usually associated with putrid odor) was not a threat but rather the "specific cause of disease" in the air (which could be odorless). Disinfectants then could effectively combat "those organic matter or organized structures, which introduced into the body, produce specific diseases (materies morbid)." In drawing out the idea of layers of "germ theories" in this period, these discussions are useful. Building on the work of Pasteur, Lister learned to prevent surgical infections by killing living airborne germs, before they could reach the wound—and, in the process, he transformed surgery. Lister's domain was the hospital, and his subject was surgical wounds. Former Civil War physicians had seen the efficacy of disinfectants in the Civil War hospitals—but what about other locales? How could this knowledge develop as a stimulus to public health?

In the postwar period, disinfections had a much wider application. They were used in houses, hospitals, and military barracks and for the purification of water, ships, the local environment, clothing, linens, and even people. However, the experiments with disinfectants, the sense of uncertainty and optimism, and the new investigative techniques among American researchers signal the beginning of the shift from concepts of disinfection based purely on sanitary theories toward concepts of disinfections with bacteriological underpinnings.[121] Bartholow observed that "to form an intelligent judgment on the action of disinfectants, we must know something of the nature and mode of action of the materies morbid." Unlike Craig, who was still debating the idea of living versus chemical theories of disease, Bartholow was sure that "the power to grow and multiply is a function of living matter. We must therefore conclude that materies morbid is living matter."[122]

During the Civil War, Bartholow's experiences seemed to confirm that each disease had a different mode or propagation—some diseases were transmitted through bodily fluids such as pus or through discharges as seen in cases of typhoid or dysentery. Cholera was most certainly transmitted through rice water discharges. He thus warned physicians to consider carefully the "sources of the virus" when applying disinfectants—a strategy certainly taught in the investigations into gangrene and erysipelas. In one revealing study in a hospital in St. Louis, it was found that of the dust collected in the wards "36 percent was of organic matter."[123] Thus, disinfectants had to "destroy the noxious gases and the volatile products of putrefactive decomposition, but especially to attack and destroy the virus of the disease, the materies morbi." And smell had very little to do with the efficacy of disinfectants, for "the destruction of foul odors will avail us little . . . our disinfectants should strike deeper, and destroy the disease matter itself."[124] The war years were important because they led to a shift in thinking about how medicine should be studied but, more importantly, revealed the potential of medical science and especially the laboratory in managing disease environments.

CHOLERA AND THE TRANSMISSION OF MEDICAL KNOWLEDGE

Craig, in conjunction with Woodward, incorporated all of the various findings, and the medical department transmitted a summary of facts and findings regarding cholera. First, Craig advocated quarantines and inspection; second, disease was treated as an importation (that men would bring it to camp and transmit through excretions). Third, in managing the disease, he utilized disinfectants to purify water supplies and neutralize the excretions from the bodies of cholera patients.[125] Disinfection was recast within developing ideas about "germs." Craig again cautioned that the "day has passed in which nauseous-smelling substances are looked upon as disinfectants. . . . To change the odor is not to disinfect." Thus, he warned that "a true disinfectant must be antiseptic; that is it must possess the power to destroy or render inert the products of decomposition of organic matter or of morbid action in the living body."[126] In his report, he variously discussed "organic germs" and "lower forms of life" as "propagating the putrefaction," and this language paved the way for the acceptance of bacteriological theories of disease, but most important was the focus on preventing the disease from developing in the first place.[127]

In 1866 cholera was a social problem but was largely "turned away" with the use of scientific medicine.[128] Craig used chemical and microscopial methods to produce knowledge about the disease, and as the leading chemist in the Surgeon General's Office, the knowledge he produced, particularly on purifying water (and even that it should be purified as a matter of policy), did much to support the efficacy of scientific methodology in the practice of medicine. Despite uncertainty about the disease itself, the medical department prided itself on measures developed to combat the spread and incidence of cholera.[129] The findings of these early investigations as contained in Circulars No. 1 and 5, which included much of the knowledge produced, along with these new management strategies, were not only transmitted to northern and southern local and state health boards but also requested by, and thus transmitted to, physicians in Vienna, Berlin, England, and Moscow.[130] Given that less than a decade earlier Silas Weir Mitchell lamented that American investigations had long been ignored by the international medical community, events suggest that American medicine had entered a new phase. Moreover, the military and civilian response to cholera highlighted the various preventative strategies, which translated into calls for boards of health similar to New York's in other North American cities.[131]

By 1875, in the Second Session of the Forty-Third Congress, the management of cholera was again a subject of discussion in the House of Representatives. This was in response to the joint resolution approved March 25, 1874, which had authorized an inquiry into the causes of epidemic cholera.[132] It also signaled the growing state involvement in public health. Once again, military and civilian physicians worked together to manage cholera. John M. Woodworth, a supervising surgeon with the Merchant Marine Hospital Service[133] (renamed the Public Health Service in 1912), in connection with medical officer Dr. E. McClellan of the Army Medical Department, was ordered to "confer with the health authorities and resident physicians of such towns (as were visited by the cholera epidemic of 1873) and to collect, as far as possible, all facts of importance with regard to such epidemic." Along with the findings of the previous investigations, the purpose of the 1875 report was to demonstrate the connection between mercantile marine transport and the importation of cholera into the United States. After an examination of the facts, an official policy mandating medical inspection (screening of merchant seamen aboard the ships), quarantine stations, a medical officer on board each ship, and a program of cleanliness and disinfection was instituted. With the rise of immigration in the Progressive Era the role of the Marine Hospital Service expanded considerably.[134]

In 1874 Elisha Harris, who had long been a student of cholera, published a treatise entitled *Conclusions concerning Cholera: Causes and Preventative Measures*. Writing on the heels of the 1873 outbreak, he reflected on how the disease had been studied and how knowledge had been produced; he claimed that "looking back on the historical records of Asiatic cholera they now appear to be entirely consistent with each other in the successive epidemics, and in all countries visited by it."[135] He recognized how difficult it had been to account for its propagation—personal contagion or contingent transportability—but suggested that there were uniform lessons that had been taught over the past few years—namely, the importance of sanitary and preventative measures that had been learned by logical deductions, empirical observation, and experiments.[136] He summarized the known facts about the disease: it originated in India, was portable and transmissible, and required circumstances favorable for transmission; regarding possible forms of transmission, it could be transmitted through infected clothing, spread by maritime communication from an infected country, exacerbated by crowds, and transmitted by water, air, and excrement.

He also noted that certain predisposing causes helped spread the disease: impaired health, lack of ventilation, emanations of soil impregnated with organic or cholera matter, contaminated water, and weakened resistance. He recognized that American medical men, along with other members of the international medical community, agreed that there was a germinal cause of cholera that acted with well waters, soil localities, and seasons to aid the spread of cholera but more work needed to be done on its specific causation. Importantly, he shared his findings with Bartholow, who then developed Harris's conclusions.[137] In the meantime, prevention, disinfectants, and water purification proved weapons against the spread of epidemic cholera. This report included the findings of the Cholera Conference at Weimar, Munich, in 1867, the Cholera Conference at Constantinople, and the International Medical Conference at Vienna (September 1873). In addition, the American response to the cholera outbreaks of 1866 and 1867 were "faithfully portrayed in the two official reports issued by the Surgeon General of the Army" and were remarkably "clear and instructive."[138]

As knowledge about communicable disease developed through these investigations, some physicians were becoming more receptive to the new "germ theory." As one example, Joseph Lister's principles became of great interest to members of the American medical department, and Lister was invited to the United States to demonstrate and outline his methods. In a letter to Assistant Surgeon A. C. Girard, of Fort Randall, Dakota Territory, Lister noted, "Your kind letter and enclosed report have reached me today; and I hasten to tell you how much pleasure they have given me. The kind reception I met with in America last year prepared me to learn before long that antiseptic treatment was taking root and bearing fruit there." As Lister further explained, "It may interest you to learn that I received a few days ago a letter from a Russian surgeon who is in chief position with the Russian army in Asia minor, and who, having learned antiseptic treatment in Edinburgh had introduced it into his University clinique at Dorsat and thence had transported it to the seat of war, taking with him the apparatus for preparing antiseptic gauze, showing that 'where there's a will there's a way.'" And, "the results he is getting are certainly[,] as he expressed it, 'herrlich.' Thus seven successive cases of gunshot wound of the knee joint almost all without inflammatory disturbance. I confess it was very gratifying to me to learn that the antiseptic treatment can really be effectually carried out in military practice."[139] Surgeon General Crane subsequently asked Girard to prepare a report on Lister's principles of surgery, which was subsequently distributed as a circular to medical officers.[140]

CONCLUSION

In 1873 cholera once again erupted in the United States. In 1875 the Surgeon General's Office, which by an act of Congress was called upon to lead the investigation, published an account of the investigations. There were no longer debates about the portability of cholera. It was observed "that cholera is a portable disease, is at the present day denied but by few observers; even among those who reject the contagiousness of the disease this fact is recognized."[141] The disease was noted to "appear wherever there are routes of human intercourse," which was amply demonstrated during the epidemiological investigations during the 1866 and 1867 outbreaks. Craig's theories were still utilized, and water was still targeted: "The popular theory at this time, and that which has the ablest supporters, is that Asiatic cholera is developed more frequently from the use of waters loaded with decaying organic matters than from any other cause."[142] As a result, the government supported investigations into various water supplies, thereby institutionalizing these findings supporting the further development of public health policy.

Though Robert Koch was not the first to see the cholera microbe, the "isolation in 1883 and 84 of what is now called *Vibrio cholera* was a watershed."[143] There was now a way to study cholera in the laboratory, to isolate the cause for the disease, and perhaps to develop effective diagnosis, treatment, and even vaccine. But these great strides were a few years away for the Civil War and American physicians who eagerly tried to master Asiatic cholera in 1866 and 1867. Through a careful record of investigations in 1866, 1867, and 1873, however, and the subsequent dissemination of this knowledge, American physicians added a valuable chapter to the international response to cholera.

In the third quarter of the nineteenth century, cholera was an international issue. There was a series of sanitary conferences around the globe that "sought consensus on cholera control."[144] The efficacy of disinfectants was variously heralded and under siege in the 1880s. The debates about managing cholera centered on how to manage the disease, with various ideas put forth, including repressive quarantines, isolation, surveillance, inspection, disinfection, and sanitation. After Koch's discovery of the vibrio in the 1880s, the Kochian model was disinfection and isolation, but even with proof of causation these findings were constantly debated (most famously, in 1892 Pettenkofer swallowed comma bacillus culture to prove it was not directly contagious—he received only a mild case of diarrhea, giving some credence to his claims).

But the new bacteriological models after 1883 complicated the response to cholera—indeed, to all infectious diseases: What if a carrier was asymptomatic? Then only quarantines would work, but all countries would have to work together. Contagious disease laws would later be created to answer these questions around the turn of the century.[145] There were no easy solutions for managing cholera (even today cholera continues to kill by the hundreds in Haiti). Much like the Civil War medical challenges, however, the investigations into cholera did not bring simplicity or clarity to disease but instead revealed new complexities but also possibilities for medicine. It was becoming clear to the physicians engaged in the Civil War or postwar investigations that to master, investigate, or understand disease, medical schools would require laboratories and microscopes, money for full-time researchers, and, above all, reform in the curriculum. The medical experiences of the Civil War and the cholera epidemic just afterward helped prepare American physicians for the transformation in medical science that was just ahead.

CHAPTER SEVEN

Postwar Reflections

I n 1867, an editorial in the *Richmond Medical and Surgical Journal* reflected on the history of medicine in the United States. The author noted that "until the last ten years, American teaching and American practice of medicine has been conspicuously devoid of individuality."[1] Part of the problem, as the editor explained, was the lack of American identity in the production of knowledge; thus "the most dogmatic aphorisms of the lecture-room, and the chief lessons from the library have, as a rule been confessedly obtained from foreign authorities." Indeed, "listeners and readers have been educated to believe, that, in professional circulation, no currency was genuine or sterling, unless it bore a European superscription." Silas Weir Mitchell recalled just before the war that one of his physiology lectures was "a more or less well stated resume 'of the best foreign books, without experiments or striking illustrations.' It was like hearing about a foreign land which we were forbidden to enter."[2]

But by 1867, however, the editor was optimistic that a "transition stage . . . is fairly and acceptably begun." It was promising that the works of American teachers "very commonly induce the respect of the most critical reviewers. . . . The records of military and civil hospitals here, are sought and read with avidity by trans-Atlantic teachers, and the facts thus obtained, are quoted with frequency and confidence."[3] Thus perhaps, as the editor suggested, Paris had "passed the era of her chief medical greatness," and while Germany was working "diligently and efficiently," there were also some American physicians who were as fully entitled to "prominence and distinction in connection with the respective departments of Medicine and Surgery."[4]

It is remarkable to consider how many changes the Civil War brought to American medicine in just four years. Former Union physicians went home, many of them to remote places such as rural Ohio, Pennsylvania, and Kentucky, to begin new medical practices or resume old ones. But these physicians took with them a vast education of unparalleled medical experience—and perhaps a new confidence. Silas Weir Mitchell noted just after the conflict that "the war trained vast numbers of country doctors and that for a long time the cases for grave operations ceased to be sent to the cities as had been usual."[5] Whether physicians had practiced in the temporary or general hospitals or in the field, they were required to write daily, weekly, and monthly reports; submit case histories, drawings, and specimens; and perform autopsies and difficult surgeries. They administered new therapeutics like bromine and even learned the importance of using these drugs prophylactically to prevent diseases in the hospitals. Physicians both relied on and benefited from the networks of knowledge that were facilitated by the Surgeon General's Office.

In the postwar period the Surgeon General's Office remained an important resource for American physicians, particularly in the growing field of American literature. Before the war, between the years 1800 and 1860, 178 medical journals were founded, which helped foster a community of American physicians, but still there were only roughly 700 subscribers and only 30 of the 178 journals were still in existence in 1860.[6] The voluminous *Medical and Surgical History of the War of the Rebellion* (all 6,000 pages of it), on the other hand, is evidence of the "many" physicians working to develop Civil War and American medicine. The six volumes of the series were published between 1870 and 1888, which likely kept the former war physicians (and contributors) interested in these publications. Indeed, many civilian physicians were encouraged to maintain a continuing association with the Surgeon General's Office, and this was an educational resource for American physicians. The publications coming out of the Surgeon General's Office were geared toward a wide array of physicians rather than merely military medical practitioners as had been common before the war.[7] For example, in the post–Civil War period, Surgeon General's Office publications addressed subjects like American medical education, hospital construction, infectious disease management, and photomicrography, making them highly relevant for the civilian practitioner.[8]

Building on this foundation and enthusiasm, John Shaw Billings was able to use government funds for the creation of a National Medical Library.[9] Not long after the end of the war, Congress began making appropriations for the library. For the first three years, Billings was given $10,000 to build the library, later set at $5,000 annually. He created the library through exchanges with universities, museums, and libraries around the world. He looked for the most up-to-date medical literature, transactions of medical and scientific societies, new and important research findings, and even

emergent specialty journals.[10] In 1874 the Government Printing Office issued a catalog of titles, which "formed three quarto volumes of about 2000
pages," and an index medicus was begun.[11] Copies were placed in medical
libraries in the United States and were made available to medical schools
and to physicians upon request. Billings noted that "although this is only
a catalogue of a single library . . . an attempt has been made to prepare, as
far as time and materials would allow, a work of practical usefulness for
bibliographical purposes to all physicians, even if they have not access to
the library itself."[12] Indeed, the museum's staff encouraged "students who
desire to avail themselves of the resources of the library in connection with
medical researches of any kind," and it was "thrown open to all medical
men who choose to use it."

By 1876 the library had 40,500 books and 41,000 pamphlets, and by the
early 1890s it was the world's largest medical library.[13] As Woodward noted,
"Although far from complete, this library is now one of the great medical
libraries of the world; . . . and even double the money expended upon it
would not have made it as valuable as it is now but for the generous assistance of the profession of this country." One of the most striking patterns
that emerges was the diligence with which American physicians built the
collection: "Many of our physicians have ransacked their own libraries to
supply us with works which, in many instances, we could not otherwise
have obtained. . . . The extent to which this has been done is the best proof
of the general desire of the medical profession of the United States that this
library should speedily become a complete library of reference on medical
subjects." The library was not for the casual reader but for the "number of
original investigators who consult it in connection with their own work."[14]

From its inception, Woodward and Billings explicitly hoped the library and museum would encourage individual researchers who might
make medical discoveries that would be "generally useful to the whole
profession. . . . Until very lately, such men had to travel to Europe for the
same purpose. It is important that this should no longer be necessary."[15]
Indeed, in 1871 the *Richmond and Louisville Medical Journal* observed, "Be-
sides several important systematic treatises and monographs of interest,
[and] collections of hospital reports that have been published in the last
five years, several courses of clinical lectures have appeared in print, and
have added to the evidence that we are no longer entirely dependent
upon foreign sources for knowledge of the progress of our art and science. The medical department has contributed its full share in this forward movement of medical literature."[16] The overarching message from

Billings and Woodward was that they were not willing to go back to the apathy of the 1850s. Americans had suffered but the lessons were not lost.

As early as 1866 some medical schools began pressuring for curricula reform placing a primacy on science-based teaching—physiology, pathology, and bacteriology, where the laboratory would slowly replace the didactic lecture. Over the next two decades medical schools like Harvard, the University of Pennsylvania, the University of Michigan, and the new Johns Hopkins would develop well-equipped laboratories, as well as methods of teaching the laboratory sciences and experimental medicine. For the generation after the war, the continuation of the Civil War medical model through the medical museum and library was important in supporting the scientific culture among American physicians. "The interest taken in this collection by the medical profession of the country is being annually more and more frequently displayed by the presentation of valuable medical and surgical specimens from all parts of the country. Such specimens are always acceptable. . . . Those which have served as the basis of original communications published in the medical journals have especial interest."[17]

RISE OF THE NATION-STATE

The influence of the medical museum and library, then, extended well beyond Washington. Physicians from all over the country were encouraged to use the museum and library and to share knowledge with physicians and researchers in America and abroad. The museum's vast collection revealed the complexities of medicine and science for the rank-and-file practitioner while also providing new opportunities. For example, those students or physicians still learning medicine in a preceptor's office or at a commercial medical school (where research material was not readily available) were encouraged to come to the capital to see, read about, and study medicine and scientific research. Or, conversely, as physicians returned home from overseas the museum and library were resources for the continuation of their education as well. And although the ranks of the profession continued to swell at all levels of practitioners for the remainder of the century, by the later 1860s many former elite Civil War physicians pressed for the reform of medical schools and medical education, which was facilitated through the medical museum in Washington. Indeed, the curators, including Joseph Woodward, George Otis, John Shaw Billings, and later Walter Reed played a central role in shaping the culture of scientific research in the final third of the decade. During the war and after there was in fact unprecedented support for medicine and health care on a national basis; however, the medical reforms that took shape with the war were able to develop only with the expanded role of the federal government and acceptance of federal authority in affairs of the state and the Civil War body.

Before the war, as David Blight has argued, the federal government did little more than deliver mail, conduct foreign policy, and issue modest tariffs.[18] However, as citizen-soldiers transitioned to patients and, in the postwar period, to veterans, the government had to redefine its responsibility toward the men who fought and died, the men who fought and lived, the men who fought and lost limbs, and the newly freed African Americans. There was an unprecedented government responsibility to provide for the casualties of the war—the freedmen and -women, soldiers, patients, veterans, and war widows—and thus a concomitant dependency on the emergent medical profession. In the postwar period, former Civil War physicians (or government-appointed physicians) were required to provide medical care for the many affected by the war. This might have meant examining patients and issuing case reports to satisfy pension requests, conducting investigations into public health threats such as cholera or smallpox, doctoring in the newly formed medical division of the Freedmen's Bureau,[19] or providing ongoing care for a variety of medical needs, from the treatment of heart disease or neurological trauma to caring for the thousands of men who lost limbs during the war.

Indeed, the disabled body became a visible and political reminder of the sacrifice and heroism of the war veterans. Photographs of amputees were widely displayed at the Army Medical Museum and postwar expositions, and short stories and poems about men with empty sleeves, phantom limbs, and peglegs increasingly began to appear.[20] The public and soldier-veterans alike viewed the amputation of a body part as a tremendous loss but also a representation of the courage exhibited by Union and Confederate soldiers during the war. As one soldier remembered, "Suffering is unpleasant; but if one must suffer it is better to do so in a good cause: therefore I had rather have my leg blown off by a rebel shell, than crushed by a locomotive, or bitten off by a crocodile."[21] But significantly, these visible hardships translated into demands for technical and financial support from the medical profession and the federal government.

In June 1862 Congress passed the "general law pension system," which formed the basis of all pension legislation until 1890.[22] The new pension programs provided support for injured veterans, war widows, children, and the dependent relatives of soldiers injured or killed while serving

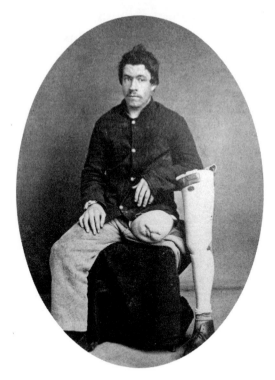

John B. Bathurst, private, Company I, 45th Pennsylvania Volunteers, suffered a gunshot wound in action at Cold Harbor, Virginia, June 4, 1864. He was admitted to Harewood General Hospital, November 2, 1865, from Douglas General Hospital after receiving a circular amputation of the left thigh at the middle third. The patient poses with a government-sponsored prosthetic leg. (Photograph courtesy of the National Library of Medicine, Washington, D.C.)

the Union. As Amy Holmes has demonstrated, from the founding of the Republic to the Civil War, the federal government spent $90 million on military pensions; however, in the fifty years following the Civil War the government spent approximately $5 billion on veterans and their dependents.[23] This amounted to a staggering 40 percent of the federal budget in 1893.[24] Moreover, Civil War veterans who had lost limbs during the war were eligible for the cost of an artificial limb ($50 for an arm and $75 for a leg) in addition to their disability pension.[25] And reflecting both need and advances in the range of prosthetic limbs between the years 1861 and 1873, 133 patents for limbs were issued, which represented a 290 percent increase from the number issued in the fifteen years prior to the war.[26]

The medicalization of the state in the postwar period was not unique in the American case but rather paralleled the situations in Europe and Britain.[27] As seen in the international response to cholera, many national governments increasingly became involved in health care systems and infectious disease management. In America, the expansion of the federal government into medical matters was transformative. The government entered, regulated, and provided support for certain aspects of the postwar

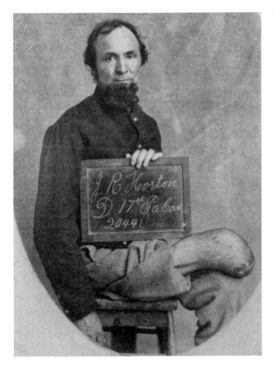

Joseph R. Horton, Company D, 17th Pennsylvania Cavalry, was wounded at the Battle of Petersburg and underwent amputation of the right leg, upper third, anteroposterior flaps, on the field. (Photograph courtesy of the National Museum of Health and Medicine, Washington, D.C.)

medical marketplace as in the Army Medical Museum, Surgeon General's Library, and Marine Hospital Service and with the creation of pension systems;[28] however, it is important to emphasize that in developing these programs and other forms of relief, the government worked closely with orthodox physicians. And the formerly low social status of the orthodox physician was elevated through this relationship.

REMEMBERING THE CIVIL WAR

The wartime medical reforms translated into tremendous support for more comprehensive medical reforms on a national basis; however, the war's impact on the individual physician was equally transformative. Discussing the effect of the war on every physician who developed through the experience is an impossible task, but examples elucidate the effect. Some physicians gained the practical experience they desperately lacked, while others realized that medicine and diseases were complex and that mastery demanded more than merely amassing clinical information. These factors worked together to create a dynamic professional environment and had a tremendous impact on some American physicians.

Years after the Civil War, Keen remembered one of the very first autopsies he performed. He always liked to refer to that experience to show just how far he had come during the war. In 1862 he thought (for a brief moment) he was dissecting a living body, yet just a year later he was performing an arterial ligation. Keen remembered: "In the years that have passed since then, other far abler surgeons, a younger generation have done more, better work. But while they have the joy and the rewards of their extensive and most important discoveries and improvements in diagnosis and technique, they never could have felt the thrill of those relatively few surgeons of my own age and generation who were among the first that ever burst into that silent sea."[29]

When Keen entered the offices of John Brinton, Jacob Da Costa, and S. W. Mitchell in 1860 as a new medical student at Jefferson Medical College, he had never so much as touched a microscope or handled a body. The war years set Keen on a very different professional course. At antebellum Jefferson Medical College, he might have performed a few dissections if he was lucky and become familiar with the basics of anatomy. But his study would have lacked the experiential opportunity that was offered by the war, which allowed him the kind of medical intervention that would help him to begin to transform American medicine but also to establish his own career. He had many professional wartime opportunities: he collected, dissected, and studied specimens, engaged in novel research projects while at Turner's Lane, pioneered experiments related to malingering, studied gangrene, and published numerous articles on his research. Keen was not atypical; these were the types of varied experiences that was Civil War medicine.

By 1865 Keen was picking up medical equipment for Jacob Da Costa in Vienna and Berlin,[30] studying microscopy with Virchow, and discussing his wartime research with Claude Bernard: "When I went to Paris as a student in the winter of 1864–65, I took a copy of *Nerves and Other Injuries* to Claude Bernard and showed him the history of this patient. It was the first confirmation in man of his experiments on animals. . . . Only those familiar with medicine can appreciate how profoundly important in anatomy, physiology, pathology, medicine, surgery and therapeutics this discovery of the function of the sympathetic nerve has been. It fundamentally altered our views and our practice in all these departments."[31]

Not every physician who served in the war developed a career path in the same way as Keen, but this new elite allowed for a hierarchy of knowledge in American medicine and a recognition of the complexities of medicine, paving the way for further medical reforms and a new reverence for scientific medicine. Looking back on his career in 1912, Keen recalled two important turning points. The first, the "one great opportunity in my life—the turning point in my surgical career"—was the successful operation for a brain tumor, one of the first in America.[32] The patient recovered, and Keen went on to operate in "two more brain cases," and along the way he gained renown for his work, which was one of the topics at the 1888 Medical Congress. As Keen noted, "the successful removal of a brain tumor, especially, so large a tumor, at a time when such operations were few in number, attracted a great deal of attention." In Keen's personal correspondence are hundreds of letters from physicians in America, Europe, and Canada asking his advice on nervous injuries, "imbeciles," "brain disease," cerebral surgery, experimentation, nerve injuries, brain disorders, and far more that stemmed from his war work.[33]

The other turning point was during the war at Turner's Lane Hospital. He suggested that his "Gunshot Wounds and Other Injuries of Nerves" published in 1864 was the "foundation of the whole modern surgery of the nervous system." As discussed in chapter 4, the development of specific methodologies relating to neurology was important, but Keen defined his medical identity through this work. The Keen of 1865 was not the Keen of 1912, but the war laid a foundation for further medical and professional development and gave physicians invaluable opportunity to develop professional authority.

John Brinton, the museum's first curator, also went on to have an illustrious career, first as a lecturer at Jefferson College and then as successor to Samuel D. Gross as professor of the practice of surgery and clinical surgery at Jefferson Medical College, a position he held until 1906. He was also a visiting surgeon and professor of surgery at St. Joseph's Hospital, Philadelphia Hospital, and Jefferson College Hospital; he was the Mutter lecturer on surgery and pathology, and he gave several lectures and addresses.[34] Like many of his wartime colleagues, he was a member of the Academy of Natural Sciences and a founding member of the American Surgical Association (with other war physicians, including Samuel Gross and Agnew Hayes), as well as a member of the Pathological Society of Philadelphia, American Medical Association, Philadelphia Surgical Club, and Philadelphia Medical Society. He helped develop *Lippincott's International Medical Magazine*, "a monthly devoted to medical and surgical science," which boasted subscribers from Vienna, Berlin, Paris, and London.[35] And he wrote the section on gunshot wounds for the surgical history of the war.

In 1896 he recalled that "various departments moved forward" as a result of the war: especially "anatomy and physiology or the two together, have led the way to more logical and truer diagnosis, to be in turn followed by a broad medical treatment or a bold operative interference."[36] For the three decades after the war, Brinton also continually pushed for the reform and development of anatomy acts. As Brinton observed, "The attention of your board is respectfully invited to the facts that the interests of medical teaching in the city of Philadelphia is seriously threatened by the scarcity of suitable material for dissection, and that scarcity is yearly increasing. It is true that by the provisions of the Anatomy Act all unclaimed bodies of persons dying are turned over to the medical college of the state to be studied"; still, with the increasing number of students, Brinton wanted to ensure there was "enough material."[37] Brinton highly valued his appointment as curator to the medical museum and was correct that his work there provided an enduring legacy, that the results of the "surgery of this war would be preserved for all time," and that the "education of future generations of military surgeons would be greatly assisted."[38] In most of his postwar addresses, he commented on the importance of the war experience for the education of both civil and military physicians.

Indeed, one important way of understanding the effect of the war is to appreciate the way in which individual physicians remembered it, as an important period in their development as physicians and an unsurpassed educational intervention. Silas Weir Mitchell recalled in 1913: "It is a record to be proud of, or I should not so willingly revert to it. If you look for that story in the histories, they are silent; if you search for it in the countless autobiographies of soldiers great or small, these too are mute except as to what the soldier did. A few forgotten books by surgeons are personal or technical, and tell us little more than the baldest story of the individual. What else there is may be found scattered through the huge volumes on the medical history of the war. We gain nowhere a sense of the immensity of the task in which as a profession we dealt with. We hear little or nothing of the unequaled capacity with which we met the call on energy and intelligence, or of the extraordinary power of the trained American to deal with the unusual."[39] He discussed some of the benefits gained through his wartime service, such as improvements in hospital ventilation and the opportunity to develop pathological anatomy, which had been anticipated by Hammond, but most of all, his tremendous satisfaction in being able to develop his interest in nervous diseases.[40]

Perhaps most poignantly, he recorded the pervasiveness of the war for the medical profession in America: "How far it taxed the average professional man of the cities—your city and mine—may be judged from the fact that in 1864 the living Fellows of the College of Physicians of Philadelphia were 174. Of these, 130 had been connected in one way or another with the service of the army or navy during four years of that bloody struggle."[41] He lamented that their contribution had not been better recognized: "We had served faithfully; we had built novel hospitals; organized such an ambulance service as had never been before seen, contributed numberless essays on diseases and wounds, and passed again into private life unremembered, unrewarded servants of duty."[42]

Mitchell's peers did, however, view his medical contributions as fundamentally important. In 1914, Talcott Williams, president of Columbia University, recalled his contribution to neurology: "The Civil War came and opened to him, as opened to many, the door of opportunity. . . . He passed through these arduous years to find, as men often do, that the patient toil which he had given to the case of one soldier and another smitten by nervous maladies had spread his name abroad." He continued: "We learn that the knowledge of his work and skill had gone to hamlets and towns where he could never have gone—and a wide public came to know that the practitioner's life had fruited in assuaging affections dependent upon the nerves. There flowed in upon him, as a result of the scientific intelligent use of large opportunity, such a practice as changed his life, and the income which had been so small in these days of struggle rose to figures which even in this day would be large, and there began for him that wider life and larger usefulness which we all know. . . . The best known use he made of his new freedom was in medical research and discovery."[43]

Like Mitchell, Woodward also received much praise for his pioneering work in microscopy, photomicrography, and cancer research. His "publications in these fields made his name famous among scientists throughout the world."[44] Woodward, along with George Otis and Joseph Barnes, received much acclaim for the *Medical and Surgical History of the War of the Rebellion*. He actively engaged in research regarding camp and hospital diseases and developed investigative methods during the war and earned status through this work. His monograph, *Outlines of the Chief Camp Diseases of the United States Armies*, was reviewed in the *American Journal of the Medical Sciences* in 1864. The reviewer was generally positive, particularly because of the "uncommon opportunities belonging to his connection with the Surgeon-General's Office."[45] While some diseases had been seen in the European armies, there were also "some peculiar features in the disorders which have affected our soldiers."[46] The reviewer suggested that Woodward's pathological views were highly influenced by Virchow, whose research "pervades in a certain sense the volume before us."[47] Less than three years after Virchow's treatise on cellular pathology was published, his doctrines were being consistently applied in Woodward's investigations, and Woodward encouraged the war physicians to become familiar with Virchow's methods. Virchow's text was placed on the army medical supply table, and there was a dialogue about using the microscope to study changes in cells within the body, tissue changes, and disease processes. Woodward's monograph explained cellular theory in the context of Civil War camp diseases, and the war provided the bodies and hospital experience for physicians to monitor "cellular abnormalities in the body." Placing a primacy on the cellular changes in organs, particularly as they were studied under the microscope, provided an important basis from which to think about disease and develop bacteriological science.

Woodward often discussed the importance of research in medicine, and in his own work he showcased the potential or demonstrated the specific techniques of investigative medicine.[48] The hundreds of photomicrographs he developed between 1864 and the 1880s were displayed in the museum, alongside the vast collection of clinical photographs. Woodward and Otis also published widely on photographic technique and engaged with issues of the day, such as the problem of "contradictory microscopic representations," which by the 1880s "filled the pages of bacteriological literature."[49] Koch, as noted earlier, suggested that photography offered the most promising rendering of disease and disease processes and might, then, "free bacteriology from the rancor of its past." But operators would first have to improve light, lenses, construction, and technique, and if done well, "the photomicrograph like the X-ray, provided a permanent record that transcended memory and subjective impression . . . a more secure path to medical truth."[50] As shown in chapter 2, Woodward worked tirelessly developing photographic standards, but equally important was the large microscopic collection in Washington with which American physicians could not only research and study the preparations but also debate the subjective versus the objective, conditions of observation, and the role of microscopy in medical education. In other words, instead of going to Europe to see investigative technique and methodology, American physicians could, in the final third of the century and beyond, make use of the museum as a research base with an unprecedented wealth of unique material.

Many Civil War physicians also returned to their local communities with a new appreciation of a science-based practice. The Minnesota Academy of Medicine provides one such example. Dr. Jacob Stewart and

Dr. Daniel Hand, both of Saint Paul, Minnesota, served as brigade surgeons in the Army of the Potomac. Hand later served as medical director of the army in North Carolina, where he treated malarial fevers and combated smallpox with policies of compulsory vaccination. When he encountered an outbreak of typhus fever among Union prisoners of war recently released from Andersonville prison, "he controlled the epidemic" by setting up hospitals in churches so that patients were clean and isolated.[51] After graduating from Harvard Medical School, Dr. George French, who settled in Minneapolis after the war, entered the Union army in July 1862. French was sent first to the general hospital in Alexandria, Virginia, and after the fall of Vicksburg, he was promoted to surgeon-in-chief, where he worked at the Confederate City Hospital and the United States Army Field Hospital at Vicksburg. French, a frequent contributor to the Army Medical Museum, mostly treated cases of acute and chronic dysentery, and he performed numerous postmortems.

During the war all three doctors had an unprecedented medical experience. They performed a variety of surgical operations, which not only gave them practical skills but also allowed them to see the importance of having a "thorough knowledge of anatomy."[52] Thus in 1868, Hand and Stewart set up a series of anatomy courses for medical students in a small stone dead house, which was adjacent to Saint Joseph's Hospital in Saint Paul. When other prominent physicians, including Dr. Alexander Stone, heard about these courses, he offered to create a preparatory medical school to supplement the anatomy courses and the apprenticeship training then common for medical students in Saint Paul. By 1878 the college was expanded into a complete medical school named the Saint Paul Medical School. Along with Drs. Hand, Stone, and Stewart, Dr. French was recruited to the faculty to lecture on genitourinary surgery. At about the same time, Dr. Wheaton, a graduate of Harvard Medical School, and Frederick Dunsmoor, a graduate of Bellevue Medical College, joined the faculty. Almost immediately, Dunsmoor transformed a local hotel into a new hospital he named the Minnesota College Hospital, which operated in conjunction with the medical school.

A variety of surgeries were performed there, including an operation to remove a large ovarian tumor, weighing sixty pounds, which was done in 1882 under carbolic acid—the first operation to be performed under Listerian antisepsis in the Twin Cities. As in the war, the sharing of this knowledge was a central educational objective, and thus Dr. French organized the Unity Club in 1884. Through this association, select physicians delivered papers on a variety of medical subjects (often accompanied by medical specimens), which were followed by a general discussion. The club eventually expanded to become the Minnesota Academy of Medicine, which was organized "for the purpose of professional research and for the association of medical men upon a basis of good fellowship, professional ability and literary merit."[53] By 1886 one of the favorite discussions concerned the methods and efficacy of antiseptic surgeries.

The important point is that Civil War physicians went home with a new appreciation of the complexities and possibilities for medicine, they recognized the importance of collaboration and the dissemination of knowledge, and they brought these ideas to another generation of American physicians. And this was not uncommon. In exactly the same period, John Shaw Billings, another prominent war physician, was mentoring the next generation of physicians in Washington.

Billings, a young contract surgeon in 1861, was regarded as the foremost authority in public hygiene and hospital construction by 1874.[54] The *Boston Medical and Surgical Journal* noted in February 16, 1871, of his essay on ventilation and warming of barracks and hospitals, "As in all recent investigations made at the Surgeon General's Office, the work has been carefully and thoroughly done and the volume adds a valuable contribution to the literature of medical sciences."[55] Billings became medical adviser to the trustees of the Johns Hopkins fund in 1876, drew the plans for the hospital and medical school, and was instrumental in securing William H. Welch and William Osler to the staff. Billings became librarian and curator of the Army Medical Museum in December 1883 and in 1889 the director of the hospital and hygiene laboratory at Johns Hopkins.[56] Perhaps most importantly, however, he had formed valuable relationships during the war that continued afterward. One of these was with Isaac Minis Hays, with whom he worked to bring the International Medical Congress to Washington in 1888. The executive congress committee consisted of Hays, Billings, Bowditch, Da Costa, Leidy, Stillé, Mitchell, and Thomson (all of whom doctored in the war) and younger physicians such as William Osler.[57]

The committee resolved to "extend on behalf of the medical profession of the United States to the International Medical Congress . . . a cordial invitation to have the next International Medical Congress at Washington DC in 1888."[58] Part of the lure of Washington was to tour the Army Medical Museum.[59] The meetings leading up to the congress were held at the museum, and members of the American Medical Association were encouraged to attend. In the correspondence from Billings to Hays, it was noted that "the work of the Congress shall be of an exclusively scientific character" and that the explicit goal was to "discuss matters of science and practice with the medical men of Europe as well as each other."[60] At the opening of the congress, Billings, as president, gave the address: "All of you are interested in medical science, not merely as a means of giving new modes of diagnosis or treatment, but also for its own sake, the sake of knowing, for the pleasure of investigation, and in the hope of helping others . . . and while the majority have devoted themselves more or less to special branches, they have not, in doing so lost interest in what may be for the general good of the whole profession."[61]

In his address he articulated the importance of the most significant and enduring medical legacy of the war, the Army Medical Museum. He observed that over the past decades, the "general government has in its turn done something for medicine and for you by founding the medical library and museum in Washington under the direction of the Medical Department of the Army."[62] He noted, however, that the "object of this address is not to boast of what we have, but to indicate what we want." There was a continuation of ideology that was shaped within the postwar development of the medical sciences. He discussed the importance of experimental pathology, pharmacology, and physiology as a basis for comparison with abnormal pathological specimens obtained from the same animals. The *American Practitioner* observed, "Those who know Dr. Billings' professional ability, zeal and industry need not be told how well he had executed his duty. In the advance which medical science is making, no inconsiderable part must be attributed more especially in reference to pathology and hygiene, to the medical department of the United States Army."[63] While the focus of the collection changed after the war, the objective was to provide support for the scientifically inclined physician, a place to learn, teach, study, and develop medical knowledge from bodies and diseases.

Physicians found identity in the museum but also pride in a new direction for American medicine, believing that "it was the bound duty of the Surgeon General's Office to undertake that scientific work of which enough has already been published to enable the medical profession throughout the world to form a judgment as to its character, and as to the fitness of the medical officers to whom it has been entrusted to accomplish the task which they have undertaken. The medical criticism of the Old World has already proclaimed the verdict, which has been altogether favorable."[64]

Meetings during the war at the Army Medical Museum or the Smithsonian to address wartime medical challenges still carried on, though the focus

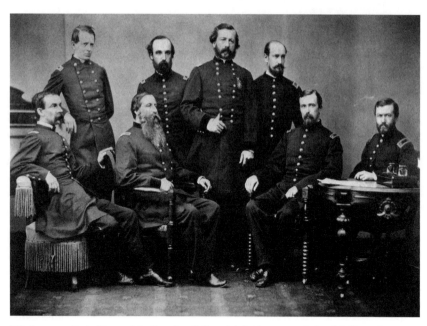

U.S. Army medical officers, 1864. Standing (left to right): Lieutenant Colonel William G. Spencer, Assistant Surgeon Alfred A. Woodhull, Surgeon General Joseph K. Barnes, Assistant Surgeon Edward Curtis; seated (left to right): Assistant Surgeons George A. Otis, Charles H. Crane, John Shaw Billings, Joseph J. Woodward. (Photograph courtesy of the National Museum of Health and Medicine, Washington, D.C.)

shifted to relevant health crises and the means to promote scientific industry or support newer developments. Through the 1870s and 1880s, Billings sent numerous letters to both civilian and military physicians asking for specimens for the museum's collection. He was pleased to receive a five-week-old fetus, for example, from Dr. A. J. Mack, a fetal skeleton and collection of hyoid bones from Dr. Matas, and two cancerous testicles from Henry Ward, which were submitted for study and analysis and contributed to the cabinet.[65] In 1883 Billings observed that "the use of the library and museum by the medical profession of this country continues steadily to increase.... The amount of correspondence connected with this work may be inferred from the fact that over two thousand letters were sent out to fill the many requests for information, books etc. which are constantly coming in."[66] In the absence of more structured medical repositories that could support medical research, the Army Medical Museum and Surgeon General's Office proved important in institutionalizing the medical developments of the war but also in supporting new ones.

In 1893 former Civil War physician George Miller Sternberg, for example, was appointed surgeon general. He had a strong commitment to medical research, especially the emerging science of bacteriology. He had discovered, for example, the pneumococcus for pneumonia in 1881 and in 1883 produced photomicrographs of the tubercle bacillus in the museum's laboratory. In 1892 he published the first American textbook on bacteriology. In 1893 he facilitated the establishment of the Army Medical School (this was also the brainchild of Hammond in 1862), and Major Walter Reed was named curator of the medical museum. The museum, library, and school functioned together and had a wealth of material, which was used for "bacteriological and chemical study in the Army Medical Museum which furnished everything essential for laboratory work."[67]

By the turn of the century, Reed led the team of researchers that discovered, through controlled experiments (on human subjects), that yellow fever was transmitted via a particular species of mosquito, rather than by direct contact. With the establishment of the yellow fever and typhoid commissions in the 1890s, which led to compulsory vaccination and other successful preventatives, the study of bacteriology, reflecting the tide of medical science, gradually overshadowed the study of pathology at the Army Medical Museum. Historians often suggest that American medical science was "launched" at Harvard Medical School in the 1870s and the Johns Hopkins and Michigan medical schools in the 1890s; however, the famous bacteriological discoveries at the medical museum in the 1890s continued the pattern of research that was established during the Civil War in 1862. The medical museum, as Hammond envisioned from its inception, was to be an institution that would support and cultivate the medical sciences in American medicine.

When Joseph Barnes was incorrectly given credit by the Adjutant General's Office for the inauguration of the *Medical and Surgical History of the War* and the Army Medical Museum, Hammond wrote a lengthy and heated demand for credit to the adjutant general: "There are few things in my professional career in which I take more pride than that the ideas of the Army Medical Museum and the *Medical and Surgical History of the Rebellion* were conceived by me, and that both were in successful operation when Dr. Barnes succeeded to the Office of the Surgeon-General."[68] Although Hammond caused a major controversy when he withdrew calomel and tartar emetic from the supply table (which was scientifically correct),[69] he ultimately went on to have a very successful and highly profitable neurology practice in New York.[70] However, his most enduring legacy to American medicine was the medical reforms initiated during the Civil War, which contributed so much to the development of American scientific medicine.

The South, on the other hand, faced a unique set of challenges. Thirty-four hundred doctors served in the Confederate army,[71] and like their northern counterparts, had a medical opportunity of unparalleled scope. Southern physicians practiced in the great military hospitals, such as Chimborazo and Winder, and they were assisted by young medical students called hospital stewards. Dr. Simon Baruch noted that "before ever treating a sick person or even having lanced a boil . . . I was put in charge of a battalion of 500 infantry, with only a hospital steward to assist me."[72] But, as noted earlier, the South was plagued by its lack of resources and lack of institutional support (as in the Army Medical Museum), which inhibited the larger development of medical knowledge production as in the northern model.

The war's effect on the South, then, was different, but no less interesting. Vaccination provides one revealing example.[73] In the North, it was common practice to contract private physicians to produce vaccine crust for the mandatory vaccination of Union soldiers.[74] There was no shortage of physicians in the North, and for a fee many were happy to produce vaccine matter in their home or school laboratories. In the South, however, there was a tremendous shortage of manpower and supplies, and the immediate objective was always to treat and manage the troops after battle. The Confederacy faced enormous difficulties procuring enough "pure" vaccine matter, and case after case of spurious vaccination (secondary infections arising from vaccination) followed routine vaccinations. Spurious vaccination became so problematic in the South that it was made a special subject of investigation.[75] The research program, initiated by Samuel Preston Moore, eventually led to new (and fascinating) ways to produce fresh vaccine (the most interesting was the "travelling laboratory" or rather the manufacture of vaccine directly from a cow).[76] Joseph Jones spearheaded these pioneering experiments, which produced invaluable research on the pathology of vaccination.[77]

The experience of doctoring in the Civil War South, then, had a striking effect on select individual southern physicians. After the war some physicians resumed their rural practices but with a new appreciation of the complexity of medicine and a profound recognition of the experience of doctoring in the war,[78] while others went on to shape medicine not only in the postwar South but also in the North.[79] The full measure of the medical and scientific development in the Civil War South has yet to be explored.[80]

The Union medical model did, however, impact the South. While the South had no comparable institution to the Army Medical Museum during the war, in the postwar period, civil and regular, northern and southern physicians were encouraged to travel to the capital to research the more than "275,000 treatises and original essays" and visit the Army Medical Museum, which by 1876 contained almost 19,000 specimens exhibiting a range of diseases and wounds. As Woodward pointed out, the specimens collected during the Civil War were almost all illustrations of military surgery and of camp diseases. However, since the war, the museum had begun to "acquire a broader scope and we now aim to make it a *National Medical Museum.*"[81]

Joseph Jones, as one example, was extremely impressed with the museum's collection and was thrilled to receive a tour in 1866.[82] Northern physicians were similarly impressed with Jones's wartime research. As the leading researcher in the Civil War South, Jones published his work in northern and southern medical journals but also official northern publications, including the United States Sanitary Commission's *Sanitary Memoirs of the War of the Rebellion* and *Surgical Memoirs of the War of the Rebellion.* American physicians had studied together before the war and again after the war, and sharing new medical knowledge was a definitive step toward reestablishing that brotherhood. Before the resumption of medical schools, medical societies, and journals in the South (many were closed during the war), the publications coming out of the Surgeon General's Office were an exceptionally valuable resource. Moreover, most American doctors went through a life-changing experience with their wartime doctoring, but there were differences in the challenges of each side, and these differences were of professional interest. In other words, the relationship between most northern and southern physicians was not acrimonious but rather collegial. Simon Baruch fondly remembered the fraternity of Union and Confederate medical men during the war, noting that it was "courteous, *yes,* brotherly." There was something remarkable about working together and "being a member of a calling that could so completely obliterate the beastly animosities of warring men."[83]

On May 5, 1867, the American Medical Association held its annual meeting in Washington: "The meeting was in all respects, happy and harmonious. Physicians from all sections from the United States were present and from all accounts, fraternization was conspicuous and complete. As has been urged before in this journal, it was eminently proper that southern physicians should attend this meeting, and no one present can regret the course pursued. Professor Gross, the president, delivered an able address and resigned the chair to W. O. Baldwin of Alabama, who was elected president for the next year. . . . The meeting is said to have been a great improvement on those of the past few years. There was less junketing and more work, and the indications are, that future meetings will contribute, once more, something of real value to the profession."[84]

CONCLUSION

It is not suggested here that because of the Civil War, American medicine was triumphing over all medical challenges in the postwar period. As discussed in the preceding chapter, there were no simple answers about disease germs, and debates between opponents and proponents of the germ theory and laboratory medicine raged for at least two decades after the war. American physicians were challenged by smallpox epidemics, yellow fever, malaria, cholera, typhoid, and typhus fever, and these diseases were on the increase with the rise of immigration in the Progressive Era. In other words, medicine was not transformed overnight. Medical reforms would continue to take shape as part of the "coming of age of American universities" in the 1870s, which variously included more money, better leadership, and increasing support for academic medicine and new ideas.[85] At the same time, states slowly began passing new anatomy laws or strengthening old ones, and the American Medical Association, state licensing boards, local medical societies, and new specialist associations had to define or redefine the larger goals of the profession in the context of their own associations. The war years, however, were important in preparing physicians for this transition. Through their wartime experience, many physicians saw the need but also the efficacy of more stringent requirements in medicine; they were exposed to new scientific techniques and gained a practical experience that could not be overestimated. Moreover, when physicians and medical students, such as William H. Welch, returned home from study overseas in the 1880s and 1890s excited about the potential of laboratory medicine, they found an environment receptive to these possibilities as well.

More than 12,000 physicians (not 100 or 200) served in the Union army[86] and then went home—they delivered babies, treated farm injuries, vaccinated patients, and treated the flu or cases of epidemic disease. Physicians had seen the value of a science-based practice in the Civil War hospitals—this might have meant being part of the bromine or disinfection debates for managing gangrene and erysipelas or cholera. Some physicians prepared multiple specimens, performed autopsies, or did countless amputations and surgeries; others managed diseases such as dysentery, tetanus, and small-pox. Physicians were daily exposed to new medical challenges, and they consulted readily with one another; they saw the possibilities of medical science and experimental methods (crude as they were in the 1860s) and the efficacy of sanitary science, which developed alongside new ideas about contagion. Some of these physicians would go to local medical society meetings, they would engage with other physicians, and during and after the war they were asking increasingly complex questions. Before the authority of the German model of medical science took shape in America, these questions and debates were facilitated through a well-tested infrastructure—not only the new Army Medical Museum and the publications of the Surgeon General's Office but also medical journals and meetings of medical societies—which got stronger through the war, along with new local public health boards, which were also formed during the war and then reshaped after.

The Civil War came at a particularly challenging period for the United States medical profession, but the time was ripe for change. With the number of medical schools and medical societies already in place in the United States, and the increasing push to reform medicine, the war years offered a unique opportunity. Hammond's reforms, beginning with Circular No. 2, paved the way for medical knowledge, study, and practice to develop. But the limitations of pathological anatomy were fairly quickly realized, prompting physicians to develop newer investigative tools, such as histology, microscopy, chemical analysis of disease processes, and physiology, which foreshadowed the importance of laboratory medicine. Civil War medicine was not the medicine of Germany, where laboratory courses were taught by full-time researchers or medical doctors. Rather wartime medicine was one stage in the larger development, stimulating and even demanding new approaches to medical study.

Physicians continually referred back to the importance and value of this early work in suggesting ways that their efforts could continue to shape medicine:

Now the museum is a valuable site for teaching lessons of the past and future, for example, the pathological conditions of most of the diseases and injuries. The wet specimens show the lesions which marked so-called typho-malarial fevers. Study these preparations in light of our recent knowledge of sepsis and bacteriology. Professors in your school will tell you to use knowledge we never had. . . . Now thanks to Joseph Lister and the outcomes of his teaching the limb fares otherwise. But the past helps us judge the present and perhaps foresee the future. Ways to study, extract information and publish what is important and what is not. But each generation is expected to know more than their predecessors.[87]

It is not the intention of this study to assert that all wars are good for medicine, but the Civil War came at a crucial stage providing an unprecedented focus on disease and patients and a growing objectivity in medical study. Elite physicians, trained in Europe or European-inspired, had long wanted to develop scientific medicine, and the wartime culture supported the intellectual current, leading to innovations in the management of disease, diagnoses, experimental medicine, research societies, and a newfound respect for the physician in charge of a specialty hospital. Indeed, one of the most important aspects of Civil War medicine was its support for new epistemological standards in medicine. The medical experience of the war contributed to new ideas about the way in which disease was understood, diagnosed, investigated, and prevented. Physicians wrote case reports and essays, and they were encouraged to publish and disseminate this knowledge through lectures and informal meetings. New ideas and patterns were structured and even institutionalized, because there was a powerful mechanism to ensure that the knowledge was transmitted, creating a community of physicians who could benefit from the wartime networks of knowledge. But "ways of knowing" were multifactorial. Every physician was encouraged to contribute to the national pathological museum and provide either analysis or descriptions of their medical cases, while some were asked to conduct specific investigations into a range of diseases, which often prompted new styles of scientific investigation and experimentation.

These differing perspectives, or rather the varied attempts to develop medical knowledge, elucidate the dynamic atmosphere in which northern physicians functioned and provide insight into the development of scientific medicine in the later nineteenth century. Of course, many physicians never looked through a microscope or engaged in research projects and were content with the more traditional clinical exam and the production of empirical knowledge. But there was an unprecedented number of physicians who wanted to engage in scientific medicine, and in the process a new language permeated medical circles and publications. They produced medical knowledge by studying the minute structures of disease processes, the blood, urine, tissues, and organs in detail and in a physical location away from the living patient, as in the investigations related to gangrene, erysipelas, and cholera.

Living bodies were also used to develop medical knowledge, as seen in the investigations relating to heart disease, neurology, prosthetic development, surgical approaches, diagnostics, and therapeutic trials, which changed basic assumptions about not only how to study disease but also how to structure medicine. Some physicians saw their own limitations in managing disease, while others were encouraged to develop their interest in a particular class of disease, and their published findings and methodology laid a foundation for medical specialism and specialized research. By the third quarter of the nineteenth century, specialist groups and societies began to appear, professional associations were taking shape, state licensing agencies were created, and state after state began passing anatomy acts.

Understanding the complex questions that physicians faced during the Civil War, the response to these challenges, and the way in which this knowledge was produced and transmitted was a crucial stage in the development of scientific medicine in the nineteenth century. The context of what constituted the medical sciences continued to evolve in the postwar period, and numerous former Civil War physicians were important as causes and beneficiaries. Somewhere along the way, their efforts to develop scientific medicine have been lost or downplayed in the larger narrative of nineteenth-century medicine, and in accounting for the medical developments in the later century, most of the attention has been lavished on the next generation of physicians who studied in Vienna and Berlin.

It is true that the Civil War did not produce one "great man," which has perhaps made it difficult to see the importance of the war for medicine as a whole. There was no Pasteur, Koch, Davaine, Schwann, Bichat, or Virchow who emerged from the Civil War hospitals and laboratories. The war's impact was different: it had an important, even transformative effect on the many physicians who took advantage of the opportunities and collectively helped to shape medicine in America. However, many Civil War physicians did go on to assume leading roles in the profession; others engaged in lively correspondence with young physicians (such as Woodward and Welch, Billings and Osler, Keen and Cushing); still others continued to develop their new specialties in the postwar period, and by 1866 there was a more receptive response to both specialization and professionalism. Whatever the specific path, the war experience was an important part of the individual and collective American medical identity in the later nineteenth century.

John Brinton recalled in 1865: "On the 9th of April, 1865, General Lee surrendered the Army of Northern Virginia, and the war was practically at an end. The news was telegraphed from Washington about ten o'clock in the evening, and our city was notified by the screeching of the whistles of the fire engines and by clamor and noise of every imaginable character. The War was over. The great experiment had been made. It had been definitely proven that the United States was a Nation."[88] The American medical profession too was on a new course. The evaluation of the Civil War case histories, medical and surgical specimens on display or in jars in the museum, publications, correspondences, and wartime reminiscences all reveal that the experience of the war had contributed to a new identity as producers of medical knowledge for many American physicians and provided an important catalyst for the development of American scientific medicine.

Appendix

TABLE 1. Summary of 2,642 Cases of Gangrene, Indicating Result and Relative Frequency

Seat of Injury	Recovery	Fatal	Undetermined	Total	Percentage of Fatality	Percentage of Relative Frequency
Flesh wounds of the head, face, and neck	5	7	n/a	12	58.3	60 = 2.2%
Fractures and penetrating wounds of the head, face, and neck	32	16	n/a	48	33.3	60 = 2.2%
Flesh wounds of the trunk	36	32	7	75	47.0	216 = 8.2%
Fractures and penetrating wounds of the trunk	44	97	n/a	141	68.7	216 = 8.2%
Flesh wounds of the upper extremities	47	50	12	109	51.5	2,366 = 89.6%
Fractures of the upper extremities	476	245	14	735	33.9	2,366 = 89.6%
Flesh wounds of the lower extremities	125	127	92	344	50.3	2,366 = 89.6%
Fractures of the lower extremities	596	568	14	1,178	48.7	2,366 = 89.6%
Aggregates	1,361	1,142	139	2,642	45.6	

Source: *Medical and Surgical History* 2:3, 824.

TABLE 2. Numerical Statement of 1,097 Cases of Traumatic Erysipelas

Seat of Injury	Cases	Recovery	Fatal	Undetermined	Regional Percentage
Head, face, and neck	154	107	44	3	14.0
Trunk	57	23	33	1	5.2
Upper extremities	457	259	180	18	41.7
Lower extremities	429	229	193	7	39.1
Aggregates	1,097	618	450	29	

Source: *Medical and Surgical History* 2:3, 852.

TABLE 3. Summary of 334 Cases of Hospital Gangrene, Giving Treatment and Results

Treatment	Total Cases	Recovered	Died	Amputations	Average Duration of Treatment	Percentage of Mortality
Bromine in different ways	152	148	4	n/a	5 days 14 hours	2.6
Pure bromine exclusively	27	25	2	n/a	2 days 22 ½ hours	2.6
Pure bromine in solution exclusively	86	84	2	n/a	6 days 11 ⅓ hours	2.6
Pure bromine after the solution failed	8	8	n/a	n/a	12 days 16 hours	2.6
Pure bromine after nitric acid failed	23	22	n/a	1	3 days 16 ⅓ hours	2.6
Bromine after other remedies failed	8	8	n/a	n/a	2 days 4 hours	2.6
Nitric acid exclusively	13	5	8	n/a	3 days 14 ⅖ hours	61.5
Other remedies exclusively	13	7	5	1	7 days 13 ⁵⁄₇ hours	38.4
Other remedies after bromine failed	4	4	n/a	n/a	n/a	n/a
Aggregates	334	311	21	2	n/a	6.2

Source: *Medical and Surgical History* 2:3, 836.

Notes

ABBREVIATIONS

APS   American Philosophical Society, Philadelphia, Pa.
CPP   Library of the College of Physicians, Philadelphia, Pa.
NARA National Archives and Records Administration, Washington, D.C.
NLM   National Library of Medicine, Bethesda, Md.
NMHM National Museum of Health and Medicine, Washington, D.C.
OHA   Otis Historical Archives, National Museum of Health and Medicine,
          Washington, D.C.

INTRODUCTION

1. W. W. Keen, "An Autobiographical Sketch by W. W. Keen," Reminiscences for His Children; 1912 with additions 1915 (unpublished handwritted draft), p. 126, APS.

2. Hacker, "A Census Based Account of the Civil War Dead."

3. Dupuy and Dupuy, *Encyclopedia of Military History*; Fox, *Regimental Losses in the American Civil War, 1861–1865*.

4. Stevens, *American Medicine and the Public Interest*, 26.

5. Ibid.

6. Ludmerer, *Learning to Heal*.

7. Kaufman, *American Medical Education*, 13.

8. Sappol, *A Traffic of Dead Bodies*, 5.

9. Stevens, *American Medicine and the Public Interest*, 26.

10. Ibid., 27.

11. Regulars tended to view competing sects (and their therapeutic practices) as "erroneous." However, allopathic treatments and therapies were also largely "erroneous." For more on nineteenth-century therapeutic practices, see Rosenberg, "The Therapeutic Revolution"; Rothstein, *American Physicians in the Nineteenth Century*; Warner, *The Therapeutic Perspective*. The term "orthodoxy" refers to the regular physicians. The so-called irregular doctors or alternative sects (Thomsonians, homeopaths, and eclectics) rose in prominence during the early nineteenth century largely due to the disastrous results of heroic medicine. See, for example, Duffy, *From Humors to Medical Science*, chap. 6.

12. Stevens, *American Medicine and the Public Interest*, 30. For more on the Paris Clinical School, see Warner, *Against the Spirit of the System*.

13. Stevens, *American Medicine and the Public Interest*, 30.

14. Warner argues that the ideals of the Paris Clinical School provided the most "powerful source of change in antebellum American medicine" and that the "allegiances to its

epistemological ideals persisted as a crucial ingredient in the reshaping of American conceptions of scientific medicine during the final third of the century." Warner, *Against the Spirit of the System*, 4.

15. Neushul, "Fighting Research," 203–24.

16. Cooter, "Medicine and the Goodness of War"; Harrison, "The Medicalization of War—The Militarization of Medicine"; Cope, "The Medical Balance Sheet of War."

17. Exceptions include, for example, Stevens, *American Medicine and the Public Interest* (the consideration of the impact of World War II on American specialization); Kelly, *War and the Militarization of British Army Medicine*.

18. Ackerknecht, *Medicine and the Paris Hospital, 1794–1848*; Bynum, *Science and the Practice of Medicine*; Cassedy, *American Medicine and Statistical Thinking*; Foucault, *The Birth of the Clinic*; Hannaway and La Berge, *Constructing Paris Medicine*; Gelfand, *Professionalizing Modern Medicine*; Russell C. Maulitz, *Morbid Appearances*; Lesch, *Science and Medicine in France*; Weisz, *The Medical Mandarins*; Duffin, "Vitalism and Organicism in the Philosophy of R. T. H. Laennec"; Jones, "American Doctors and the Parisian Medical World, 1830–1840"; Jones, "American Doctors in Paris, 1820–61"; Smith, "Gerhard's Distinction between Typhoid and Typhus"; Warner, *Against the Spirit of the System*; Warner, "The Selective Transport of Medical Knowledge."

19. Bonner, *Becoming a Physician*; Ludmerer, *Learning to Heal*; Rothstein, *American Physicians in the Nineteenth Century*.

20. Rosenberg, *Explaining Epidemics*.

21. Booth, "Clinical Research."

22. There was much confusion about the results of the experiments due to the "lack of opportunity for American practitioners to observe the disease." Smith, "Gerhard's Distinction between Typhoid and Typhus," 379.

23. Warner, "Physiology," 48–71.

24. Warner, "The Rise and Fall of Professional Mystery," 114. On the eve of the Civil War, regular medicine was still struggling to set the agenda within what Warner has described as a "medical market-place that was remarkably open."

25. Smith, "Austin Flint and Auscultation in America," 129–49.

26. Beginning with William Osler's essays on the impact of the Paris School (see *An Alabama Student and Other Biographical Essays*), there has been an industry looking at the growth (or, more frequently, lack of growth) of hospital medicine in the antebellum era. The American medical community had an almost insignificant proportion of university-educated M.D.s; virtually all practitioners were trained by apprenticeships. One result was a deficit of general education and a lack of widespread conviction in the possibility of scientific progress in medical care. By the 1820s, many leaders were recognizing that competition was harming U.S. medical schools and that the spread of M.D. degrees was not necessarily a reflection of progress in medicine. See Shryock, *The Development of Modern Medicine*, for the first generation of social history. Kett, *The Formation of the American Medical Profession*, was among the best monographs to look at the role of professional organization, but Kett did not find a profession posed for progress. Attention has been given to the generation of medical tourists who went to the Paris hospitals. Russell Jones did yeoman's work to identify them, and John Warner has made a strong case for their leadership, but ultimately Warner follows Rothstein and gives credit to the German tourists and the power of the new science. But

neither the Rothstein nor the Warner narrative, with the exception of reports on a select few, such as Henry Pickering Bowditch, can account for the timing of the social change, which happened before the doctors came home and achieved professional prominence and influence.

27. See, for example, Bynum, *Science and the Practice of Medicine*, 114. Bynum notes, the "clinical opportunities of Paris attracted many ambitious young doctors; however it was the laboratories of the German universities that left their mark"; Ackernecht, *A Short History of Medicine*, 224, notes that "the recovery of medicine in the last decades of the nineteenth century coincided with the rise of leadership of men trained in Germany"; Bonner, "The German Model of Training Physicians in the United States, 1870–1914"; Weisz, *Divide and Conquer*.

28. Blustein, *Preserve Your Love for Science*, 75. She noted almost twenty years ago that the "full measure of the war had yet to be taken." For the past decade, historians have begun to look at the larger impact of the Civil War on American medicine. See, for example, Devine, "Producing Knowledge"; Bollet, *Civil War Medicine*; Rutkow, *Bleeding Blue and Gray*; Schmidt and Hasegawa, *Years of Change and Suffering*; Flannery, *Civil War Pharmacy*; Long, *Rehabilitating Bodies*; Schultz, *Women at the Front*. See also Margaret Humphreys's forthcoming work, *The Civil War and American Medicine*.

29. See, for example, some standard texts of the period that neglect to analyze or include the role of the Civil War: Ackerknecht, "Anti-contagionism between 1821–1867"; Cassedy, *Medicine in America*; Haller, *American Medicine in Transition*; King, *Transformations in American Medicine*; Morantz-Sanchez, *Sympathy and Science*; Rosenberg, *The Cholera Years*; Rothstein, *American Physicians in the Nineteenth Century*; Rothstein, *American Medical Schools and the Practice of Medicine*; Rosen, *A History of Public Health*; Sappol, *A Traffic of Dead Bodies*; Shryock, *American Medical Research*; Warner, *Against the Spirit of the System*.

30. Bruce, *The Launching of American Science*; G. Jones, "Sanitation in the Civil War"; Shryock, "A Medical Perspective on the Civil War."

31. See, for example, Adams, *Doctors in Blue*; Brooks, *Civil War Medicine*; Cunningham, *Doctors in Gray*; Denney, *Civil War Medicine*; Freemon, *Gangrene and Glory*.

32. Green, *Chimborazo: The Confederacy's Largest Hospital*; Rosenberg, *The Care of Strangers*; Lein-Schroeder, *Confederate Hospitals on the Move*; Johns and Page, "Chimborazo Hospital and J. B. McCaw, Surgeon in Chief."

33. See, for example, Faust, "Altars of Sacrifice"; Schultz, *Women at the Front*; Austin, *The Woolsey Sisters of New York*; Giesberg, *Civil War Sisterhood*; Clinton and Silber, *Battle Scars*; Hilde, *Worth a Dozen Men*.

34. Glatthaar, "The Costliness of Discrimination"; Freemon, "The Health of the American Slave Examined by Means of Union Army Medical Statistics"; Humphreys, *Intensely Human*; Steiner, *Disease in the Civil War*; Downs, *Sick from Freedom*.

35. Flannery, *Civil War Pharmacy*; Smith, *Medicines for the Union Army*.

36. Duncan, *The Medical Department of the United States Army in the Civil War*; Dupree, *Science in the Federal Government*; Freemon, "Lincoln Finds a Surgeon General"; Gillett, *The Army Medical Department*; Haller, *Farmcoats to Ford*; Henry, *The Armed Forces Institute of Pathology*; Maxwell, *Lincoln's Fifth Wheel*.

37. There is consensus among historians that the war proved a stimulus for the development of public health in America. See Brieger, "Sanitary Reform in New York City"; Leavitt,

"Public Health and Preventative Medicine"; Duffy, *The Sanitarians*, 110–24; Kramer, "The Effect of the War on the Public Health Movement"; Wintermute, *Public Health and the U.S. Military*.

38. Nudelman, *John Brown's Body*; Laderman, *The Sacred Remains*; Faust, *This Republic of Suffering*; Schantz, *Awaiting the Heavenly Country*; Rable, *God's Almost Chosen Peoples*.

39. Figg and Farrell-Beck, "Amputation in the Civil War"; Kuz and Bengston, *Orthopaedic Injuries and Treatment during the Civil War*; Berman, "Civil War Embalming"; Rutkow, *Bleeding Blue and Gray*.

40. Blustein, "To Increase the Efficiency of the Medical Department," 26. Blustein suggests that the "research sponsored by the Medical Department provided a basis for later development of medical sciences in the United States on a significant scale," but she is proposing further directions for research and thus does not go into detail or demonstrate exactly how knowledge was produced during the war, how individual physicians benefited from the opportunity of the war, and if there was an epistemological departure as a result of the war.

41. Warner, "Physiology," 60.

42. Ibid.

43. Sappol, *A Traffic of Dead Bodies*, 316–19.

44. Ibid., 5.

45. *Congressional Globe*, 37th Cong., 2nd Sess., 1861–62, 997.

46. The Wilson Bill (introduced by Free-Soil Republican Henry Wilson), signed into law April 16, 1862, placed central authority for medicine with the Army Medical Department, which was designed to ensure that professional standards were enforced. See Blustein, "To Increase the Efficiency of the Medical Department," 28–29; Flannery, "Another House Divided."

47. A. M. Woodman to Joseph Barnes, Nov. 23, 1863, Office of the Surgeon General, Letters Received, 1818–1870, entry 12, RG 112, NARA.

48. Ibid.

49. Smith, "Military Medical History," 19.

50. For example, Cassedy discusses the "commercial factor" in nineteenth-century medicine. The physician had to "cope with office records and with the collection of accounts, though he did not do very well at either." He was in "competition for patients with one or more sectarian practitioners, and sometimes made less money than they did." Cassedy, *Medicine in America*, 58–59. See also Starr, *The Social Transformation of American Medicine*, 81–85.

51. Quoted in Breeden, *Joseph Jones, M.D.*, 172.

CHAPTER 1

1. See Rothstein, *American Physicians in the Nineteenth Century*, 55–62.

2. During the summer months of 1861 the sick list routinely averaged close to 30 percent. See Adams, *Doctors in Blue*, 14. The evacuation of troops off the field (lack of an effective ambulance system), preventative medicine, and immediate care in the hospitals were reported as "disastrous." Many of the recruits came from rural or isolated areas and were thus vulnerable to myriad contagious diseases to which they had no immunity.

3. J. T. Calhoun "Narrative of Service," in John Brinton's Manuscripts, 1861–1865, vol. 2, entry 628, RG 94, NARA.

4. Ibid.

5. The department consisted of the surgeon general, thirty surgeons, and eighty-three assistant surgeons; of these, twenty-four surgeons were southern and left the army when the South seceded. See Adams, *Doctors in Blue*, 4.

6. Quoted in Gillett, *The Army Medical Department*, 154.

7. Finley found the purchase of medical books to be an extravagance and refused to spend money on new surgical equipment. Adams, *Doctors in Blue*, 4. Finley sealed his own fate when he refused to cooperate with members of the Sanitary Commission, feeling they were merely "mischief-makers" intruding on the medical department's turf.

8. Gillett, *The Army Medical Department*, 155.

9. Frederick Law Olmsted to Henry Whitney Bellows, Sept. 25, 1861, in *The Papers of Frederick Law Olmsted: Defending the Union*, 202.

10. *The Sanitary Commission of the United States Army: A Succinct Narrative of Its Works and Purposes*, 5.

11. Ibid. See also Adams, *Doctors in Blue*, 6–7.

12. *The Sanitary Commission of the United States Army: A Succinct Narrative of Its Works and Purposes*, 24–27.

13. *Congressional Globe*, 37th Cong., 2nd Sess., 1861–62, 995.

14. Ibid. For more on these debates, see Maxwell, *Lincoln's Fifth Wheel*, 118–29.

15. Hammond studied medicine in William Van Buren's office prior to attending the University Medical College of New York. William Van Buren (a former army surgeon and professor at the University of the City of New York) was a prominent member of the Sanitary Commission and its executive committee. He had a personal friendship with Hammond and was instrumental in garnering support for Hammond's appointment.

16. When Hammond reentered the army, he did so at the rank of first lieutenant (assistant surgeon), the bottom of the promotion list. He was not given credit for his ten years of service.

17. Of the eight original members of the Sanitary Commission, three were primarily scientists. See Dupree, *Science in the Federal Government*, 129.

18. See "William Hammond: Biographical Directory," in *The Papers of Frederick Law Olmsted: Defending the Union*, 96–97. See also "Dr. William A. Hammond," *Harper's Weekly*, Nov. 21, 1863, 748.

19. Letter from William Welch to Edwin Stanton, Apr. 15, 1862, Papers of William Hammond, Personal Papers of Medical Officers and Physicians, box 244, entry 561, RG 94, NARA.

20. Olmsted to John Strong Newberry, Nov. 16, 1861, in *The Papers of Frederick Law Olmsted: Defending the Union*, 229.

21. Blustein, "To Increase the Efficiency of the Medical Department," 25. See also Freemon, "Lincoln Finds a Surgeon General."

22. Silas Weir Mitchell, "The Medical Department in the Civil War: Address before the Physicians Club Chicago, Ills. 1902/March/25," Silas Weir Mitchell Papers, box 17, ser. 7, p. 9, CPP. This draft speech was later published as *The Medical Department in the Civil War: Address delivered before the Physicians' Club of Chicago, February 25, 1913*.

23. Blustein, "To Increase the Efficiency of the Medical Department," 24.

24. By 1888 the government had, in addition to the cost of the building that housed the new Army Medical Museum, put more than $50,000 into the museum. See Billings, "Medical Museums."

25. Circular Letter issued by Hammond, July 27, 1862, Central Office Correspondence, Letters and Endorsements Sent, 1818–1946, vol. 32, p. 25, entry 2, RG 112, NARA.

26. "Information for Persons Desirous of Entering the Medical Staff of the Army," issued by the War Department, Jan. 1860, Circulars and Circular Letters of the Surgeon General's Office, 1861–85, box 1, pp. 5–8, entry 63, RG 112, NARA. Volunteer physicians were examined at the state level, while regulars and those seeking promotion were examined by a national examining board appointed by the secretary of war, Edwin Stanton. See also Gillett, *The Army Medical Department*. Several acts of Congress beginning in August 1861 increased the organization of the regular medical staff. These included provisions for a surgeon general, medical inspector general of hospitals, and sixteen medical inspectors, as well as surgeons, assistant surgeons, volunteer regimental assistant surgeons, acting staff surgeons, acting assistant surgeons, and a corps of medical cadets.

27. "Information for Persons Desirous of Entering the Medical Staff of the Army," Circulars and Circular Letters of the Surgeon General's Office, p. 5–8, entry 63, RG 112, NARA.

28. Ibid.

29. Ibid.

30. Hammond came up with a complicated point system in which the twelve branches of the exam were allotted 100, 80, 50, or 30 points, for a maximum or perfect score of 1,200. If the candidate scored 400 points, he was generally awarded the rank of surgeon, and a score of 300 was needed to become an assistant surgeon.

31. J. B. Brown to LeConte, Jan. 22, 1864, John LeConte Papers, APS.

32. See J. B. Brown to John LeConte, Dec. 11, 1863, ibid., discussing the reforms and the fears of some regarding the merging of volunteers and regulars.

33. Most of these letters can be found in Office of the Surgeon General, Letters Received, 1818–1870, entry 12, RG 112, NARA.

34. Flannery suggests that "when the process got down to the state level, most boards appointed associates and cronies through liberal interpretations of these requirements." See Flannery, "Another House Divided," 486. This may have been true, but the evidence overwhelmingly suggests that the exams were a source of stress and numerous physicians worried about taking them and performing well.

35. Joseph Woodward Papers, RG 363, OHA, NMHM.

36. Quoted in Conway and Stark, *Plastic Surgery at the New York Hospital*, 54.

37. Billings, "Medical Reminiscences of the Civil War," 115.

38. Ibid., 116.

39. Papers of Lavington Quick, Personal Papers of Medical Officers and Physicians, box 471, entry 561, RG 94, NARA.

40. Papers of Roberts Bartholow, Personal Papers of Medical Officers and Physicians, box 38, entry 561, RG 94, NARA.

41. "Thesis of Joseph Woodward on Hospital Gangrene," May 30, 1861, Medical Records, 1814–1919, D file, box 15, entry 623, RG 94, NARA.

42. Ibid.

43. John H. Brinton to Meylert, Dec. 27, 1862, Letterbooks of the Curators, RG 15, OHA, NMHM.

44. Warner, *Against the Spirit of the System*, 215–17.

45. See Rosenberg, *The Care of Strangers*.

46. Ibid., 93.

47. See, for example, Stevens, "Sweet Charity."

48. Register of Surgical Operations, 1862–1865, 1875–82, Christian Street General Hospital, Philadelphia, Pa., vol. 4, entry 559, RG 94, NARA.

49. John Shaw Billings to Mr. L. Casella, May 1864, Medical Records, 1841–93, box 28, D file, entry 623, RG 94, NARA.

50. See Whitman, *The Wound Dresser*, 36.

51. Ibid., 18.

52. Ibid., 43.

53. Ibid. See also Clark, "Inspection of Military Hospitals," 443–44.

54. Warren Webster, "The Army Medical Staff: An Address Delivered at the Inauguration of the Dale General Hospital, Feb. 22, 1865, Worcester, Massachusetts," pamphlet #6065, Historical Collections, Reynolds Library, University of Alabama, Birmingham.

55. Brown, *Medical Department of the U.S. Army from 1775–1883*, 225.

56. Riggs Bank was the first home of the museum. In 1863 the museum moved to Corcoran School House on H Street, in 1866 the museum moved to Ford's Theatre (which the government took over after Lincoln's death), and by 1887 the Army Medical Museum and Surgeon General's Library moved to a new location on the national mall. See "Chronology of Events concerning the Army Medical Museum and Surgeon General's Library," 1–5. Courtesy of the OHA, NMHM.

57. George A. Otis, "Notes on the Contributions of the Army Medical Museum," Feb. 7, 1878, Special Scientific and Historical Reports, 1814–1919, file A, no. 41, entry 629, RG 94, NARA.

58. For more on the Army Medical Museum, see Rhode, "'The extent of these materials is simply enormous'"; Goler and Rhode, "From Individual Trauma to National Policy"; Rhode and Connor, "Curating America's Premier Medical Museums" and "A Repository for Bottled Monsters and Medical Curiosities"; Herschbach, "Fragmentation and Reunion"; McCleary, "Science in a Bottle." The medical museum was an important site of knowledge production in the nineteenth century—it was attached to both medical schools and hospitals, of varying sizes.

59. This was not a new impulse in American medicine. As one example, in 1857 the Pathological Society of Philadelphia organized by Samuel Gross, Addinell Hewson, and S. Weir Mitchell, was formed with the aim of promoting the study of pathology through the exhibition and study of specimens.

60. Circulars and Circular Letters of the Surgeon General's Office, Circular No. 2, issued, May 21, 1862, box 1, p. 23, entry 63, RG 112, NARA.

61. Harris, "Army Medical Museum," 306–7.

62. "Report of the Committee on Military Affairs of the Senate of the United States," made to that body on Feb. 19, 1878, Central Office Correspondence, Letters and Endorsements Sent, 1818–1946, entry 2, RG 112, NARA.

63. Billings, "Medical Museums," 129.

64. L. A. Edwards to W. L. Wells, June 16, 1862, General Central Office Correspondence, Letters and Endorsements Sent, 1818–1946, vol. 30, p. 128, entry 2, RG 112, NARA. Dr. W. L. Wells of Philadelphia noted how much he wanted the opportunity to doctor in the war and hoped to obtain a post of acting assistant surgeon to the new military hospital in West Philadelphia, but he was informed that there was no vacancy. He was, however, offered a contract for general service. See also Blustein, *Preserve Your Love for Science*, 34.

65. Da Costa to Hammond, May 9, 1862, Papers of J. M. Da Costa, Personal Papers of Medical Officers and Physicians, box 144, entry 561, RG 94, NARA.

66. Benjamin Woodward to Hammond, Aug. 23, 1862, Personal Papers of Medical Officers and Physicians, box 657, entry 561, RG 94, NARA.

67. Benjamin Woodward to Barnes, Mar. 11, 1863, ibid. Benjamin Woodward discusses here the benefits associated with hospital medicine, including his development in the areas of microscopy and pathology.

68. Samuel Gross to Surgeon General Finley, Dec. 8, 1861, Personal Papers of Medical Officers and Physicians, box 235, entry 561, RG 94, NARA. He was paid, however. He initially had two contracts with the Surgeon General's Office at $80 each per month. The second contract was annulled, and he then received the standard contract of $100 per month. See Letter to W. S. King from C. H. Alden, Aug. 14, 1862, Central Office Correspondence, Letters and Endorsements Sent, 1818–1946, vol. 32, p. 254, entry 2, RG 112, NARA.

69. Gross to Finley, Feb. 4, 1862, Personal Papers of Medical Officers and Physicians, box 235, entry 561, RG 94, NARA.

70. Samuel Gross to William Hammond, May 7, 1862, Office of the Surgeon General, Letters Received, 1818–1870, box 36, entry 12, RG 112, NARA.

71. Rothstein, *American Medical Schools and the Practice of Medicine*, 49.

72. Ibid., 50.

73. See Rothstein, *American Physicians in the Nineteenth Century*, 110–11.

74. W. W. Keen, "An Autobiographical Sketch by W. W. Keen," Reminiscences for His Children; 1912 with additions 1915, p. 31, APS.

75. Joseph R. Smith to Roberts Bartholow, July 12, 1862, Central Office Correspondence, Letters and Endorsements Sent, 1818–1946, vol. 30, p. 438, entry 2, RG 112, NARA. Smith noted that Bartholow was authorized to hire as many medical men from Newton University Hospital as he may have needed.

76. Quoted in Hasegawa, "The Civil War's Medical Cadets," 5. For a contemporary account of medical officers, cadets, and hospital stewards, including their pay, duties, responsibilities, and the different opportunities offered an individual physician or students, see Grace, *The Army Surgeon's Manual*.

77. Letter dated Nov. 25, 1864, Joseph Woodward Letterbooks, RG 28, OHA, NMHM.

78. Ibid.

79. John Brinton to C. M. McDougall, Jan. 15, 1863, Letterbooks of the Curators, RG 15, OHA, NMHM.

80. The medical, surgical, and microscopial sections of the catalog were published in 1867. The surgical section by Surgeon A. A. Woodhull, the medical section by J. J. Woodward, and the microscopial section by Surgeon E. Curtis. By 1876 the museum's collection had doubled in size. See Woodward, "The Medical Staff of the U.S. Army," 21.

81. See the appendixes of the six volumes of the *Medical and Surgical History* for a detailed list of contributors, including which specimens, photographs, and case histories the individual physicians contributed.

82. *Medical and Surgical History*. For a list of reporters and operators, see 2:2, I–XVI.

83. Woodward and Otis, *Circular No. 6*, 2.

84. This is a small sample. The war's impact was ubiquitous. Most journals at the time devoted at least a third if not half of the contents to war-related medical articles. See especially *American Medical Times, American Journal of the Medical Sciences, Boston Surgical Reporter*.

85. See, for example, Hammond, *Military Medical and Surgical Essays*. Contributors included William H. Van Buren, Elisha Harris, Austin Flint, Stephen Smith, Valentine Mott, and Richard Hodges.

86. Letter to Hammond from Blanchard and Lea, Apr. 11, 1863, Office of the Surgeon General, Letters Received, 1818–1870, box 12, entry 12, RG 112, NARA.

87. Silas Weir Mitchell, "The Medical Department in the Civil War: Address before the Physicians Club Chicago, Ills. 1902/March/25," Silas Weir Mitchell Papers, box 17, ser. 7, p. 20, CPP.

88. This book has relied on a broad range of case files, which indicate how the many different and complementary opinions shaped the discourse and official action taken by the medical department.

89. In the prewar period it was common for the scientific sessions to be open to visitors; however, only society members could attend the private sessions (which generally discussed goals of the profession, business, etc.).

90. According to Marks, "Those who aspired to transcend the limitations of individual investigators turned to surveying a large number of physicians about their experience"; this type of investigation "enjoyed a brief flurry of interest in England and the United States between the 1860s and the 1890s." See Marks, *The Progress of Experiment*, 43–44. He does not mention the war. But he does demonstrate that because collective investigation suggested an equality of observers, the findings were eschewed by critics who suggested that not all were qualified to make "reliable and pertinent" observation. During the war there were fewer critics of collective investigation. It was new and considered a valuable and necessary tool for keeping track of the medical activities of the thousands of doctors and patients who served during the war. The elite used the opportunity to train the less experienced physician.

91. Circulars and Circular Letters of the Surgeon General's Office, 1861–1885, entry 63, RG 112, NARA. See also Grace, *The Army Surgeon's Manual*, part III, "General Orders of the Medical Department," and part VI, "Circulars."

92. Circular No. 5, issued June 9, 1862, Washington, D.C., Circulars and Circular Letters of the Surgeon General's Office, 1861–1885, p. 38, entry 63, RG 112, NARA.

93. Ibid.

94. For the history of case reporting, see Epstein, *Altered Conditions*; Fissell, "The Disappearance of the Patient's Narrative and the Invention of Hospital Medicine"; Iacovetta and Mitchinson, *On the Case*; Sappol, "The Odd Case of Charles Knowlton."

95. For example, many elite physicians kept casebooks, particularly while in Paris. See Warner, *Against the Spirit of the System*. See also Reiser, "Creating Form Out of Mass."

96. Circular No. 10, issued Aug. 10, 1862, Washington, D.C., Circulars and Circular Letters of the Surgeon General's Office, 1861–1885, p. 58, entry 63, RG 112, NARA.

97. W. W. Keen, "Surgical Reminiscences of the Civil War," in *Addresses and Other Papers*, 423–24.

98. Hammond, Circular No. 10, issued Aug. 10, 1862, Washington, D.C., Circulars and Circular Letters of the Surgeon General's Office, 1861–1885, p. 58, entry 63, RG 112, NARA.

99. Billings, "Medical Museums," 31.

100. Woodward, "The Medical Staff of the United States Army and Its Scientific Work," 10.

101. RG 94, entries 621–23, file A (1841–93) and D file (1814–1919), NARA, and RGs 13, 15, 21, 28, 124, OHA, NMHM, have the best collection of unpublished Civil War case histories and specimen reports.

102. Woodward and Otis, *Circular No. 6*, 1.

103. Ibid., 2.

104. Walt Whitman pointed out that a "large number of visitors to the hospitals do no good at all, while many do harm. . . . The surgeons have great trouble from them. Some visitors go from curiosity—as to a show of animals." See Whitman, *The Wound Dresser*, 33. A resolution of the Senate passed July 19, 1861, said that all newspapers were to publish the name and location of each hospital, and the number of sick and wounded of the various regiments, along with the name of the surgeon in charge, in an attempt to make wartime medicine transparent. See Circulars and Circular Letters of the Surgeon General's Office, 1861–1885, p. 42, entry 63, RG 112, NARA.

105. Circular No. 2 also asked that physicians detail the conditions requiring operations, especially amputations and exsections, along with details relating to all "important cases," which were to be reported in full. Circular No. 6 issued by Hammond, July 14, 1862, asked that medical officers in charge of hospitals "make special and careful examination of all convalescents under their charge, and cause all who are fit for duty to be returned at once to their regiments." See Circulars and Circular Letters of the Surgeon General's Office, 1861–1885, p. 52, entry 63, RG 112, NARA.

106. The nonhuman elements or microorganisms drove the development of scientific medicine. Latour, for example, favors a complex theoretical model that stresses the role of nonhuman elements in the process of knowledge formation ("actants"—described as autonomous figures that constitute the material world, such as microbes, technologies, and ideas). Networks of actants emerge that can both depend on and influence each other and can shape ideas. See Latour, *The Pasteurization of France*.

107. Special Orders No. 98, May 3, 1862, assigned Woodward and Brinton to "special duty" in the Office of the Surgeon General. See Hammond to Woodward, May 18, 1862, Central Office Correspondence, Letters and Endorsements Sent, 1818–1946, entry 2, RG 112, NARA.

108. Circular Letter, June 9, 1862, Central Office Correspondence, Letters and Endorsements Sent, 1818–1946, vol. 30, p. 124, entry 2, RG 112, NARA.

109. Joseph Woodward Papers, RG 363, OHA, NMHM.

110. John H. Brinton Manuscript Collection, box 1, RG 124, OHA, NMHM. See also Brinton, *Personal Memoirs*, xvi.

111. John H. Brinton, Sept. 25, 1862, Letterbooks of the Curators, RG 15, OHA, NMHM.

112. He sent orders to Surgeon Lavington Quick, U.S V., Baltimore; Acting Assistant Surgeon Edward Hartshorne, Philadelphia; Acting Assistant Surgeon George Shrady, New

York; Surgeon Middleton Goldsmith, Louisville; Surgeon F. J. Carpenter, Cincinnati; Assistant Surgeon F. L. Town, Nashville; Surgeon John Hodgen, St. Louis; and Surgeon H. S. Hewitt, Army of the Mississippi. Those selected were generally respected surgeons with interest and experience in pathological studies. See also Lamb, *History of the U.S. Army Medical Museum*, 13.

113. Ibid.

114. Ewing, "Experiences in the Collection of Museum Material from Army Camp Hospitals."

115. Brinton, *Personal Memoirs*, 185–86.

116. Woodward to Barnes, June 21, 1864, Outgoing Correspondence, RG 21, OHA, NMHM. By 1864 the government had a financial arrangement with the Adams Express Company.

117. Brinton to R. G. Wood, Oct. 13, 1862, Letterbooks of the Curators, RG 15, OHA, NMHM (to be discussed at length in chapter 5).

118. Report by Brinton to the Surgeon General's Office, 1863, box 1, Curatorial Records: Circulars and Reports, RG 6, OHA, NMHM.

119. Ibid.

120. Joseph K. Barnes Papers, Personal Papers of Medical Officers and Physicians, box 34, entry 561, RG 94, NARA. Barnes replaced Joseph R. Smith, who had been standing in for Hammond, on Sept. 3, 1863. For more on Hammond's removal as surgeon general, see Blustein, *Preserve Your Love for Science*; Freemon, "Lincoln Finds a Surgeon General"; Gillett, *The Army Medical Department*.

121. "Medical Officers Who Have Made Contributions of Worth to the Science of Medicine," Armed Forces Medical Library Document Section, MS B 281, NLM.

122. Circular Letter issued by Joseph Barnes, Feb. 1864, Circulars and Circular Letters of the Surgeon General's Office, 1861–1885, entry 63, RG 112, NARA. See also Billings, "Medical Museums," 134–36.

123. Brinton to R. G. Wood, Oct. 13, 1862, Letterbooks of the Curators, RG 15, OHA, NMHM.

124. See John H. Brinton, "Address to the Members of the Graduating Class of the Army Medical Museum: Closing Exercises of the Session 1895–96, Army Medical School," 599–605, John H. Brinton Manuscript Collection, box 1, RG 124, OHA, NMHM.

125. Ibid.

126. Woodward and Otis, *Circular No. 6*, 7.

127. In particular, in the attempt to understand epidemic diseases physicians were asked to note in the case reports symptoms of the disease, the treatment of those diseases, and the appearances disclosed at the postmortem. See Circular No. 9, issued June 30, 1862, Circulars and Circular Letters of the Surgeon General's Office, 1861–1885, p. 58, entry 63, RG 112, NARA.

128. Woodward, "The Medical Staff and the United States Army," 8.

129. Billings, "On Medical Museums," 18.

130. See Lamb, *History of the U.S. Army Medical Museum*, 76 (he quotes Woodward).

131. John H. Brinton, "Address to the Graduating Class of Jefferson Medical College, April 27, 1892," 2, John H. Brinton Manuscript Collection, box 1, RG 124, OHA, NMHM.

132. Edward H. Smith to William Hammond, Feb. 3, 1863, Reports of Diseases and Individual Cases, file A, entry 621, RG 94, NARA. He also submitted six case studies of wounds

of the right leg, left thigh, inferior maxilla, right shoulder, right tibia, and left humerus after conducting the studies in Ward D at Satterlee General Hospital.

133. Billings, "On Medical Museums," 28. Thus while there were great limitations to medical research before the war, this was an important intervention. See also Ludmerer, *Learning to Heal*, 27–28.

134. "Report of the Surgeon General's Office, Nov. 10, 1862, for Edwin Stanton, Secretary of War," vol. 3 (Jan. 2, 1852–Apr. 25, 1863), entry 46, RG 112, NARA.

135. C. Wagner to John Brinton, Dec. 26, 1862, Incoming Correspondence, RG 13, OHA, NMHM.

136. C. Wagner to John Brinton, Jan. 11, 1863, ibid.

137. C. Wagner to George Otis, Apr. 21, 1865, ibid.

138. Prof. Frances Bacon: Case of General Sherman, Specimen AMM 3604, New Haven, Conn., Jan. 14, 1863, Medical Records, 1814–1919, D file, no. 44, entry 623, RG 94, NARA.

139. James H. Armsby to Joseph Woodward, Nov. 8, 1865, Incoming Correspondence, RG 13, OHA, NMHM.

140. W. W. Keen, "An Autobiographical Sketch by W. W. Keen," Reminiscences for His Children; 1912 with additions 1915, p. 28, APS.

141. Ibid., 29.

142. Ibid., 108.

143. Ibid., 31–32.

144. Ibid.

145. W. W. Keen to John H. Brinton, May 2, 1863, Medical Records, 1814–1919, D file, box 1, entry 623, RG 94, NARA.

146. Ibid.

147. R. Weir to Hammond, Dec. 12, 1862, Incoming Correspondence, RG 13, OHA, NMHM.

148. A. B. Campbell to Hammond, May 9, 1863, Office of the Surgeon General, Letters Received, 1818–1870, box 21, entry 12, RG 112, NARA.

149. Woodward to Alfred Stillé, Jan. 20, 1865, Joseph Woodward Letterbooks, RG 28, OHA, NMHM.

150. Ibid.

151. Woodward to Surgeon M. K. Taylor, Sept. 2, 1864, ibid. Autopsies were similarly important in illustrating to physicians that disease states were specific: similar entities in every body, place, time, region, and locale (in contrast to the individual approach to each patient that dominated before the war).

152. Joseph Woodward to W. L. Faxon, Apr. 4, 1865, ibid.

153. Woodward to Assistant Surgeon Henry Stone, June 14, 1864, ibid.

154. Letter dated May 25, 1864, ibid. Woodward's emphasis.

155. Woodward, "The Medical Staff of the U.S. Army," 22.

156. "Proceedings of Societies," *Cincinnati Lancet and Observer* 8 (1865): 129.

157. Jonathan Letterman to William Hammond, Aug. 8, 1863, Special Scientific and Historical Reports, 1814–1919, box 8, entry 629, RG 94, NARA. Jonathan Letterman, Medical Director of the Army of the Potomac, by General Order, Aug. 2, 1862, established the ambulance and evacuation system, supply system, and field hospital, which became basic models all over the world. See "Medical Officers Who Have Made Contributions of Worth to the Science of Medicine," MS B 281, NLM.

158. Jonathan Letterman to John Brinton, Dec. 4, 1863, Medical Records, 1814–1919, D file, box 1, entry 623, RG 94, NARA.

159. Hartshorne would later go on to do important work related to heart disease. See chapter 4.

160. Henry Hartshorne Papers, CPP.

161. Interestingly, in the 1850s Hartshorne, Joseph Leidy, and S. Weir Mitchell tried to establish a "biological society" for the development of medical science. But it was unable to survive due to the lack of support for scientific medicine already discussed. The war allowed all three of these physicians to pursue and develop their interests in scientific medicine.

162. Henry Hartshorne Papers, CPP.

163. Ibid.

164. Ibid.

165. "Medical Officers Who Have Made Contributions of Worth to the Science of Medicine," MS B 281, NLM.

166. See Chapman, *Order Out of Chaos*, 64–65. Billings also suggests that his introduction to Leidy and the introduction to the microscope were "educational factors of major moment in his subsequent career."

167. Mitchell to Fielding Garrison, Sept. 22, 1913, Silas Weir Mitchell Papers, CPP. Mitchell was also instrumental in securing a position for Billings at the University of Pennsylvania as professor of hygiene.

168. "Medical Officers Who Have Made Contributions of Worth to the Science of Medicine, 7–8, MS B 281, NLM.

169. Ibid.

170. Reports of Diseases and Individual Cases, 1841–1893, box 20, file A, entry 621, RG 94. NARA.

171. Ibid.

172. Ibid.

173. Ibid.

174. See *Medical and Surgical History*, 3:69, for the published case history.

175. Two hundred operations involving trephining (making a hole in the skull in order to reach and remove bullets or bone fragments) were attempted during the Civil War, with a 43 percent survival rate. It was rarely done for closed head injuries at that time. See Bollet, *Civil War Medicine*, 168; Rutkow, *Bleeding Blue and Grey*. For statistics on cranial operations, see *Medical and Surgical History*, 1:193.

176. Cliffburne Hospital, "Special Cases: Surgical," reported by John Shaw Billings, Reports of Diseases and Individual Cases, 1841–1893, file A, nos. 43 and 89, entry 621 RG 94, NARA.

177. Ibid.

178. Ibid.

179. Narrative of Service, John Shaw Billings, Chancellorsville and Gettysburg, Reports of Diseases and Individual Cases, 1841–93, file A, no. 79, entry 621, RG 94, NARA.

180. Ibid.

181. For the best general history of the Civil War, see McPherson, *Battle Cry of Freedom*.

182. Narrative of Service, John Shaw Billings, Chancellorsville and Gettysburg, RG 94, NARA.

183. Ibid.

184. In 1863 repairing serious intra-abdominal wounds was still very new, and surgeons had either to rely on European or American textbooks or to invent new procedures for performing these operations. Surgeons had more success treating these injuries when the intestine was not injured. For more on treating abdominal wounds, see Bollet, *Civil War Medicine*, 173.

185. Narrative of Service, John Shaw Billings, Chancellorsville and Gettysburg, RG 94, NARA.

186. Ibid.

187. Ibid.

188. Ibid.

189. This was a narrative of service; however, many of his cases were recorded in his casebook.

190. Ibid.

191. Quoted in Chapman, *Order Out of Chaos*, 75.

192. Joseph Woodward Papers, RG 363, OHA, NMHM. Just before being assigned duty in Washington, Billings led an expedition to Haiti in which he rescued 371 freed slaves who had been "resettled there and swindled in the process." See Rogers, *Selected Papers of John Shaw Billings*, 3.

193. He prepared a reorganization plan for the Marine Hospital Service, later renamed the Public Health Service, setting public health on a new course; prepared long reports on army hospitals and army hygiene; planned a hospital for the soldiers' home in Washington; became active in the affairs of the American Public Health Association; was elected member of the National Academy of Sciences; built the Library of the Surgeon General's Office; and designed the new hospital, which opened in 1889. He was the chief medical adviser to the president of the university, Daniel Coit Gilman. Billings designed the curriculum and emphasized the history of medicine, keeping records, and the use of physiological and pathological laboratories, which were, in part, based on the Army Medical Museum laboratory. See Rogers, *Selected Papers of John Shaw Billings*, 1–11. See also Special Correspondence, 1862–1887, RG 26, OHA, NMHM.

194. Bynum, *Science and the Practice of Medicine*, 116.

195. Approximately 12,000 physicians served during the war as listed in the 1860 census. See Blustein, *Preserve Your Love for Science*, 25. However, as the war went on, many more physicians served in various capacities. See Silas Weir Mitchell Papers, CPP.

196. Warner, *Against the Spirit of the System*, 109.

197. Billings, "Medical Museums," 134–36.

198. Woodward and Otis, *Circular No. 6*, 139.

199. Billings, "On Medical Museums," 30.

200. See U.S. Army Surgeon General's Office: Correspondence Acknowledging Receipt of Circulars 1–7, box 1, MS C 7, NLM. These were sent to libraries, museums, universities, medical schools, and journals and reflect the confidence among American physicians that donating this material conferred.

201. Joseph Henry to Isaac Minis Hays, Aug. 12, 1865, Isaac Hays Papers, box 1, APS. Henry, who was secretary of the Smithsonian Institution, "specifically recognized the connection of science and warfare." Henry promised that the institution would "continually render

active cooperation and assistance." This assistance ranged from manufacturing "disinfecting liquid" in the chemical laboratory or holding lectures and seminars at the Smithsonian to receiving material for transfer to the Army Medical Museum or hospitals. For more on the Smithsonian Institution during the war, see Dupree, *Science in the Federal Government*, chap. 7.

202. Woodward, "The Army Medical Museum at Washington," 233–39.

203. A report from Dr. Meusal of Gotha, Germany. See Lamb, *History of the U.S. Army Medical Museum*, 73.

204. George A. Otis, "Notes on the Contributions of the Army Medical Museum," Feb. 7, 1878. George Otis was an ideal choice to lead the surgical section of the museum. He obtained his medical degree from the University of Pennsylvania in 1851 and soon after sailed for Paris, where he spent a year studying with Louis, Piorry, Desmarres, Nelaton, Jobert, Velpeau, Cruveilhier, and Andral. He was interested in operative surgery, particularly ophthalmic surgery. See, for example, George A. Otis Papers, RG 226, OHA, NMHM.

205. John Brinton to Joseph Barnes, Aug. 24, 1863, Letterbooks of the Curators, RG 15, OHA, NMHM.

206. Quoted in editorial, *Richmond Medical and Surgical Journal* (Jan. 1867): 66.

207. U.S., Army Surgeon General's Office Correspondence: Acknowledging Receipt of Circular nos. 1–7, MS C 7, NLM.

208. Editorial, *Medical and Surgical Reporter* (Philadelphia, July 2, 1870): 18.

209. Editorial, *Medical Gazette*, 1871, Library of the Surgeon General's Office: Data Relevant to the Library, box 3, MS C 185, NLM.

210. Blight, *Race and Reunion*, 6. See also Faust, *This Republic of Suffering*; Neff, *Honoring the Civil War Dead*.

211. Quoted in editorial, *Richmond Medical Journal* (Jan. 1867): 66.

CHAPTER 2

1. Warner and Rizzolo, "Anatomical Instruction and Training," 403.

2. Sappol suggests that "anatomy conferred authority and legitimacy because it worked: it expanded the technical repertoire and proficiency of medicine." See *A Traffic of Dead Bodies*, 95. For anatomy and medical authority, see also Maulitz, *Morbid Appearances*; MacDonald, *Human Remains*.

3. See Warner, *Against the Spirit of the System*, 13.

4. Ibid., 44.

5. Ibid.

6. See, for example, Circular No. 6: Original and Rough Proof of Circular No. 6, War Department, Reports on the Extent and Nature of the Materials Available for the Preparation of a Surgical History of the Rebellion, Surgeon General's Office, Washington, Nov. 1, 1865," entry 64, RG 112, NARA. By illustrating these cases in the medical history of the war, it was intended as a diagnostic aid and a record of the war but also a recognition of the achievements of the war doctors.

7. Quoted in Ackerknecht, *A Short History of Medicine*, 147.

8. See Reports of Diseases and Individual Cases, 1841–93, file A and bound manuscripts, box 2, no. 1, entry 621, RG 94, NARA. Further, in October 1862, Hammond requested that

surgeons in charge of general hospitals submit reports on cases of special interest, including autopsy reports in "accordance with orders sent out in Circular No. 2."

9. Though Warner does not consider the Civil War, his article discusses the "reciprocal influence between approaches to dissection and concepts of professionalism." See Warner and Rizzolo, "Anatomical Instruction and Training."

10. For medical narrative, see Mattingly and Garro, *Narrative and the Cultural Construction of Illness and Healing*. For identity formation through dissection, see Sappol, *A Traffic of Dead Bodies*. Many homeopathists had formerly been members of the orthodoxy and also dissected bodies; however, the different ways the body was used during the war supported the development of science as practiced by the regulars.

11. John H. Brinton to John L. LeConte, Nov. 15, 1863, Medical Records, 1814–1919, D file, entry 623, RG 94, NARA.

12. The standardized form consisted of six: secto cadaveris (hours after death, rigidity of body, degree of embonpoint, other former wounds or disease, state of body as to composition); head (scalp, calvaruium, meninges, medullary substance); chest (pleural cavities, pericardium, lungs, heart); abdomen (peritoneal cavity, solid viscera, liver, spleen, kidneys, hollow viscera, stomach, intestine, bladder, and ureters); blood in veins and heart, and urine in bladder and before death if possible; remarks (in which there was a large space for impressions). See Medical Records, 1814–1919, D file, box 4, entry 623, RG 94, NARA.

13. Quoted in Rable, *Fredericksburg! Fredericksburg!*, 307.

14. For an excellent account of field hospitals and transport of the wounded in the wake of Fredericksburg, see Rable, *Fredericksburg! Fredericksburg!*, 312–13.

15. "Cases of Post Mortem and Examinations Made at Field Hospital 15th Army Corps by order of Dr. John Woodworth, Medical Inspector of the Army of the Tennessee during the Atlanta Campaign," Reports of Diseases and Individual Cases, 1841–93, box 16, entry 621, RG 94, NARA.

16. "Case of John W. Thompson," submitted by Geo. W. Wilson, ibid.

17. Numerous projectiles, along with bones and wet specimens, were sent to the Army Medical Museum to give a more rounded story of the war.

18. "Case 2792: Gunshot fracture of the Scapula; death of sloughing and exhaustion," submitted by H. M. Bellows, Assistant Surgeon, U.S. Army, "History of Pathological Specimens Forwarded to the Army Medical Museum," Reports of Diseases and Individual Cases, 1841–93, file A, no. 171, RG 94, NARA. Hypostatic congestion refers to the congestion of a dependent part of the body or an organ due to gravitational forces, such as venous insufficiency.

19. Ibid.

20. Ibid.

21. "Case of Henry Johnson," submitted by Frederick Hohly, Surgeon of the 37th Ohio Volunteers, ibid.

22. Ibid.

23. For a brief but well-done discussion of Civil War hospitals, see Schultz, *This Birth Place of Souls*, 1–51.

24. John LeConte Papers, Correspondence, APS.

25. The hospital was opened on June 9, 1862, in honor of Surgeon Satterlee (oldest surgeon in the service in the United States at the time and medical purveyor of New York). Satterlee

was a large pavilion hospital (the largest military hospital while in operation) and had a capacity of 3,519. For a brief history of the hospital, see West, *History of U.S.A. General Hospital*.

26. "Reports of Surgical Cases at Kennedy's, Keen's and Smith," Reports of Diseases and Individual Cases, 1841–1893, no. A-15, entry 621, RG 94, NARA.

27. Today we might have a different understanding of postoperative pneumonia.

28. "Specimen Histories, Douglas Hospital," submitted by Assistant Surgeon William Thomson, June 1863, Reports of Diseases and Individual Cases, 1841–1893, file A, no. 103, entry 621, RG 94, NARA.

29. Ibid.

30. Sappol, *A Traffic of Dead Bodies*, 53.

31. Quoted in Sappol, "The Odd Case of Charles Knowlton," 463. Sappol suggests that the "paradigmatic medical science was anatomy, the study of human bodies based on the dissection of cadavers."

32. *Medical and Surgical History*, 3:818–19. There were 509 cases of tetanus among the Union forces (89 percent fatal).

33. Joseph Leidy, "Post Mortem Examinations at Satterlee Hospital," Reports of Diseases and Individual Cases, 1841–1893, no. A-17, entry 621, RG 94, NARA.

34. Case 123, Zach Banbier, private, Company K, 136th New York, ibid. Before the war, Leidy conducted research into whether there was bacteria present in the intestine, which he conclusively demonstrated.

35. Joseph Woodward Papers, RG 363, OHA, NMHM.

36. Joseph Leidy, "Post Mortem Examinations at Satterlee Hospital," case 136, Henry A. Fellows, private, Company C, 12th New York Cavalry. Reports of Diseases and Individual Cases, 1841–1893, no. A-17, entry 621, RG 94, NARA.

37. Case Report Submitted by W. W. Keen from Satterlee Hospital, Reports of Diseases and Individual Cases, 1841–1893, file A, no. 210, entry 621, RG 94, NARA.

38. *Medical and Surgical History*, 3:762.

39. Case Report Submitted by W. W. Keen from Satterlee Hospital.

40. Ibid.

41. Ibid.

42. Ibid.

43. He also routinely made woodcuts of photographs of the brain. See J. C. Dalton to Keen, Feb. 22, 1863., W. W. Keen Correspondence, box. 1, CPP.

44. "Clinical Notes on Cases Seen at the Douglas Hospital at Washington, D.C. during the late Civil War," submitted by William F. Norris, CPP.

45. Pyemia is an infection that spread into the bloodstream and was referred to during the war as either pyemia or blood poisoning. The disease was easily recognizable and was characterized by red, hot, swollen, and very sore skin. In trying to ascertain the cause of the disease, many physicians employed the microscope to understand the nature of symptoms we know now were primarily caused by bacterial infection.

46. "Clinical Notes on Cases Seen at the Douglas Hospital at Washington, D.C. during the late Civil War," submitted by William F. Norris, CPP.

47. Ibid.

48. The number and range of cases that he submitted illustrate his desire to master the diseases that ravaged the internal body (both as related to cause of death and otherwise).

49. H. Wood, "Synopsis of Autopsies made at Lincoln General Hospital," *Proceedings of the Pathological Society of Philadelphia* (Jan. 1865): 133–42.

50. "Report of Surgical Cases by R. B. Bontecou," Reports of Diseases and Individual Cases, 1841–1893, file A, no. 449, entry 621, RG 94, NARA.

51. Ibid.

52. Ibid.

53. This is a 300-year-old story, and the work of Liebig, Virchow, Pasteur, Koch, and Lister, among others, makes up a very tiny but significant part of the story. For one of the best syntheses of the history of medicine, see Bynum, *Science and the Practice of Medicine*.

54. For the development of the laboratory in medicine, see Cunningham and Williams, *The Laboratory Revolution in Medicine*; Bynum, *Science and the Practice of Medicine*; Geison, *The Private Science of Louis Pasteur*; Brock, *Robert Koch*.

55. Tangible proof was not presented until 1883, when Robert Koch conducted a clinical trial among 120 patients with tuberculosis. Physicians examined matter coughed up from the lungs and found TB bacilli in all the cases. This proof did much to support the possibility that disease could be combated by using the existence of the microorganisms as the starting point for treatment or diagnosis. See Reiser, *Medicine and the Reign of Technology*, 88.

56. See Worboys, *Spreading Germs*, for a very well done and accessible elucidation on the multiple "germ theories" of the period.

57. See Breeden, *Joseph Jones, M.D.*, 205.

58. Some historians suggest the "laboratory revolution" in medicine depended on a central agent of technology: the microscope. See Davis, *Medicine and Its Technology*; Maulitz "The Pathological Tradition"; Bracegirdle, "The Microscopial Tradition"; Reiser, *Medicine and the Reign of Technology*.

59. Circular No. 12, Oct., 20, 1862, "Directions Concerning the Manner of Obtaining and Accounting for Medical and Hospital Supplies for the Army with a Standard Supply Table," Circulars and Circular Letters of the Surgeon General's Office, 1861–1885, p. 114, entry 63, RG 112, NARA.

60. Circular Letter Issued by William Hammond, Mar. 23, 1863, ibid.

61. Ibid.

62. Reiser, *Medicine and the Reign of Technology*, 79. There were also concerns over how specific diseases should be diagnosed and recorded. See La Berge, "Dichotomy or Integration?," 275–312.

63. Woodward to Dr. H. Wintz, Nov. 26, 1865, Joseph Woodward Letterbooks, RG 28, OHA, NMHM.

64. Benjamin Woodward, for example, used his own, which was an Oberhauser, and he had a Roisis on loan; but he asked for a new microscope from the government since his were "not as good" as he needed. See Benjamin Woodward to John H. Brinton, Jan. 2, 1863, Medical Records, 1814–1919, D file, no. 196, entry 623, RG 94, NARA. Goldsmith also asked for a new microscope since the one he ordered from Paris "had not yet arrived." Letter from Goldsmith to Brinton, Mar. 8, 1863, ibid.

65. During the war, microscopes were employed mostly in clinical observation, with the exception of the Army Medical Museum and a few select laboratory researchers who used the microscope primarily as a research tool. See Woodward to Dr. H. Wintz, Nov. 26, 1865,

Joseph Woodward Letterbooks, RG 28, OHA, NMHM. It was quite common in the 1860s and 1870s to use the microscope to settle diagnostic questions. See Reiser, *Medicine and Reign of Technology*, 80.

66. Elliot Cous, Assistant Surgeon, Mount Pleasant Hospital, to Hammond, Mar. 24, 1863, Office of the Surgeon General, Letters Received, 1818–1870, box 65, entry 12, RG 112, NARA.

67. Elias J. Marsh, Judiciary Square Hospital, Washington, to Hammond, Jan. 7, 1863, ibid.

68. Adam Hammer, Assistant Surgeon, United States Volunteers, General Hospital New House of Refuge, Saint Louis, Mo., to Hammond, Dec. 30, 1862, box 42, ibid.

69. C. A. Cowgill, Stanley General Hospital, New Berne, N. Carolina, to Hammond, June 23, 1863, box 21, ibid.

70. D. L. Huntington, Post Hospital, Monroe, Va., to Hammond, Feb. 10, 1863, box 22, ibid.

71. Roberts Bartholow, "A Report on Camp Measles," *American Medical Times* 8 (1864): 231–32.

72. Papers of Middleton Goldsmith, Personal Papers of Medical Officers and Physicians, box 223, entry 561, RG 94, NARA. He was appointed superintendent of hospitals at Louisville, Ky., Feb. 1863.

73. Middleton Goldsmith to Hammond, Nov. 4, 1862, Office of the Surgeon General, Letters Received, 1818–1870, box 36, entry 12, RG 112, NARA.

74. Papers of Middleton Goldsmith, Personal Papers of Medical Officers and Physicians, box 223, entry 561, RG 94, NARA. He was assigned duty as assistant medical director in Louisville, Oct. 3, 1862.

75. Middleton Goldsmith to Hammond, Nov. 4, 1862, Office of the Surgeon General, Letters Received, 1818–1870, box 36, entry 12, RG 112, NARA.

76. See Bynum, *Science and the Practice of Medicine*, 123.

77. Virchow's *Cellular Pathology* was not a treatise but rather a record of twenty lecture-demonstrations given by Virchow in February, March, and April of 1858 to an audience interested in the state of medical science and disease theories at the time, and the focus was on the cells. Other conferences leading up to this one had focused on the tissues and/or organs, and this singular focus on the cell was of particular interest in the 1850s. See introduction by Rather in *Cellular Pathology*, vii.

78. Bynum, *Science and the Practice of Medicine*, 123–24. See also Rather, in Virchow, *Cellular Pathology*, xv.

79. Rudolph Virchow, "Cells and Cellular Theory," Lecture One, Feb. 10, 1858, in *Cellular Pathology*, 27–50. Virchow's student, Julius Cohnheim, further developed Virchow's ideas, particularly the study of disease processes in the various stages of disease. See Worboys, *Spreading Germs*, 32.

80. Woodward, review of *Cellular Pathology* by Rudolph Virchow, 465.

81. The Army Medical Museum was clearly devoted to research, but some hospitals were also equipped with rudimentary laboratories for research, or basic research was conducted in the autopsy rooms of the hospitals. For example, Lincoln Hospital had an operating room, a cupboard for instruments including a microscope, and a "Dead House and Pathological Department" divided into three rooms, for bodies, postmortem, and plaster casts. Operators were employed at $100 per month for surgical cases and for the preparation of pathological specimens. See Circular No. 6: Original and Rough Proof of Circular No. 6,

Surgeon General's Office, Washington, Nov. 1, 1865, entry 64, RG 112, NARA. See handwritten report entitled "The Organization of Lincoln Hospital."

82. See Ackerknecht, *A Short History of Medicine*, 157. See Bynum, *Science and the Practice of Medicine*, 114–17. Between 1880 and the First World War more than 15,000 American physicians studied in Germany, and thus there was naturally a strong German influence in the United States.

83. Woodward to Rudolph Virchow, May 14, 1864, Joseph Woodward Letterbooks, RG 28, OHA, NMHM.

84. Ibid.

85. Ibid.

86. Rather, "Cellular Pathology," introduction, xxi.

87. Woodward to Rudolph Virchow, May 14, 1864, Joseph Woodward Letterbooks, RG 28, OHA, NMHM.

88. Ibid.

89. Ibid.

90. See Reiser, *Medicine and the Reign of Technology*, 79.

91. Woodward, Circular No. 6: Original and Rough Proof of Circular No. 6, 156. Woodward's handwritten rough draft.

92. Ibid.

93. Ibid., 159. Beale, as a professor at King's College, also pioneered differential staining techniques, but Woodward criticized Beale for making errors by "confining his observations on the tissues of his preparations soaked in carmine and mounted in glycerin instead of extending them to the equally careful study of other methods." Ibid., 159. In his 1858 book *The Microscope in Its Applications to Practical Medicine*, Beale described the cell as a perfectly closed sac containing a nucleus, which in turn usually contained a clear bright spot, the nucleolus; see Beale, chap. 4. Woodward may have seen Beale's work firsthand. On June 16, 1865, he sent J. W. Queen to England to exchange a section of the scalp and ulcerated intestine prepared with moderate magnifying power. Woodward also asked for "specimens showing the termination of the nerves, the structure of cartilage of connective tissue," and Queen was authorized to "pay whatever he demands within reason." See, for example, Woodward to Queen, June 16, 1865, Joseph Woodward Letterbooks, 1865, RG 28, OHA, NMHM.

94. Woodward to Rudolph Virchow, May 14, 1864, Joseph Woodward Letterbooks, RG 28, OHA, NMHM.

95. Ibid.

96. George Otis to Joseph Barnes, July 1, 1864, Curatorial Records: Circulars and Reports, box 1, RG 6, OHA, NMHM.

97. Quoted in Henry, *The Armed Forces Institute of Pathology*, 90.

98. Woodward's effort to develop investigative medicine represents a specific cast of mind. There was a strong sense in the mid- to late nineteenth century that microscopic expertise could transform medicine—once microscopy was effectively mastered. As "evidence of increasing specialization within medical science," Rudolph Albert von Kolliker gave up "his joint chair in physiology and comparative anatomy in 1864 to concentrate his energy on microscopial work," believing his findings would transform medicine. See Bynum, *Science and the Practice of Medicine*, 100–101. Woodward similarly suggested that

mastery of microscopy, photomicrography, and histology would lead to better diagnosis and treatment for Civil War soldiers.

99. Joseph Woodward Papers, RG 363, OHA, NMHM.

100. Woodward, "The Army Medical Museum," 237.

101. Davis, *Medicine and Technology*, 146.

102. Maddox is best known for producing the first workable dry plates using gelatin as the medium to hold the silver bromide. See, for example, Capa, *The International Center of Photography Encyclopedia of Photography*, 317; Lenman, *The Oxford Companion to the Photograph* (includes a short biography on Richard Leach Maddox).

103. Woodward to Maddox, thanking him for the photomicrographs he presented to the museum, Nov. 10, 1866, Joseph Woodward Letterbooks, RG 28, OHA, NMHM.

104. Woodward requested that the apparatus "consist of a heavy base board of black walnut, at the end of which is to be an arrangement for clamping fast the microscope of your make which is in use here (it is no. 36) at the other end a platform on which a four by four photographic camera box can slide. This box must have a draw of eight inches; its front is to be made to receive the eye piece end of the microscope with or without the eyepiece by a joint which will exclude light. The following points require care: The center of the ground glass of the camera to be centered with the microscope. The camera to slide back and forth without lateral motion and so that it can be clamped in the position required, the ground glass meanwhile being always perpendicular to the axis of the microscope. The whole to be made of black walnut oiled." Woodward to M. Zentmeyer, Nov. 19, 1864, Joseph Woodward Letterbooks, RG 28, OHA, NMHM.

105. There was to some extent an obsession with the "means of production," perhaps because the objects were so difficult to see, manage, and understand. For more on the idea on technological apparatus and the scientific gaze, see Cartwright, *Screening the Body*.

106. Woodward to the New York Microscopial Society, May 20, 1868, Joseph Woodward Letterbooks, RG 28, OHA, NMHM.

107. Diatom resolution test included looking at Pleurosigma angulatum or Frustulia rhomboids to check the quality of their lenses and microscope expertise.

108. Woodward to M. Zentmeyer, Jan. 28, 1864, Joseph Woodward Letterbooks, RG 28, OHA, NMHM.

109. Woodward to R. L. Maddox, Mar. 25, 1867, ibid.

110. Woodward to M. Wales, June 25, 1866, ibid.

111. Woodward to R. L. Maddox, Nov. 10, 186, ibid.

112. Woodward to R. L Maddox, June 17, 1867, ibid.

113. Woodward to A. M. Edwards, Feb. 15, 1866, ibid.

114. Woodward to Heinrich Frey, Aug. 31, 1866, ibid.

115. Woodward to T. Murmich, June 26, 1866, ibid.

116. Woodward to Keen, Mar. 25, 1867, ibid.

117. William Olser, as one example, often wrote John Shaw Billings and asked to see and draw specific specimens. See letters to Billings, Incoming Correspondence, RG 13, OHA, NMHM.

118. Rufus King Brown to Woodward, May 28, 1866, Joseph Woodward Letterbooks, RG 28, OHA, NMHM.

119. Woodward to A. M. Edwards, Dec. 18, 1867, ibid.

120. Civil War physicians often used the terms "diarrhea" and "dysentery" to mean the same thing (though dysentery was often differentiated by the blood in the stools). *Medical and Surgical History*, 4:401–2, 799–800.

121. Woodward and Otis, *Circular No. 6*, 118.

122. Woodward to Virchow, May 14, 1864, Joseph Woodward Letterbooks, RG 28, OHA, NMHM.

123. Woodward, "On the Use of Aniline in Histological Researches," 109.

124. Woodward and Otis, *Circular No. 6*, 147.

125. Ibid., 151.

126. Bynum, *Science and the Practice of Medicine*, 126.

127. Woodward and Otis, *Circular No. 6*, 151.

128. Woodward, Circular No. 6: Original and Rough Proof of Circular No. 6, 150–160. Woodward's handwritten rough draft.

129. In the years after the war, Woodward remained, however, skeptical about bacteria in the cause of disease. For Woodward's skepticism of bacteria, see Henry, *The Armed Forces Institute of Pathology*, 66–68. For more on medical progress and technology, see Bynum, *Science and the Practice of Medicine*, 148.

130. Woodward and Otis, *Circular No. 6*, 148.

131. The new dye industry was developed in Germany in 1862, and as a result synthetic colors were used to stain tissues and organs for microscopic examination. Woodward made these discoveries independently. See Henry, *The Armed Forces Institute of Pathology*, 34.

132. It is significant that in this article he devotes two paragraphs to his earlier method, which he found less effective (it involved cutting sections of intestines, which were soaked and dried). He found after drying they changed shape, that it was difficult to cut good sections without the follicles chipping off and that the sections often became disfigured by the oil drops. This again could be effective for new researchers or less experienced physicians to use as a guide.

133. Woodward to H. E. Brown, Nov. 26 1865, Joseph Woodward Letterbooks, RG 28, OHA, NMHM.

134. Woodward, "On the Use of Aniline in Histological Researches," 110.

135. Ibid.

136. Being able to use different colors for different sections provided the contrast Woodward wanted when studying tissues.

137. Woodward, "On the Use of Aniline in Histological Researches."

138. Ibid., 107.

139. Henry, *The Armed Forces Institute of Pathology*, 36.

140. Woodward, "On the Use of Aniline in Histological Researches," 113.

141. He used a freezing microtome manufactured by R & J Beck, 1865. Quick freezing techniques did not become common until well into the 1880s, though they had been used in Europe since the 1820s.

142. Woodward and Curtis created a photomicroscopic apparatus and first used sunlight as the source of illumination, which was reflected by a heliostat. The light passed through a copper ammoniosulfate solution light filter before passing through the specimen. The image was projected through the microscope, the eyepiece now a concave lens, onto a movable plate holder. He later pioneered the use of artificial light sources (magnesium and

electric lights). See Rapkiewicz, Hawk, Noe, and Berman, "Surgical Pathology in the Era of the Civil War."

143. Woodward and Otis, *Circular No. 6*, 146.

144. Ibid., 148.

145. Fox and Lawrence, *Photographing Medicine*, 23.

146. Reiser, *Medicine and the Reign of Technology*, 87.

147. Quoted in ibid., 87. See also Daston and Galison, *Objectivity*, 164.

148. For more on "objectivity" in the nineteenth century, see Daston and Galison, *Objectivity*, especially chaps. 2, 3, 4.

149. Woodward to Dr. Sam Jones, Microscopial Society, Dec. 12, 1865, Joseph Woodward Letterbooks, RG 28, OHA, NMHM. This letter outlines the types of experiments they were performing at the museum. He notes that he found yellow the best "because a very short exposure does the work."

150. Woodward, "The Army Medical Museum," 237.

151. Thomson Photomicrographs, RG 330, OHA, NMHM.

152. Woodward to J. C. Derby, Aug. 23, 1866, Joseph Woodward Letterbooks, RG 28, OHA, NMHM. Woodward notes that the photomicrographs should be "displayed on a table, under glass, a space of 10 feet long by 4 inches wide." See also "International Exposition of 1876, Medical Department Photographs," RG 76, OHA, NMHM; and Curatorial Records: Expositions," RG 12, OHA, NMHM; Otis, *Photographs of Surgical Cases and Specimens*.

153. *The Toner Lectures*. Most of these lectures were reprinted or reviewed in numerous national and international medical journals. Woodward's article, for example, was published and/or reviewed in the *Edinburgh Medical Journal*, 1874; *Philadelphia Medical Times*, 1873–74; *Atlanta Medical and Surgical Journal*, 1873–74; and *American Journal of the Medical Sciences*, 1874.

154. *The Toner Lectures*.

155. Joseph Woodward, "On the Structure of Cancerous Tumors, and the Manner in Which Adjacent Parts Are Invaded, delivered March 28, 1873," in *The Toner Lectures*, 2.

156. *The Toner Lectures*.

157. Joseph Woodward, "On the Structure of Cancerous Tumors, and the Manner in Which Adjacent Parts Are Invaded, delivered March 28, 1873," in *The Toner Lectures*. See also Joseph Woodward's Photomicrographs, RG 83, OHA, NMHM.

158. Joseph Woodward, "On the Structure of Cancerous Tumors, and the Manner in Which Adjacent Parts Are Invaded, delivered March 28, 1873," in *The Toner Lectures*. For a complete list of the 74 photomicrographs exhibited during the lecture, see pp. 37–40. The photomicrographs illustrate with remarkable thoroughness the atlas of cancer of the breast.

159. Ibid., 35.

160. Toward the end of the century, medical schools began reforming their curriculums by adding courses (e.g., clinical medicine, microscopy, anatomy, physiology, comparative osteology, pathological anatomy, surgery) that had been traditionally covered in private courses. Faculties were also expanded to meet the new needs of the schools. For more on medical education in the later nineteenth century, see Numbers, *The Education of American Physicians*. See also Rothstein, *American Physicians in the Nineteenth Century*.

161. Woodward, Circular No. 6: Original and Rough Proof of Circular No. 6, 156. Woodward's handwritten rough draft.

CHAPTER 3

1. Extract from a Report of Hospitals at Nashville, Tenn., Apr. 30, 1863, Frank H. H. Hamilton, Med. Inspector, USA, Medical Records, 1814–1919, D file, box 3, entry 623, RG 94, NARA.

2. For more on the hospitalism crisis in the nineteenth century, see Loudon, *Death in Childbirth*.

3. Professor William Pepper, University of Pennsylvania, noted that erysipelas meant "to draw near or to approach," which was intended to designate its migratory peculiarities. He also referred to it as St. Anthony's fire to illustrate the inflammation of the skin and redness. Herbert Marshall Howe Papers, from his personal notebook, "Notes upon the Lectures Delivered by Prof. William Pepper on the Theory and Practice of Medicine, 1863," CPP.

4. As a result of the extensive mortality that resulted from these diseases, Hammond ordered select physicians to investigate erysipelas, gangrene, and pyemia. See, for example, Medical Records, 1814–1919, D file, entry 623, RG 94, NARA, especially boxes 3–15, for case histories and reports fulfilling Hammond's directive. See also Special Order 182, Curatorial Records: Circulars and Reports, 1863–1864, RG 6, OHA, NMHM.

5. *Medical and Surgical History*, 5:824.

6. By the 1890s these diseases were known to be infectious. Bacteria appeared in clusters resembling a string of beads. Types of this bacteria cause common diseases such as pneumonia (and so spread early in hospitals). *Staphylococcus aureus* may also cause gangrene and often works with strep A. Other aerobic and anaerobic pathogens may be present, including Bacteroides, Clostridium, Peptostreptococcus, Enterobacteriaceae, Coliforms, Proteus, Pseudomonas, and Klebsiella, making the disease very virulent (these pathogens have been isolated as causes of necrotizing fasciitis or flesh-eating disease, a modern-day equivalent).

7. Bollet, *Civil War Medicine*, 201. This may have been due to the fact that several organisms worked together to produce a particularly deadly infection. As a result of the various organisms, the clinical course often varies from patient to patient.

8. Ibid.

9. *Medical and Surgical History*, 5:823.

10. The most common cause identified is *Streptococcus pyogenes*.

11. Lavington Quick Papers, "Symptoms, Diagnosis, Pathology and Treatment for Erysipelas," Personal Papers of Medical Officers and Physicians, box 471, entry 561, RG 94, NARA.

12. Ibid.

13. See also "Notes upon the Lectures Delivered by Prof. William Pepper on the Theory and Practice of Medicine, 1863," Herbert Marshall Howe Papers, CPP.

14. This chapter is concerned with how physicians learned and developed medical knowledge; thus, case reports and essays are examined and at times quoted in detail. There remains room, however, for greater study of the patient perspective.

15. In her excellent study, Susan Lederer examines the history of human experimentation within a transforming medical science in the later nineteenth century. See Lederer, *Subjected to Science*. But the mind-set about how to produce knowledge shifted for some physicians during and because of the war, which she does not consider. Many of the physicians

that she does examine, including Keen and Roberts Bartholow, began using humans as investigative material during the war. This chapter aims to give greater historical reflection on the development of investigative medicine in the nineteenth century, particularly therapeutic investigations.

16. Jordan Goodman, Anthony McElligott, and Lara Marks argued that the "concept of usefulness is the point of contact between human experimentation, knowledge and the state." See Goodman et al., *Useful Bodies*, 2. During the Civil War, the government similarly laid claim to the bodies of soldiers for its own needs. Circulars were issued supporting and sanctioning the investigation of the body, clinical trials were funded, and this knowledge was widely transmitted. There was also a new social responsibility. Patients were no longer treated at home but rather in the newly formed government hospitals, and the public expected a certain efficacy from the medical profession.

17. Many physicians had never seen a well-marked case of gangrene, although between 1840 and 1860 there were well-documented cases of erysipelas. See Loudon, *Death in Childbirth*, 71–72.

18. "Thesis of Joseph Woodward on Hospital Gangrene," May 30, 1861, Medical Records, 1814–1919, D file, box 15, entry 623, RG 94, NARA.

19. See McPherson, *Battle Cry of Freedom*, 474–75.

20. It was estimated that 108,049 wounds, or 76 percent, were caused by the minié ball. See *Medical and Surgical History*, 3:696.

21. "Circular and Letter in Regard to Hospital Gangrene," Mar. 14, 1863, Medical Records, 1814–1919, D file, box 15, no. 253, entry 623, RG 94, NARA. See also Special Order 182, Curatorial Records: Circulars and Reports, 1863–1864, RG 6, OHA, NMHM.

22. "Circular and Letter in Regard to Hospital Gangrene," Mar. 14, 1863, Medical Records, 1814–1919, D file, box 15, no. 253, entry 623, RG 94, NARA.

23. Mitchell, "The Medical Department in the Civil War: Address before the Physicians Club Chicago, Ills. 1902/March/25," Silas Weir Mitchell Papers, box 17, ser. 7, p. 7, CPP.

24. Goldsmith, "A Report of Hospital Gangrene in Nashville and Murfreesboro," July 12, 1863, Reports of Diseases and Individual Cases, 1841–93, file A, no. 261, entry 621, RG 94, NARA.

25. Goldsmith, *A Report on Hospital Gangrene, Erysipelas and Pyaemia*, 17.

26. Woodward, *Outlines of the Chief Camp Diseases*, 13–27. The classification "zymotic" was introduced by William Farr in the 1840s (though he drew on Justus von Liebig's chemical theories of disease), and the label covered most infectious and contagious diseases. Disease was thought to be caused by some organic particle that was ingested and, when combined with the internal body, started a process of decay. These ideas would lay the foundation for bacteriology to develop, especially the idea that "small entities of life" could cause disease. See Waller, *The Discovery of the Germ*, 55–57.

27. The idea of predisposition is important—it is mentioned in a number of case reports.

28. For the pioneering study on disease theories and anticontagionism, see Ackerknecht, "Anti-contagionism between 1821–1867."

29. See, for example, Pelling, "Contagion, Germ Theory, Specificity."

30. This "ambiguous" term encompassed the idea that poisons could come either from another person or from the environment. See Worboys, *Spreading Germs*, 38.

31. Virchow, "Cells and Cellular Theory," Lecture One, Feb. 10, 1858, in *Cellular Pathology*, 27–50.

32. For more on the historical development of disease theories, see Pelling, "Contagion, Germ Theory, Specificity," 309–34.

33. Laudable pus meant the quality of pus, for example "yellow color, creamy and inodorus" versus infected or ichorous pus, which smelled foul and was thinner and blood tinged, signaling a serious infection. See Bollet, *Civil War Medicine*, 200.

34. W. W. Keen, USA General Hospital, West Philadelphia, Ward 2, "Clinical Observations on Hospital Gangrene, 1862," Reports of Diseases and Individual Cases, 1841–93, file A, no. 265, entry 621, RG 94, NARA.

35. Ibid.

36. "Circular and Letter in Regard to Hospital Gangrene," Mar. 14, 1863, Medical Records, 1814–1919, D file, box 15, no. 253, entry 623, RG 94, NARA.

37. Daniel Morgan, Assistant Surgeon, USA General Hospital, Indiana, "Surgical Report of Hospital and Surgical Cases," Reports of Diseases and Individual Cases, 1841–93, file A, box 5, no. 269, entry 621, RG 94, NARA.

38. Ibid.

39. Middleton Goldsmith, "Report of Hospital Gangrene in Nashville and Murfreesboro," July 12, 1863, Reports of Diseases and Individual Cases, 1841–93, file A, no. 261, entry 621, RG 94, NARA.

40. Ibid. See also Goldsmith, *A Report on Hospital Gangrene, Erysipelas and Pyaemia*, 6–7.

41. Goldsmith, *A Report on Hospital Gangrene, Erysipelas and Pyaemia*, 6. The Vienna physician Ignac Semmelweis advocated washing hands in chlorine to prevent the spread of puerperal sepsis in obstetric cases. There were a number of comparisons and studies linking puerperal fever and erysipelas in Europe and the United Kingdom between the years 1850 and 1900 (most began after 1860). See Loudon, *Death in Childbirth*, 72–76.

42. See Watson, *Liberty and Power*.

43. Benjamin Butler's quarantine measures in New Orleans were another matter. See Bell, *Mosquito Soldiers*; Butler, "Some Experiences with Yellow Fever and Its Prevention."

44. Carter, *The Rise of Causal Concepts of Disease*, 39.

45. Goldsmith, *A Report on Hospital Gangrene, Erysipelas and Pyaemia*, 10.

46. Ibid.

47. In 1867 Lister published his ground-breaking paper "On the Antiseptic Principle in the Practice of Surgery," which explained that surgical infections were caused from small "germs" floating in the air. He thus used carbolic acid to prevent infection during and after surgery. Civil War physicians were able to redefine their debates, hygienic models, and management practices along Listerian lines (without changing their approaches). See chapter 6. See also Waller, *The Discovery of the Germ*, 92.

48. See Waller, *The Discovery of the Germ*, 92. See also Goldsmith, *A Report on Hospital Gangrene, Erysipelas and Pyaemia*, 6.

49. He was not the first American to make this connection. Oliver Wendell Holmes published a paper after confirming the contagious disorder (puerperal sepsis) was spread by the midwife or attendant. But this work was highly contested until Pasteur actually proved that deaths from puerperal fever were due to the *Streptococcus pyogenes* organism (also the cause

of erysipelas). See Carter, *The Rise of Causal Concepts*, 40–44; Loudon, "Childbirth." See also Parsons, "Puerperal Fever, Anticontagionists, and Miasmatic Infection, 1840–1860."

50. Carter, *The Rise of Causal Concepts of Disease*, 56.

51. He also advanced the idea that there could be some kind of catalysis in the body, which he believed to be lactic acid in the blood.

52. See *Medical and Surgical History*, 6:846, for the report of C. H. Cleveland of Church Hospital, Memphis, Tenn.

53. As Pelling has shown, however, in the nineteenth century it was possible to "transpose the ontological idea to the cellular level, so that disease could be seen as invasive within the interior environment of the body." See Pelling, "Contagion, Germ Theory, Specificity," 315.

54. Goldsmith, *A Report on Hospital Gangrene, Erysipelas and Pyaemia*, 43. The staphylococcus bacteria formed pus organisms in the blood to produce pyemia. It had "constitutional" symptoms such as fever, chills, and nausea.

55. Ibid., 44. From midcentury and well into the late nineteenth century, physicians spoke of "autoinoculation" or "autointoxication" absorption of the "products" of wounds then infecting the body. These theories were also developed in the bacteriological era as physicians debated whether disease could be caused by the absorption of breakdown products of intestinal bacteria. See Bynum, *Science and the Practice of Medicine*, 130. Loudon suggests that "it seemed futile to suggest that puerperal fever could be attributed to a single cause, yet this is just what Semmelweis was suggesting for puerperal fever when he insisted it was due to the absorption of morbid or decaying matter." Loudon, *Death in Childbirth*, 70. Without proper evidence, however, Semmelweis lost his most ardent supporters. During the war, however, physicians were learning, were communicating what they saw, and most importantly were part of shared experiences and investigations. Goldsmith's views were received favorably by a number of physicians.

56. Goldsmith to Brinton, Mar. 17, 1863, Medical Records, 1814–1919, D file, box 15, no. 193, entry 623, RG 94, NARA.

57. "Circular and Letter in Regard to Hospital Gangrene."

58. Woodward, "Report on the Microscopial Appearance of Hospital Gangrene in the Annapolis General Hospital," Feb. 19, 1863, Reports of Diseases and Individual Cases, 1841–93, file A, no. 295, entry 621, RG 94, NARA.

59. Ibid.

60. Like Virchow, Woodward believed inflammatory pus cells came from other cells.

61. Woodward, "Report on the Microscopial Appearance of Hospital Gangrene in the Annapolis General Hospital." His report was accompanied by four microscopic drawings demonstrating the various stages of putrefactive decomposition and changes, masses of so-called cell formations, and cells in various stages of enlargement and multiplication.

62. Tho. E. Jenkins, "On the Chemical and Physical Character of Sloughs resulting from Hospital Gangrene," Mar. 19, 1863, Medical Records, 1814–1919, D file, box 3, no. 252, entry 623, RG 94, NARA. Similarly, the southern physician J. Chambliss conducted numerous tests on the chemical properties of hospital gangrene in which he mixed nitric acid with gangrenous matter, preserved in a solution of distilled water and submitted to physician-scientist Joseph Jones for further analysis. He noted that he had "tried this experiment with matter taken from this and other wounds affected with gangrene," and his experiments continually produced a "pink colored precipate." He compared the solution with

so-called healthy pus, which produced a white coagulate, and tested the matter taken from the body of a decayed rat. Jones conducted separate experiments to test for the presence of the disease but found the results were not uniform. The development of chemical experimentation was important in garnering support for laboratory-style medicine. See *Surgical Memoirs of the War of the Rebellion*, 274–75.

63. Jenkins report to Goldsmith, reprinted in Goldsmith, *A Report on Hospital Gangrene, Erysipelas and Pyaemia*, 22.

64. Benjamin Woodward wrote a paper entitled "Iodine and Its Possibilities in Medicine," *Northwestern Medical and Surgical Journal*, June 1857. See Litvin, *The Young Mary, 1817–1861*, chaps. 4–6, for a list of Woodward's early writings. See also Benjamin Woodward Papers, Personal Papers of Medical Officers and Physicians, box 657, entry 561, RG 94, NARA.

65. Probably the result of a less serious staphylococcal infection versus a more serious streptococcal infection. Bollet, *Civil War Medicine*, 200.

66. Ben Woodward to John Brinton, "Notes on the Pus and Ichor of Hospital Gangrene," Jan. 2, 1863, Medical Records, 1814–1919, D file, box 3, no. 205, entry 623, RG 94, NARA.

67. The role of pus, white corpuscles, inflammation, and cells as observed in diseased states was the subject of much debate in the second half of the nineteenth century. Woodward's investigations again reveal the dynamism that characterized Civil War medicine. For more on the debates concerning the "nature of pus," see Bynum, *Science and the Practice of Medicine*, 122–27.

68. Ben Woodward to John Brinton, "Notes on the Pus and Ichor of Hospital Gangrene." Woodward advocated treatment for gangrene; however, depending on the severity of the wound, he did suggest that tissues could regenerate due to their vitality.

69. Ibid. Associated here with extensive swelling of the tissues.

70. As the disease spread into the bloodstream, other infection sites would or could arise in the body.

71. Goldsmith, *A Report on Hospital Gangrene, Erysipelas and Pyaemia*, 16.

72. Letter entitled "Letters and Experiments on Hospital Gangrene and concerning Pathological Specimen," from Ben Woodward, U.S. Hospital, Tullahoma, Tennessee, to John Brinton, Jan. 2, 1863, Medical Records, 1814–1919, D file, box 15, no. 196, entry 623, RG 94, NARA. See also letter entitled "Private Letter," from Ben Woodward, U.S. Hospital, Tullahoma, Tennessee, to John Brinton, Dec. 31, 1863, D file, box 15, entry 623, RG 94.

73. He treated the patient with bromine successfully; but very little concern was expressed for the patient in this letter.

74. Ben Woodward, "Letters and Experiments on Hospital Gangrene and concerning Pathological Specimen."

75. Ben Woodward to Joseph Barnes, Mar. 11, 1863, Papers of Benjamin Woodward, Personal Papers of Medical Officers and Physicians, box 657, entry 561, RG 94, NARA.

76. Goldsmith, *A Report on Hospital Gangrene, Erysipelas and Pyaemia*, 16.

77. This technique, also known as debridement, consisted of applying the remedy to the diseased surfaces but also just beyond to the sound parts so that the disease could not spread. It was very painful, and patients were often given anesthetic during the application of the remedy.

78. For an example of creosote use, see Pryer, "Hospital Gangrene in the DeCamp General Hospital."

79. For more on the development of controlled experiments in the later nineteenth century, see Marks, *The Progress of Experiment*.

80. The most significant was Goldsmith, *A Report on Hospital Gangrene, Erysipelas and Pyaemia*. This report was ninety-four pages and gave detailed information on the pathology of these diseases, how to treat the diseases in each stage, and testimonials about the efficacy of bromine.

81. For more on specificity in disease and therapeutics, see Warner, *The Therapeutic Perspective*.

82. Hinkle, "Remarks on the Use of Permanganate Potassa in the Treatment of Hospital Gangrene," Reports of Diseases and Individual Cases, 1841–93, file A, no. 263, entry 621, RG 94, NARA.

83. Ibid.

84. The government purchased the solution from Henry Bower, a chemist from Philadelphia.

85. Hinkle, "Remarks on the Use of Permanganate Potassa."

86. The solution used by him (and eventually furnished by the government) was from two to four drachms of the concentrated solution added to a pint of water, the stringents varying in accordance with the severity of the case.

87. He accepted the ontological connection between the lesion and disease, which was uncommon in the nineteenth century. See Pelling, "Contagion, Germ Theory, Specificity," 315.

88. He found that by applying the concentrated solution with a hair pencil and then soaking lint dressings with the solution for twenty-four hours, he could control the hemorrhage.

89. Hinkle, "Remarks on the Use of Permanganate Potassa."

90. Ibid. This also suggests wider acceptance of Semmelweis's ideas and theories of disease transmission.

91. Ibid.

92. Frank Hinkle's Case Report, Jarvis General Hospital, Case Three, Charles McElroy, Company K, 17th Connecticut Volunteers, from Reports of Diseases and Individual Cases, 1841–93, file A, no. 263, entry 621, RG 94, NARA.

93. Bartholow, "Pathology and Treatment of Hospital Gangrene: Turpentine as a Local Application."

94. See Atlee, "Two Cases of Pyemia of Purulent Infection"; Lea, "On the Transformation of Alkaline Sulphites in the Human System"; DeRicci, "Therapeutic Value of the Alkaline and Earthy Sulphites," 236.

95. Joseph Woodward to Joseph Barnes, Mar. 28, 1865, Office of the Surgeon General, Letters Received, 1818–1870, box 109, entry 12, RG 112, NARA.

96. Lea, "On the Transformation of Alkaline Sulphites in the Human System," 82.

97. When discussing specific chemical formulas, he referenced Liebig's work.

98. "Relation of Scientific Research to Medical Science," *Richmond Medical Journal* (1866): 25. Excerpt from the *Annual of Scientific Discovery*.

99. Bromine worked by inhibiting the further growth of the bacteria rather than directly killing them (as antibiotics do).

100. "Hospital Gangrene," Reports of Societies, New York Academy of Medicine, May 20, 1863, *American Medical Times* (Sept. 12, 1863): 123.

101. Goldsmith, *A Report on Hospital Gangrene, Erysipelas and Pyaemia*, 26, 45.

102. "Article IV, 'Erysipelas,'" *Cincinnati Lancet and Observer* (Feb. 1863): 83–86. As Waller has pointed out, how could diffuse clouds of poison or miasma single out individual practitioners? Waller, *The Discovery of the Germ*, 61.

103. "Article IV, 'Erysipelas,'" *Cincinnati Lancet and Observer* (Feb. 1863): 83–86.

104. Goldsmith, *A Report on Hospital Gangrene, Erysipelas and Pyaemia*, 24.

105. Ibid., 28.

106. Goldsmith to Brinton, Mar. 17, 1863, Medical Records, 1814–1919, D file, box 15, no. 193, entry 623, RG 94, NARA.

107. Goldsmith, *A Report on Hospital Gangrene, Erysipelas and Pyaemia*, 23.

108. Benjamin Woodward to J. T. Head, Medical Director of Hospitals in Louisville, from Nov. 15, 1862, "Special Report on the Use of Bromine in preventing the spread of Erysipelas," Medical Records, 1814–1919, D file, no. 235, entry 623, RG 94, NARA.

109. Ibid.

110. Ibid.

111. This report was first read before the Louisville Society of Army Surgeons and nicely illustrates how the medical environment of the war stimulated both new knowledge and the transfer of this knowledge so that other physicians could practically test the results. He believed that bromine worked by antagonizing certain animal poisons.

112. It also foreshadowed Lister's famous discovery of antisepsis, the method he invented to kill germs during surgical operations, which entailed applying chemicals to the body (though Lister was targeting and killing "living germs"). See Lister, "On a New Method of Treating Compound Fracture, Abscess, etc., with Observations on the Conditions of Suppuration," *Lancet* 1 (1867): 357–59.

113. Benjamin Woodward to J. T. Head, "Special Report on the Use of Bromine in Preventing the Spread of Erysipelas."

114. Goldsmith to Hammond on using bromine for gangrene and erysipelas, Reports of Diseases and Individual Cases, 1841–93, file A, box 18, no. 290, entry 621, RG 94, NARA.

115. Special order of William Hammond, Mar. 28, 1863, Curatorial Records: Circulars and Reports, 1863–1864, RG 6, OHA, NMHM. See also Reports of Diseases and Individual Cases, 1841–93, file A, box 18, no. 253, entry 621, RG 94, NARA.

116. J. H. Brinton to W. Hammond, "Report on the Prevalence of Hospital Gangrene and Erysipelas in the Cities of Louisville and Nashville and on the Treatment Adopted," Apr. 16, 1863, Reports of Diseases and Individual Cases, 1841–93, file A, box 18, no. 253, entry 621, RG 94, NARA.

117. Ibid.

118. Ibid.

119. Ibid. See also Goldsmith to J. H. Brinton, Mar. 8, 1863, Medical Records, 1814–1919, D file, box 3, no. 250, entry 623, RG 94, NARA.

120. Goldsmith to Hammond, Mar. 22, 1863, Reports of Diseases and Individual Cases, 1841–93, file A, box 18, no. 193, entry 621, RG 94, NARA.

121. Ibid.

122. Goldsmith, *A Report on Hospital Gangrene, Erysipelas and Pyaemia*, 28–29. See also Goldsmith to Hammond, Mar. 22, 1863, Reports of Diseases and Individual Cases, 1841–93, file A, box 18, no. 193, entry 621, RG 94, NARA.

123. Statistical analyses of patients treated with bromine demonstrated that patients undergoing a course of treatment with the agent often improved and/or healed under treatment. See appendix tables 1–3.

124. Geo. R. Weeks, "Report on Hospital Gangrene as Observed in General Hospital in Louisville, Ky.," in Goldsmith, *A Report on Hospital Gangrene, Erysipelas and Pyaemia*.

125. Goldsmith, *A Report on Hospital Gangrene, Erysipelas and Pyaemia*, 32. In fact, the *Medical and Surgical History* records only 135 cases of hospital gangrene from July 1864 to June 1865 as compared to a year earlier, when 1,611 cases were reported. See *Medical and Surgical History*, 3:825.

126. "Editorial Abstracts and Selections," *Cincinnati Lancet and Observer* (1863): 701–4.

127. "Reports of Societies: New York Academy of Medicine, May 20, 1868," *American Medical Times* (Sept. 1863): 109.

128. Ibid.

129. Ibid.

130. Ibid., 123.

131. Ibid.

132. "Proceedings of the Cincinnati Academy of Medicine," *Cincinnati Lancet and Observer* 6 (1863): 347–48.

133. Bromine and bromide of potassium have the same properties. When chlorine gas is bubbled into a solution of bromide of potassium, some of the bromide ions are oxidized to bromine. Bromine can be displaced from bromide of potassium using a solution of chlorine.

134. Roberts Bartholow, "Experimental Investigations into the Actions and Uses of the Bromide of Potassium," *Cincinnati Lancet and Observer* 8 (1865): 658–73.

135. The issue of consent was not discussed in his paper. Since he performed experiments on himself first, however, the subsequent experiments on his patients were deemed more acceptable. Lederer notes that, "although not always possible, the obligation to try a new drug or procedure on oneself before applying it to patients was an acceptable feature of medical research in the mid-nineteenth century." For more on the development of experimentation, self-experimentation, and consent in the later nineteenth century, see Lederer, *Subjected to Science*, 18.

136. Bartholow, "Experimental Investigations," 662–64. But the numerous debates about the miraculous properties of the agent led him to search for other ways bromine, and its properties, could be used. He then conducted experiments to test the theory that bromide of potassium was a hypnotic or sedative in the search for a way to treat spasmodic and nervous affections of the respiratory organs. Bromides were a class of sedatives used to treat various nervous disorders, especially epilepsy.

137. J. H. Hollister, "Bromine and Its Compounds," *Richmond Medical and Surgical Journal* (Apr. 1867): 340–45.

138. "Tabular Statement of Hospital Gangrene and Gangrenous Erysipelas in Hospital and Private Practice, Embraced within a Period of Eleven Years, from 1865–1876," in von Tagen, *Biliary Calculi: Perineorrhaphy*, 154. Moreover these findings were compared with the bromine trials at Satterlee General Hospital in West Philadelphia and at Fredericksburg and City Point, Virginia, in the summer and fall of 1863 and in 1864. The wartime hospital records were used as a guide for physicians adopting or conducting trials with bromine just after the war; ibid., 152–53.

139. R. F. Weir, U.S. Army General Hospital, Frederick, Maryland, "Remarks on Hospital Gangrene," Mar. 1863, Reports of Diseases and Individual Cases, 1841–93, file A, no. 288, entry 621, RG 94, NARA; Cullen, "Observations on the Influence of the Present War upon Medicine and Surgery."

140. Hartshorne, *Essentials of the Principles and Practice of Medicine*, 323.

141. Quoted in Parsons, "Puerperal Fever, Anticontagionists, and Miasmatic Infection," 445.

142. Goldsmith to Hammond, Aug. 26, 1863, Medical Records, 1814–1919, D file, box 15, no. 193, entry 623, RG 94, NARA.

143. Letter from Goldsmith to Brinton, Mar. 22, 1863, ibid.

CHAPTER 4

1. In the early nineteenth century, specialism was a hallmark of the charlatan. Regular physicians were required to have a well-rounded view of all aspects of medicine: therapeutics, diagnosis, the body—that is, all parts of the human body, not just the eye or ear, for example. Stevens argues that in the early nineteenth century the "self-styled specialist (bonesetter, pile doctor, or clap doctor) was often little different from a quack; and the energies of the medical profession had long been devoted to stamping out such phenomena," because their actions undermined the general practitioner. See Stevens, *American Medicine and the Public Interest*, 44.

2. Mitchell, Morehouse, and Keen, *Gunshot Wounds and Other Injuries of Nerves*, 143.

3. For example, American Ophthalmological Society, 1864; American Ontological Society, 1868; American Neurological Association, 1875; American Dermatological Association, 1876; American Gynecological Association, 1876; American Laryngological Association, 1879; American Surgical Association, 1880; American Association of Genito-Urinary Surgeons, 1886; American Orthopedic Association, 1887; American Pediatric Society, 1888; American Laryngological, Rhinological and Otological Society, 1895; American Academy of Ophthalmology and Otolaryngology, 1896; American Gastroenterological Association, 1897; American Proctological Society, 1899; American Urological Association, 1902. See Rothstein, *American Physicians in the Nineteenth Century*, 213; Stevens, *American Medicine and the Public Interest*, 46.

4. The development of the various specialisms was uneven. Neurology, for example, established a foundation to investigate and diagnose neurological disorders, and a significant record of this work was published and later consulted by medical professionals around the world. Developments in "plastic operations," on the other hand, were less common and left a smaller body of work, yet still laid a foundation for specialized study.

5. Mitchell, "The Medical Department in the Civil War: Address before the Physicians Club Chicago, Ills. 1902/March/25," Silas Weir Mitchell Papers, box 17, ser. 7, p. 20, CPP.

6. Ibid.

7. Thomas McFadden, Ohio, Post Hospital Camp Chase, to Hammond, Aug. 23, 1863, Office of the Surgeon General, Letters Received, 1818–1870, box 66, entry 12, RG 112, NARA.

8. Mitchell, Morehouse, and Keen, *Gunshot Wounds and Other Injuries of Nerves*, iii.

9. There is an important economic factor here: physicians were being paid by the state to treat national troops who needed general care but also, in many cases, specialized care.

Being paid for this expertise sanctioned this work during the war, and in the process a record of experience was amassed and published.

10. Mills Madison, Medical Directors Office, St. Louis, Mo., Jan. 22, 1864, Office of the Surgeon General, Letters Received, 1818–1870, box 66, entry 12, RG 112, NARA.

11. John Brinton to Joseph LeConte, Oct. 29, 1862, John LeConte Papers, APS.

12. LeConte published more than 200 papers on coleoplera, which were republished in Europe, and described about 270 species of scarabaeoidea. He studied medicine at the College of Physicians and Surgeons in New York but did not practice medicine until the Civil War. John LeConte Papers, APS.

13. Ibid.

14. John LeConte to John Brinton, Nov. 17, 1863, Letters and Memorandums from John Brinton, Medical Records, 1814–1919, D file, box 1, entry 623, RG 94, NARA.

15. John M. Cuyler to John LeConte, Dec. 9, 1863, John LeConte Papers, APS.

16. John L. LeConte also formed lifelong associations through his work in the war. He conducted a number of experiments with Joseph Woodward on all forms of specimens at the request of Joseph Henry. They studied, microscopically, certain fabrics, foodstuffs, calf-hair goods, anthropological specimens, and bodies. See John LeConte Papers, 1875–1876, APS. There is a nice series of letters between Woodward, LeConte, and Joseph Henry (all of the work was ordered by the Smithsonian and undertaken at the Army Medical Museum). The reports were later published in various medical and other journals, including the *Boston Wool Manufacturers Association Quarterly*, which illustrates the diversity of interest.

17. Letter from John M. Cuyler to John LeConte, Jan. 3, 1864, John LeConte Papers, APS.

18. W. W. Keen, "Surgical Reminiscences of the Civil War," in *Addresses and Other Papers*, 437.

19. John Campbell, Department of Lusquemhama Medical Director's Office to the Surgeon General's Office Oct. 6, 1863, Office of the Surgeon General, Letters Received, 1818–1870, box 21, entry 12, RG 112, NARA.

20. George Rosen has similarly shown that the creation of "specialized hospitals provided centers for the transmission and development of knowledge and skills connected with the special field of practice." See Rosen, *The Specialization of Medicine*, 39. Rosenberg, "Social Class and Medical Care in Nineteenth-Century America," also illustrates the importance of specialized departments in the general dispensaries to accommodate professional goals and in the development of medical careers.

21. Mitchell, "The Medical Department in the Civil War: Address before the Physicians Club Chicago, Ills. 1902/March/25," Silas Weir Mitchell Papers, box 17, ser. 7, p. 36, CPP.

22. See Ludmerer, *Learning to Heal*, 191–206. See also Stevens, *American Medicine and the Public Interest*, 39.

23. Rothstein, *American Physicians in the Nineteenth Century*, 212.

24. Weisz, *Divide and Conquer*, 70–83.

25. Fye, *The Development of American Physiology*, 60.

26. Fye does, however, suggest that Mitchell's wartime work was important but secondary to his interest in physiology. Fye, *The Development of American Physiology*, 68.

27. Fye, "S. Weir Mitchell, Philadelphia's Lost Physiologist," 188–202.

28. Reprinted from *Nature*, Jan. 1, 1914, Silas Weir Mitchell Papers, CPP.

29. *Smithsonian Contributions to Knowledge*, 1860, 150. For a complete list of his publications, see Silas Weir Mitchell Papers, ser. 7.5, "Analytical Catalogue of Work," CPP.

30. Silas Weir Mitchell, "Report on the Progress of Physiology and Anatomy." Quoted in Fye, *The Development of American Physiology*, 59.

31. Rothstein, *American Physicians in the Nineteenth Century*, 209.

32. Mitchell, Morehouse, and Keen, *Gunshot Wounds and Other Injuries of Nerves*, 32–33.

33. Circular No. 26, Issued by Joseph K. Barnes, Nov. 24, 1863, Circulars and Circular Letters of the Surgeon General's Office, 1861–85, p. 296, entry 63, RG 112, NARA.

34. Report, John Brinton to Joseph Barnes, Sept. 16, 1864, Reports of Diseases and Individual Cases, 1841–93, file A, entry 621, RG 94, NARA.

35. For more on Turner's Lane Hospital, see Blustein, *Preserve Your Love for Science*; Freemon, "The First Neurological Research Center"; Stone, "W. W. Keen: America's Pioneer Neurological Surgeon."

36. Mitchell, "The Medical Department in the Civil War: Address before the Physicians Club Chicago, Ills. 1902/March/25," Silas Weir Mitchell Papers, box 17, ser. 7, p. 36, CPP.

37. Ibid.

38. Starr, *The Social Transformation of American Medicine*, 90–91. As Starr notes, the "AMA [American Medical Association] was so embroiled in political squabbles" prior to the war that the more scientifically minded members often formed their own societies or research groups. Yet they did not have the institutional support or government resources that physicians found during the war.

39. William H. Welch, "S. Weir Mitchell: Physician and Man of Science," in *Silas Weir Mitchell: Memorial Addresses and Resolutions*, 109. He never abandoned his interest in physiology. For example, in reference to the knee jerk, the contraction of certain muscles was seen by Mitchell as a physiological contraction in response to a blow upon the body (tendon tap results in the reply of a jerky kick). See Silas Weir Mitchell Papers, CPP.

40. Keen, "Tribute to S. Weir Mitchell," in *Silas Weir Mitchell: Memorial Addresses and Resolutions*, 16.

41. Ibid.

42. Mitchell, Morehouse, and Keen, *Gunshot Wounds and Other Injuries of Nerves*, 13.

43. Mitchell, Morehouse, and Keen, *Circular No. 6*, 1. Quoted also in Canale, "'The Firm,'" 134.

44. This was first published in 1864 and expanded in 1871.

45. Silas Weir Mitchell Papers, ser. 7.5, CPP.

46. Mitchell, Morehouse, and Keen, *Gunshot Wounds and Other Injuries of Nerves*, 11.

47. Because of the scope of cases during the war, very particular headings were adopted to organize the research. Ibid., 12.

48. R. Weir to Joseph Barnes, May 28, 1864, Office of the Surgeon General, Letters Received, 1818–1870, box 67, entry 12, RG 112, NARA.

49. Mitchell, "The Medical Department in the Civil War: Address before the Physicians Club Chicago, Ills. 1902/March/25," Silas Weir Mitchell Papers, box 17, ser. 7, p. 36, CPP.

50. "Special Cases in USA General Hospital, 16th and Filbert Street," Reported by George Morehouse, Oct. 31, 1862, Reports of Diseases and Individual Cases, 1841–93, file A, entry 621, RG 94, NARA.

51. Keen, "Surgical Reminiscences of the Civil War," 435–36.

52. Ibid.

53. Welch, "S. Weir Mitchell: Physician and Man of Science," 117.

54. Canale, "'The Firm,'" 133. After the war, through experiments with animals, Mitchell found success suturing the divided end of nerves to recover nerve function.

55. Mitchell, Morehouse, and Keen, *Gunshot Wounds and Other Injuries of Nerves*, 11–12.

56. Ibid., 137–38.

57. Ibid.

58. Ibid., 9. For a description of Turner's Lane Hospital, see Bokum, *Wanderings North and South*.

59. Silas Weir Mitchell Papers, ser. 7.5., CPP.

60. It is also important to note that before the war Mitchell and other elite physicians pursued scientific experimentation almost as a hobby; during the war, the experiments and work had immediate and significant clinical relevance, which Mitchell commented on frequently.

61. Hammond, as Blustein has shown, also adopted a "conventional lesion-oriented pathology" in his program of neurology; she noted of Hammond's work that "with a new and rather vague functionalism rooted in his physiological experience . . . the neurologist could consistently hold out hope for recovery only if the disorder were functional rather than the result of organic damage." See Blustein, *Preserve Your Love for Science*, 127.

62. For example, shock may have manifested specific functional disorders (headache, confusion, spasms, and dizziness), symptoms similar to those of a brain tumor, but there would be no organic symptom (i.e., tumor). This distinction was important, and Mitchell developed specific methodologies, including clinical research, autopsy, and microscopial investigation, to understand and classify these different neural maladies.

63. Mitchell, Morehouse, and Keen, *Gunshot Wounds and Other Injuries of Nerves*, 20.

64. Turner's Lane Hospital Case and Follow up Studies, 1863–1892, Silas Weir Mitchell Papers, CPP.

65. Mitchell, Morehouse, and Keen, *Gunshot Wounds and Other Injuries of Nerves*, 13.

66. Turner's Lane Hospital Case and Follow up Studies, Silas Weir Mitchell Papers, CPP.

67. Blustein, *Preserve Your Love for Science*, 128. She shows that Hammond was among the first to introduce the works of Duchenne and Remak in the United States. See also Mitchell, Morehouse, and Keen, *Gunshot Wounds and Other Injuries of Nerves*, 137. They discuss Duchenne's theories.

68. In discussing electricity, Mitchell referred to its controversial status when he said that "one of them, and the most efficient, is perhaps the most overrated and underrated of all the medical armamenta. Need we add that we refer to electricity?" See Mitchell, Morehouse, and Keen, *Gunshot Wounds and Other Injuries of Nerves*, 136.

69. *New York Medical Journal*, early 1870, quoted in Blustein, *Preserve Your Love for Science*, 129.

70. Mitchell, Morehouse, and Keen, *Gunshot Wounds and Other Injuries of Nerves*, 142.

71. Ibid., 136. Electricity, however, gradually fell into disfavor (especially by the 1880s). See Blustein, *Preserve Your Love for Science*, 131.

72. Especially for use in cases of spinal and local disease to restore function. By recommending the local use of massage, he clearly reconciled localized pathology in his work, but

his simultaneous emphasis on functionalism illustrates the coexistence of functionalism and organic localism.

73. For a full description of his treatments, which were perfected during and after the war, see Mitchell, *Fat and Blood*. The entire book deals with therapeutics for neurological disorders, was highly popular as a guide in America and Europe, and was reprinted more than ten times.

74. Ibid., 67.

75. Mitchell, Morehouse, and Keen, *Gunshot Wounds and Other Injuries of Nerves*, 140.

76. Ibid.

77. Turner's Lane Hospital Case and Follow up Studies, Silas Weir Mitchell Papers, CPP.

78. Ibid.

79. Ibid.

80. Ibid.

81. Merritte Weber Ireland, "Biographical Sketches of Jefferson Medical College Graduates who Served in the Civil War," MS B 169, NLM.

82. Whether it was a "nerve concussion" or a "direct wound," each disease presented different and ultimately well-defined symptoms—once again, a benefit of having so many cases to study and compare.

83. Mitchell, Morehouse, and Keen, *Gunshot Wounds and Other Injuries of Nerves*, 36.

84. Ibid.

85. Ibid.

86. Turner's Lane Hospital Case and Follow up Studies, Silas Weir Mitchell Papers, CPP.

87. Ibid.

88. Mitchell, Morehouse, and Keen, *Gunshot Wounds and Other Injuries of Nerves*, 17.

89. Ibid., 18.

90. Ibid.

91. But he generally found that with paralysis of the nerves, motion was more frequently impaired then sensation.

92. Ibid., 18–19. He did reconcile his views to the anatomy of the brain, noting that "all of our anatomical views incline us to the belief that the two orders of nerves are intimately blended in the large nerves." This troubled him because, if this were so, he wondered, why would one set escape the loss of function which the missile inflicted on the other? This work was so interesting because it challenged Mitchell's basic assumptions about the body's function, while also outlining specific research (or problem) areas for future neurologists to investigate.

93. Turner's Lane Hospital Case and Follow up Studies, Silas Weir Mitchell Papers, CPP.

94. Ibid.

95. *Medical and Surgical History*, 5:725.

96. Mitchell, Morehouse, and Keen, *Gunshot Wounds and Other Injuries of Nerves*, 146.

97. Ibid., 147.

98. Ibid.

99. A counterirritant, excited in a part of the body to produce an irritation, designed to relieve one existing in another part of the body.

100. Mitchell, "The Medical Department in the Civil War: Address before the Physicians Club Chicago, Ills. 1902/March/25," Silas Weir Mitchell Papers, box 17, ser. 7, p. 39, CPP.

101. Ibid.

102. Turner's Lane Hospital Case and Follow up Studies, Silas Weir Mitchell Papers, CPP.

103. Being discharged did not mean being cured. Cases that did not respond to treatment could be discharged (sometimes to general hospitals where other conditions needed to be treated).

104. Mitchell, Morehouse, and Keen, *Gunshot Wounds and Other Injuries of Nerves*, 62–63.

105. For a discussion of malingering, see Devine, "Producing Knowledge."

106. Turner's Lane Hospital Case and Follow up Studies, Silas Weir Mitchell Papers, CPP.

107. Mitchell, Morehouse, and Keen, *Gunshot Wounds and Other Injuries of Nerves*, 37.

108. Ibid.

109. Ibid.

110. See Aminoff, *Brown-Séquard*, 125–26.

111. In 1864 Brown-Séquard delivered a lecture at the Smithsonian Institution; see "Notes of a Lecture by Dr. Brown-Séquard Delivered at the Smithsonian June 14, 1864," Reports of Diseases and Individual Cases, 1841–93, file A, no. 344, entry 621, RG 94, NARA. In 1864 Brown-Séquard spoke to a gathering of military and civilian physicians about nerve diseases, among other things, and offered suggestions on how best to manage wartime nervous diseases. This lecture illustrates once again the depth and the international scope of medical teaching during the Civil War. He had achieved some acclaim on his work on nervous diseases after his book of lectures was published: *Course of Lectures on the Physiology and Pathology of the Central Nervous System*. Like Mitchell, Keen, and Morehouse, Brown-Séquard was interested in spinal injuries, which he suggested may have been caused by peripheral injury (pressure of bone or bone fragments on the spinal cord after being shot) rather than direct injury to the spine.

112. Mitchell, Morehouse, and Keen, "On the Antagonism of Atrophia and Morphia," 67–76.

113. For example, in 1874 the British Medical Association appointed a committee to investigate the antagonism of medicines, and the results were published in the *British Medical Journal*, Jan. 25, 1875. See Bartholow, *On the Antagonism between Medicines*, 19.

114. Bartholow, *On the Antagonism between Medicines*, 15. The only significant work published prior to this in America was by Dr. William H. Mussey of Cincinnati, who examined the antagonism between opium and belladonna; Dr. C. C. Lee of Philadelphia, who examined the same subject; and Dr. William Norris, who in 1862 used cases to illustrate the antagonism. All of the authors examined opium and belladonna poisoning, in which one drug was used to counterbalance the effects of the other.

115. Ibid., 10.

116. Ibid.

117. Ibid.

118. Mitchell, Morehouse, and Keen, "On the Antagonism of Atrophia and Morphia," 68.

119. Ibid.

120. One of Robert Koch's postulates was the reproduction of a typical pathological manifestation of a disease in an animal.

121. Mitchell, Morehouse, and Keen, "On the Antagonism of Atrophia and Morphia," 68 (though they did mention how much they liked to study the toxicological effects of poisons on cold-blooded creatures). But ultimately they wanted to see the influence of medicinal properties "upon the being to whom finally it is to be of medicinal value."

122. Ibid., 71.

123. Ibid., 76.

124. Ibid., 75.

125. Reprinted in *Nature*, Jan. 1, 1914, Silas Weir Mitchell Papers, ser. 7, CPP.

126. Mitchell, "Influence of Nerve Lesions on Local Temperatures," 351.

127. Ibid.

128. Mitchell, "Relation of Pain to Weather," 305.

129. Letter to Silas Weir Mitchell from John K. Mitchell Sept. 4, 1893, box 11, ser. 4, Silas Weir Mitchell Papers, CPP.

130. Follow up Studies on Patients with Nerve Injuries, Oct. 1892, box 11, ser. 4, Silas Weir Mitchell Papers, CPP.

131. Ibid.

132. This letter nicely illustrates the great status that Mitchell had achieved during the war.

133. "Case of Richard D. Dunphy Age 52," box 11, ser. 4, Silas Weir Mitchell Papers, CPP.

134. "Case of Wesley Jones," ibid. Mitchell was fascinated with the effects of amputation on the body and mind. In 1871 he published "Phantom Limbs," in which he discussed the "neuralgias" and "spasmodic maladies" suffered by Civil War amputees. He also discussed the soldier's feeling of having a "constant or inconstant phantom of the missing member." His most famous article, perhaps, was published in the *Atlantic Monthly* in 1866, "The Case of George Deadlow" in which he describes "phantom limb syndrome."

135. Letter to Silas Weir Mitchell from John K. Mitchell Sept. 4, 1893, box 11, ser. 4, Silas Weir Mitchell Papers, CPP.

136. Mitchell, "The Medical Department in the Civil War: Address before the Physicians Club Chicago, Ills. 1902/March/25," Silas Weir Mitchell Papers, box 17, ser. 7, p. 40, CPP.

137. This was not recognized as a psychiatric syndrome, however, until 1980. For the best study of PTSD during the Civil War, see Dean, "'We will all be lost and Destroyed,'" and Dean, *Shook over Hell*.

138. Mitchell, "Stumps and Spasmodic Disorders: Chorea of Stumps," 100.

139. Silas Weir Mitchell is remembered by some as a pioneer for his innovative approaches to the treatment of nervous disorders and by others for his difficult treatment of hysteria. The most famous example comes from Charlotte Perkins Gilman, who wrote in 1892 "The Yellow Wallpaper." She was diagnosed with "temporary nervous depression" with a "slight hysterical tendency" (p. 6). Her physician was Silas Weir Mitchell, who prescribed his famous "rest cure" which consisted of taking to bed, being secluded from the family, not working or reading, and drinking only fatty dairy products. Her husband, also a physician, confined her to a room in their summer home that had yellow wallpaper, described by Gillman as "repellent, almost revolting" (p. 9). The story follows her descent into madness as a result of her confinement. See Gillman, *The Yellow Wallpaper and Other Stories*.

140. Mitchell, "The Medical Department in the Civil War: Address before the Physicians Club Chicago, Ills. 1902/March/25," Silas Weir Mitchell Papers, box 17, ser. 7, p. 36, CPP.

141. See, for example, Wooley, *The Irritable Heart of Soldiers*.

142. Papers of J. M. Da Costa, Personal Papers of Medical Officers and Physicians, box 144, entry 561, RG 94, NARA.

143. Ibid. His contract lasted from May 15, 1862, until May 11, 1865.

144. Letter to John Campbell, Oct. 21, 1864, ibid.

145. Letter from B. Knickerbocker to Barnes, Oct. 7, 1863, ibid.

146. Da Costa, *Medical Diagnosis*, v.

147. Ibid., vi.

148. Da Costa, "On Irritable Heart."

149. Ibid., 17. He also remarked that he had seen many of the same cases in his private practice.

150. Da Costa, "On Functional Valvular Disorders of the Heart," 17.

151. This was also called "muscular exhaustion" or "Soldiers Heart," and after the war in honor of Da Costa, "Da Costa's Syndrome." The World Health Organization classes this disorder as somatoform autonomic dysfunction (a type of psychosomatic disorder); but Da Costa approached the disease as a physiological abnormality. See Bollet, *Civil War Medicine*, 322.

152. There were cases attributed to drills and double-quick movements of camp life, or when the soldier was debilitated with diarrhea or typhoid fever, and some were diagnosed with overaction of the heart during or after a battle. *Medical and Surgical History*, 3:862. A number of soldiers, for example, were treated for heart disease after the "continued exertion, anxieties and excitement of the seven days' fight from Richmond to Harrison's Landing, Va."

153. Da Costa, "On Irritable Heart," 17.

154. Ibid.

155. Ibid. He also remarked that it was not just observed among troops engaged in actual war, but "soldiers kept long under drill were also liable to functional derangement of the heart with palpitation."

156. *Medical and Surgical History*, 3:862.

157. Da Costa, "On Irritable Heart," 19.

158. Ibid., 22.

159. Da Costa also comments on the fact that irritable heart probably occurred among men in the southern army. He reasoned that "men of the same race, transformed into soldiers under much the same circumstances," and enduring "more privations, should not have escaped" this affection. Ibid., 19.

160. Ibid.

161. Ibid.

162. Da Costa, "On Functional Valvular Disorders of the Heart," 17–34.

163. *Medical and Surgical History*, 3:864.

164. Ibid.

165. Ibid.

166. Hartshorne, "On Heart Disease in the Army," 89.

167. Ibid.

168. Though Da Costa examined functional heart disease as a physiological abnormality, it was primarily associated with mental stress.

169. Da Costa, "On Functional Valvular Disorders of the Heart," 17.

170. Ibid., 18.

171. Ibid., 21.

172. See *Medical and Surgical History*, 3:864.

173. Wooley, *The Irritable Heart of Soldiers*, 13.

174. Ibid.

175. Da Costa "On Irritable Heart," 31.

176. Ibid., 31–32.

177. See Wooley, *The Irritable Heart of Soldiers*, 1–20.

178. He understood that enlarged heart was the result of mitral valve function and dysfunction, or inflammation of the valve, or thickening and hardening of the heart muscle, but he did not know the underlying causes of mitral regurgitation. We know today it is caused by degenerative disease (valve prolapse) or is a consequences of coronary disease—both are treated by sophisticated operations involving valve repair or valve replacement. Da Costa spent much of his investigations trying to understand the symptoms and the role of different murmurs in leading to valvular disease. Da Costa "On Irritable Heart," 18.

179. Quoted in Wooley, *The Irritable Heart of Soldiers*, 17.

180. Ibid.

181. Da Costa, "On Irritable Heart," 52.

182. Ibid.

183. Da Costa "On Functional Valvular Disorders of the Heart," 34.

184. Although as Keen remarked, chloroform had been used as early as 1846 in the Massachusetts General Hospital (on Oct. 16, 1846). See Keen, "Surgical Reminiscences of the Civil War," 430.

185. Anesthesia was first used in the United States on September 30, 1846, by dentist William Thomas Greene Morton. He administered sulfuric ether prior to performing a dental extraction, and two weeks later he gave a public demonstration at the Massachusetts General Hospital, October 16, 1846. It was demonstrated that ether could render a patient insensible to pain. See Ellis, *The Case Books of Dr. John Snow*, ix. See also Pernick, *A Calculus of Suffering*, 3–5.

186. See Pernick, *A Calculus of Suffering*, 4–5.

187. Gross, *A Manual of Military Surgery*, 81–82.

188. Bollet, *Civil War Medicine*, 78.

189. Buck also invented a device for treating fractures of the femur known as "Bucks Extension," a splint used as a surgical aid in the treatment of fractures. See *Medical and Surgical History*, 6:348. He also sat on the Council of Hygiene and Public Health to give recommendations on how to reform the unsanitary conditions in New York. See Rosen, *A History of Public Health*, 220–21.

190. Quoted in Conway and Stark, *Plastic Surgery at the New York Hospital*, 48.

191. *Medical and Surgical History*, 2:379.

192. Ibid., 368–81. There were six cases of reparative surgery made to the eyelids, five for the nose, three for the cheek, twelve on the lips, palate, or mouth, four on the chin, and one instance of blepharoplasty and an unsuccessful case of staphylorraphy (p. 379). There were, however, many more reconstructive surgeries performed, and the unpublished case reports can be found in Reports of Diseases and Individual Cases, 1841–93, file A, entry 621, and Medical Records, 1814–1919, D file, entry 623, RG 94, NARA. See also RGs 13, 15, 21, 28, 82, 124, OHA, NMHM.

193. At least twenty-one different surgeons submitted case reports of plastic operations to the *Medical and Surgical History*. See, for example, Register of Surgical Operations, Harvey, U.S.A. General Hospital, 1864–1865, vol. 3, entry 559, RG 94, NARA. See also "Performing a Plastic Operation," Report from USA General Hospital, Rolla, Mo., H. Culbertson Surgeon, U.S.V., Reports of Diseases and Individual Cases, 1841–93, file A, box 12, no. A-484, entry 621, RG 94, NARA.

194. A rating of "total disability" entitled the patient to a higher pension than those designated as "one-half disabled." Because of the physical deformities suffered by this class of patients, the government required physicians to rate their level of patient disability. *Medical and Surgical History*, 2:379.

195. The authors were referring to his successful facial reconstruction of a patient who had suffered massive facial trauma. Ibid., 379.

196. Bernard and Huette, *Illustrated Manual of Operative Surgery and Surgical Anatomy*, 271–72.

197. Conway and Stark, *Plastic Surgery at the New York Hospital*, 4.

198. Ibid., 10.

199. Ibid.

200. Charles McDougall to Hammond, June 19, 1863, Office of the Surgeon General, Letters Received, 1818–1870, box 13, entry 12, RG 112, NARA. This letter promises to follow up on Buck's operations and have the case histories and photos sent to the museum.

201. Ibid.

202. Conway and Stark, *Plastic Surgery at the New York Hospital*, 56. The case in question was that of Carleton Burgan, considered one of Buck's greatest triumphs, which was subsequently published in the *Medical and Surgical History*. Burgan was horribly disfigured, but after a series of operations his face was reconstructed (an artificial roof for the mouth, a nose piece, a cup that covered the lower teeth, and a practicable jaw were created). The patient went on to marry, have a family, and find work.

203. Gurdon Buck to William Sloan, June 18, 1863, Office of the Surgeon General, Letters Received, 1818–1870, entry 12, RG 112, NARA.

204. It was actually considered the most important monograph on the subject until after World War I.

205. A double lip switch operation was first performed by a Danish surgeon in 1848. Buck pioneered his version of this surgery during the Civil War. See Conway and Stark, *Plastic Surgery at the New York Hospital*, 6.

206. A Case of Autoplastic Surgery Applied to the Face by Gurdon Buck MD, Surgeon to the New York Hospital, St. Luke's Hospital, Reports of Diseases and Individual Cases, 1841–93, file A, box 14, no. 509, entry 621, RG 94, NARA.

207. Ibid.

208. Ibid.

209. Ibid.

210. *Medical and Surgical History*, 2:379.

211. See Weisz, *Divide and Conquer*, 76–83; Stevens, *American Medicine and the Public Interest*, chap. 2.

212. Whitman, *The Sacrificial Years*, 14.

CHAPTER 5

1. Today the Uniform Anatomical Gift Act of 1968 provides for the procurement of unclaimed bodies by medical schools, and each state has its own version of the statute. For more on American anatomy legislation, see Sappol, *A Traffic of Dead Bodies*, 123–24.

2. Ibid., 4.

3. Ibid.

4. Ibid., 5. Sappol has demonstrated how the failure of the passage of these acts led to a veritable "traffic of dead bodies" or a climate in which body snatching was compelled to flourish.

5. See ibid.; Humphrey, "Dissection and Discrimination"; Schultz, *Body Snatching*; Richardson, *Death, Dissection, and the Destitute*; Savitt, "Use of Blacks for Medical Experimentation and Demonstration in the Old South"; Fett, *Working Cures*.

6. Hacker, "A Census Based Account of the Civil War Dead," 310.

7. Ibid., 311.

8. Whitman, *The Wound Dresser*.

9. Whitman, *Specimen Days and Collect*, 106.

10. Ibid.

11. Lowenfels, *Walt Whitman's Civil War*, 285.

12. Quoted in Rable, *Fredericksburg! Fredericksburg!*, 315. Indeed, as Rable observes of the dying and wounded soldiers, "Their wounds proved their valor, but so did their endurance of pain."

13. Whitman, *Specimen Days and Collect*, 45.

14. Schantz, *Awaiting the Heavenly Country*, 2.

15. Rable, *God's Almost Chosen People*, 167.

16. Faust demonstrates that battle sites were a "focus of wonder and horror" and became "crowded with civilians immediately after the cessation of hostilities"; some civilians were looking for loved ones, some were embalmers, still others just wanted to "gratify their morbid curiosity." Faust, *This Republic of Suffering*, 85. For attitudes about the nature of the overwhelming death associated with the war, see Neff, *Honoring the Civil War Dead*.

17. For antebellum death rituals and attitudes about death, see Washington, *Medical Apartheid*; Nudelman, *John Brown's Body*; Laderman, *The Sacred Remains*; Faust, *This Republic of Suffering*; Schantz, *Awaiting the Heavenly Country*.

18. Abigail L. Johnston to Mr. W. H. Sigston, Warden Master, Jan. 16, 1863, Office of the Surgeon General, Letters Received, 1818–1870, box 11, entry 12, RG 112, NARA.

19. In particular, the establishment of the Graves Registration Service, the designation of national cemeteries for soldiers that died in the service of the country, and the government burial of fallen union soldiers. See Laderman, *The Sacred Remains*, 119.

20. Capt. E. L. Hartz to the Quarter Master General, Jan. 19, 1863, Office of the Surgeon General, Letters Received, 1818–1870, box 11, entry 12, RG 112, NARA.

21. Laderman, *The Sacred Remains*, 113. The strides made in embalming during the war would contribute significantly to the development of the funeral industry and the professionalization of the undertaker. See Faust, *This Republic of Suffering*, 92.

22. A number of preservatives were used, including permanganate of potassa, arsenic, zinc, various salts, and chloride.

23. See Bollet, *Civil War Medicine*, 465.

24. Quoted in Laderman, *The Sacred Remains*, 114. See also Faust, *This Republic of Suffering*, 96. Faust demonstrates that "public discomfort with embalmers appeared most often in regard to the issue of money and the unsettling commodification of the dead that their business represented."

25. Faust, *This Republic of Suffering*, 97.

26. Embalming companies were formed, and they ran numerous advertisements in local papers offering their services—and most promised that their methods would leave the body looking lifelike and "marble like in character." Drs. Brown and Alexander to Hammond, Nov. 26, 1862, Office of the Surgeon General, Letters Received, 1818–1870, box 11, entry 12, RG 112, NARA.

27. Ibid.

28. Davis, *The Embattled Confederacy*, 9.

29. Davis, *Shadow of the Storm*, 9. Davis also notes that there were hundreds of photographers who could capture the images of war.

30. For more on Civil War photography, see Frassanito, *Gettysburg*, 21; Burns, *Early Medical Photography in America*; Goler and Rhode, "From Individual Trauma to National Policy."

31. Frassanito, *Gettysburg*, 27.

32. See Gardner, *Gardner's Photographic Sketchbook*, 38–41. Gardner's images literally capture the thousands of dead bodies after the Battle of Antietam. They lie dead all over the fields. Some scenes are profound, for example, the Confederate dead in the "Bloody Lane" (see pp. 49, 50, 59). Many of these images were printed in *Harper's Weekly*, providing a stark view of the reality and destructiveness of the war. Gardner also published his "Photographic Sketchbook of the War Vol. I," immediately following the war.

33. For the "harvest of death," see Gardner, *Gardner's Photographic Sketchbook*, 81, pl. 36.

34. Whitman, *Specimen Days and Collect*, 79.

35. Ibid.

36. Ibid.

37. Ibid., 80.

38. See Faust, *This Republic of Suffering*. Her book examines "the work of death," how it was managed, risked, endured, understood, and prepared for and its long-term effect on society. See also Neff, *Honoring the Civil War Dead*. For changes in death and body, see Long, *Rehabilitating Bodies*.

39. Faust, *This Republic of Suffering*, 268. Some people turned to embalming to separate the distance from the living and dead, but more practically, Congress passed a resolution to establish national cemeteries intended to memorialize the dead—but this was a transformation in the way death was handled by Americans. Faust, 99–101. See also Laderman, *The Sacred Remains*, chap. 9, in which he discusses the federal government's handling of the remains of Union soldiers. See also Laderman, *The Sacred Remains*, 103.

40. Laderman, *The Sacred Remains*, 10.

41. For example the elite physician Valentine Mott was convinced about anatomical study and dissections as the cornerstone of medical education, but this was after he worked with prominent anatomists in Europe (Abernathy, Bell, Cooper, and Monro). He also maintained a large collection of specimens for teaching aids. See Schultz, *Body Snatching*, 49. Schultz also acknowledges that Mott was a "body snatcher par excellence." Valentine Mott, however, volunteered to serve in the war for the experience of working with soldiers and developing techniques as a surgeon. He was the first surgeon to tie both carotid arteries and wrote articles and a monograph on how to arrest hemorrhage from wounds. See Valentine Mott Correspondence, NLM.

42. As I read through the autopsy reports, I was struck by how empirical and short they were or how some lacked confidence early in the war. But by 1863 specific diseases based on symptoms were more easily recognized. One can see the confidence develop through the war. See, for example, U.S.A. Gen. Hospital Newton University, Baltimore, Md., Apr. 21, 1864, C. W. Jones Case of Elmer H. Dudley, private, Company K, 16th, AMM specimen no. 2231; Hiram C. Weber, age 26, private, Company G, 3rd Mc. Regt. Vol., AMM 2785; H. C. Yarrow, AMM 806: Case of Compound Comminuted Fracture of the Leg, Followed by Traumatic Tetanus and Death, Charles Fees, age 22, private, Company B, 14th Regiment, U.S. Infantry, Medical Records, and Reports on Diseases and Individual Cases, files A and D, entries 621–23, RG 94, NARA.

43. There was an important class dimension to the project, however. Woodward noted of the museum's collection in 1871 that "mention must also be made of a shelf in which side by side specimens derived from the mutilated limbs of seven general officers. Need it be said that no critical eye could distinguish them from the similar mutilations of subalterns or of private soldiers?" Woodward, "The Army Medical Museum," 236. There is a racial dimension as well. When the war ended in 1865 the doctors at the AMM turned to the black bodies in the newly formed Freedmen's hospital for continued access to bodies.

44. Quoted in Lamb, *History of the U.S. Army Medical Museum,* 36.

45. Sappol argues that doctors were not the sole authority in antebellum America; they competed with ministers, "who also asserted moral conclusions about the life lived, and relations between the two authorities were tricky." But medical officials were gaining authority in antebellum America, as Sappol demonstrates, and this study suggests that the war was central in this transformation. See Sappol, *A Traffic of Dead Bodies,* 41.

46. Otis to Crane, Nov. 2, 1869, Outgoing Correspondence, RG 21, OHA, NMHM.

47. Henry, *The Armed Forces Institute of Pathology,* 56.

48. Brinton, *Personal Memoirs,* 189.

49. Woodward, "The Army Medical Museum," 235.

50. Bagger, "The Army Medical Museum," 294.

51. Ibid., 295.

52. Ibid.

53. Mr. Mivart publishing in *Nature* (London), Aug. 11, 1870, 290. Quoted in Henry, *The Armed Forces Institute of Pathology,* 62.

54. Ibid.

55. Alberti, *Morbid Curiosities*; Sappol, *A Traffic of Dead Bodies,* chaps. 6–8.

56. Quoted in Henry, *The Armed Forces Institute of Pathology,* 88.

57. Ibid., 56.

58. Homeopathists remained influential in some large cities for the remainder of the century, particularly in the Northeast, and some eclectics were successful in small towns and villages. However, regulars emerged as the largest and most influential group after the war. See also Rothstein, *American Physicians in the Nineteenth Century,* 177.

59. At first they wanted a new fireproof building and $5,000 more per annum. But eventually there were demands for money for the new Army Medical School and continued funds for the Surgeon General's Library.

60. S. D. Gross, Austin Flint, and O. W. Holmes, "The Army Medical Museum and Library," *Proceedings of the American Medical Association* (July 1883): 3.

61. Henry, *The Armed Forces Institute of Pathology*, 76–77. Congress appropriated $5,000 annually for the museum, which was eventually raised to $10,000. Brinton, *Personal Memoirs*, 182. See also "Army and Navy News: Congressional Appropriations," *American Medical Times* (1864): 30; "The Army Medical Museum and Library," *Proceedings of the American Medical Association*, July 1883, 3.

62. Smart, "The Army Medical Museum and the Library of the Surgeon General's Office," 578.

63. Quoted in Henry, *The Armed Forces Institute of Pathology*, 88.

64. John H. Brinton, "Address to the Members of the Graduating Class of the Army Medical Museum: Closing Exercises of the Session 1895–96, Army Medical School," 599–605, John H. Brinton Manuscript Collection, box 1, RG 124, OHA, NMHM.

65. Quoted in Lamb, *History of the U.S. Army Medical Museum*, 4.

66. Library of the Surgeon General's Office: Data Relevant to the Library in the Annual Reports of the Surgeon-General's Office, box 3, NLM.

67. Ibid.

68. Editorial, *Medical Record of New York*, Apr. 1, 1871.

69. See Alotta, *Civil War Justice*.

70. Davis, *The Guns of '62*, 250.

71. Hanging was usually assigned to men found guilty of rape, pillaging, or robbery. The firing squad was used for deserters, murders, and mutineers. Alotta, *Civil War Justice*, 37.

72. Ibid., 188. There was usually a $5 reward for the capture of a deserted soldier.

73. Ibid. Alotta found that 54.31 percent were either foreign born or black, and the numbers suggest that "ethnic and racial factors did influence who was chosen to set the example by execution" (ibid., 187).

74. Davis, *The Guns of '62*, 252.

75. Quoted in Alotta, *Civil War Justice*, 67.

76. Ibid.

77. Brinton, *Personal Memoirs*, 191.

78. During his investigations at Antietam, he studied "battlefield rigidity" and the "instantaneous rigor of death" and published his observations in the *American Journal of the Medical Sciences* (Jan. 1870): 87. His observations were also reprinted in European medical journals. See Brinton, *Personal Memoirs*, 207, and Brinton Manuscripts, entry 628, RG 94, NARA. See also John H. Brinton Manuscript Collection, RG 124, OHA, NMHM.

79. Brinton, *Personal Memoirs*, 181.

80. Ibid.

81. Lamb, *History of the U.S. Army Medical Museum*, 36. See also chapter 2.

82. George Otis to Professor Flowers, Nov. 14, 1864, Curatorial Records/Annual Reports, RG 2, OHA, NMHM. See also George Otis to Professor Flowers, Nov. 14, 1864, Outgoing Correspondence, RG 21, OHA, NMHM. Flowers had previously been exchanging specimens with Professor Baird of the Smithsonian, and Otis comments that the AMM would perhaps have more specimens of particular interest.

83. Flowers to Otis, Dec. 23, 1864, Incoming Correspondence, RG 13, OHA, NMHM.

84. Foucault, The *Birth of the Clinic*, 196.

85. Ibid., introduction.

86. Brinton, *Personal Memoirs*, 182.

87. John H. Brinton, "Address to the Members of the Graduating Class of the Army Medical Museum: Closing Exercises of the Session 1895–96, Army Medical School," 599–605, John H. Brinton Manuscript Collection, box 1, RG 124, OHA, NMHM.

88. Ibid.

89. Brinton, *Personal Memoirs*, 182.

90. Ibid., 190. Brinton also relates the same story in his address to the members of the graduating class of the Army Medical Museum. See John H. Brinton, "Address to the Members of the Graduating Class of the Army Medical Museum: Closing Exercises of the Session 1895–96, Army Medical School," 599–605, John H. Brinton Manuscript Collection, box 1, RG 124, OHA, NMHM.

91. John Brinton to Joseph Barnes May 14, 1864, Letterbooks of the Curators, RG 15, OHA, NMHM.

92. Letters sent Feb. 11, 1863, ibid.

93. Surgeons Lavington Quick, Edward Hartshorne, George Shrady, Middleton Goldsmith, F. J. Carpenter, F. L. Town, John Hodgen, H. S. Hewitt, and W. W. Keen were authorized to collect specimens. Lamb, *History of the U.S. Army Medical Museum*, 13.

94. Brinton to Keen, Sept. 25, 1862, Letterbooks of the Curators, RG 15, OHA, NMHM.

95. Moss became the first "assistant curator" to the museum, and then a curator charged with working on the specimens. See Brinton, *Personal Memoirs*, 185.

96. Brinton to William Moss, Jan. 5, 1863, Letterbooks of the Curators, RG 15, OHA, NMHM.

97. Ibid.

98. John H. Brinton, "Address to the Members of the Graduating Class of the Army Medical Museum: Closing Exercises of the Session 1895–96, Army Medical School," 599–605, John H. Brinton Manuscript Collection, box 1, RG 124, OHA, NMHM.

99. Letters were dated Oct. 11, 1862, Letterbooks of the Curators, RG 15, OHA, NMHM.

100. Letters sent to heads of general hospitals, Sept. 25, 1862, ibid.

101. Letters were dated July 28, 1862, ibid.

102. Letters were dated Aug. 7, 1862, ibid.

103. Letter from Brinton, Dec. 1, 1862, ibid.

104. Letter from Brinton, Dec. 20, 1862, ibid.

105. "Report to the Medical Director from Surgeon L. Guild," May 23, 1863, Medical Records, 1861–1889, file F, entry 624, RG 94, NARA.

106. He then went to a number of battlefields, including Antietam, Fredericksburg, and Malvern Hill, for the express purpose of collecting specimens. Brinton to Dr. Schenck, Dec. 28, 1862, Letterbooks of the Curators, RG 15, OHA, NMHM.

107. Brinton, *Personal Memoirs*, 182.

108. Special Order 116, issued May 22, 1863, granted the use of the schoolhouse located on H Street North between 13th and 14th Streets owned by Mr. Corcoran for use of the Army Medical Museum. Brinton, *Personal Memoirs*, 183.

109. Brinton to January, Dec. 28, 1862, Letterbooks of the Curators, RG 15, OHA, NMHM.

110. Brinton to Dewitt C. Peters, Baltimore General Hospital, Jan. 5, 1863, ibid.

111. Letter sent from Brinton, Dec. 22, 1862, ibid.

112. J .T. Calhoun, "History of Five Specimens Forwarded to the AMM with Suggestions as to the Preservations of Specimens in Field Service," Reports of Diseases and Individual Cases, 1841–1893, file A, no. 336, entry 621, RG 94, NARA.

113. Report from John Lidell to John Brinton, June 8, 1864, Medical Records, 1814–1919, D file, box 14, entry 623, RG 94, NARA.

114. Woodward to Surgeon Barker, USA Invalid Bureau, Mar. 10, 1864, Joseph Woodward Letterbooks, RG 28, OHA, NMHM.

115. H. K. Neff to Brinton, Sept. 24, 1863, Letterbooks of the Curators, RG 15, OHA, NMHM.

116. Surgeon General's Office to Dr. R. S. Kenderdine, Philadelphia, Aug. 25, 1862, Central Office Correspondence, Letters and Endorsements Sent, 1818–1946, vol. 32, entry 2, RG 112, NARA.

117. Charles McDougall to S. W. Gross, Feb. 23, 1863, copied to Brinton, Letterbooks of the Curators, RG 15, OHA, NMHM. Wood, one of the founders of Bellevue Medical College in New York, was undoubtedly looking to enhance his medical museum.

118. Ibid.

119. Ibid.

120. Charles McDougall to Hammond, Feb. 24, 1863, Incoming Correspondence, RG 13, OHA, NMHM.

121. Hammond to Bontecou copied to Brinton, Feb. 23, 1863, ibid.

122. Like Gross, he blames the destruction or loss of specimens on "negroes" in charge of the dead house—but considering Bontecou's numerous publications, many of which relied on wet specimens, I think this is probably unlikely. For Bontecou's casebook, see Reports of Diseases and Individual Cases, 1841–93, file A, entry 621, RG 94, NARA.

123. Hammond to Bontecou, copied to Brinton, Feb. 23, 1863, ibid. He eventually submitted 101 specimens.

124. Brinton to Hammond, June 2, 1863, Curatorial Records: Circulars and Reports, box 1, RG 6, OHA, NMHM.

125. Brinton to Thomas Markoe, Mar. 4, 1863, Letterbooks of the Curators, RG 15, OHA, NMHM. Emphasis in original.

126. Ibid.

127. Thomas Markoe to Brinton, May 27, 1863, ibid.

128. Ibid.

129. James Armsby to Brinton, Dec. 21, 1865, ibid.

130. Brinton to J. W. Mintzer, June 6, 1863, ibid.

131. Alexander Hoff to Professor Alden, Mar.–Dec. 20, 1862, Alexander Henry Hoff Papers, 1821–1876, MS C 484, NLM.

132. Ibid.

133. Hammond to J. E. Ebersole, July 26, 1863, Letterbooks of the Curators, RG 15, OHA, NMHM.

134. Brinton to George Cogwell, June 5, 1863, ibid.

135. H. K. Neff, Huntington, Penn., to Brinton, June 21, 1864, Incoming Correspondence, RG 13, OHA, NMHM.

136. J. W. Mintzer to Brinton, June 9, 1863, ibid.

137. Ibid.

138. Quoted in Rable, *God's Almost Chosen People*, 184.

139. "Specimen Histories," Histories of Pathological Specimens, prepared and forwarded by William Thomson from Douglas Hospital, Medical Records, 1814–1919, D file, box 28, entry 623, RG 94, NARA.

140. Ibid.

141. Ibid.

142. These occur only infrequently and can be found in case histories largely in Medical Records, files A and D, entries 621–23, RG 94, NARA.

143. Mason Cogswell, Assistant Surgeon, U.S. Volunteers, "Remarks on the Monthly Report of Sick and Wounded in US General Hospital in Albany, New York," Aug. 1864, Reports of Diseases and Individual Cases 1841–93, box 4, entry 621, RG 94, NARA.

144. Submitted by Assistant Surgeon H. Stone, "Case of Pyemia Subsequent to an Operation of Resection of the Radius after Being Wounded Sept. 17, 1862 at Antietam," Medical Records, 1814–1919, D file, no. 147, entry 621, RG 94, NARA.

145. J. T. Calhoun, "History of Five Specimens Forwarded to the AMM with Suggestions as to the Preservations of Specimens in Field Service," Reports of Diseases and Individual Cases, 1841–93, file A, no. 336, entry 621, RG 94, NARA.

146. John H. Brinton, "Address to the Members of the Graduating Class of the Army Medical Museum: Closing Exercises of the Session 1895–96, Army Medical School," 599–605, John H. Brinton Manuscript Collection, box 1, RG 124, OHA, NMHM.

147. Letter from Lorin Leray, Dec. 29, 1883, Incoming Correspondence, RG 13, OHA, NMHM.

148. Some former soldiers wrote the museum and gave the number of their specimens or history of the wound, along with photographs of themselves, which often showed the missing part in question; they then asked for a photograph of the specimen. The tone of the letters was often friendly, deferential, and not demanding (as I first thought they might have been). See Incoming Correspondence, RG 13, OHA, NMHM. Most letters came in the 1870s and 1880s. The pension records at NARA and the Searcher Reports at the NMHM also contain these types of letters. In some cases, it was to show their entitlement to a pension.

149. Bagger, "The Army Medical Museum," 296.

150. For an interesting history on Daniel Sickles, see Hessler, *Sickles at Gettysburg*.

151. Woodward, "The Army Medical Museum," 236.

152. Ibid., 233. See also Frederickson, *The Inner Civil War*, 199. Fredrickson demonstrates that both during and after the war there was a "decline in the prestige of traditional religion" (in which opposition to dissection had generally been couched) and a developing interest in new scientific ideas, principally Darwinism.

153. Brinton, *Personal Memoirs*, 187.

154. Woodward, "The Army Medical Museum," 233.

155. Brinton, *Personal Memoirs*, 188.

156. Woodward to Charles Greenleaf, Nov. 4, 1864, Joseph Woodward Letterbooks, RG 28, OHA, NMHM.

157. Ibid.

158. Interestingly, the other main institutional body, the Sanitary Commission, also had an important function, and it used the support of the government to develop preventative medicine (central goal) and relief for the soldiers and the organization of medical professionals (administrators, doctors, nurses, volunteers). In terms of the work of individual physicians, there was much overlap between the Army Medical Museum and the Sanitary Commission. See *The Sanitary Commission of the United States Army: A Succinct Narrative of its Works and Purposes*.

159. Editorial, *American Medical Times* 6 (May 23, 1863): 249.

160. John Brinton, Report to the Surgeon General, Washington, D.C., Jan. 10, 1863, Curatorial Records: Circulars and Reports, RG 6, OHA, NMHM.

161. "Report from Brinton on the Inspection of Books, Registrars of the U.S. Hospitals, Nov. 21, 1863," submitted to Hammond and medical inspectors, hospitals, Medical Records, 1814–1919, D file, entry 623, RG 94, NARA. Original emphasis.

162. "History of Pathological Specimens Forwarded to the AMM, U. S. A General Hospital, Broad and Cherry Street, Philadelphia, Penn., submitted by William Keating, Assistant Surgeon USA," Reports of Diseases and Individual Cases, 1841–93, file A, no. 171, entry 621, RG 94, NARA.

163. Ibid.

164. "History of Pathological Specimens Prepared and Forwarded by William Thomson from Douglas Hospital, 1864," Reports of Diseases and Individual Cases, 1841–93, file A, no. 171, entry 621, RG 94, NARA.

165. Ibid.

166. "History of Pathological Specimens Forwarded to the AMM, U.S.A General Hospital, Broad and Cherry Street, Philadelphia, Penn., submitted by I. Eagleton, Assistant Surgeon USA," Reports of Diseases and Individual Cases, 1841–93, file A, no. 171, entry 621, RG 94, NARA.

167. Ibid.

168. Calhoun, "History of Five Specimens Forwarded to the AMM."

169. Ibid.

170. Ibid.

171. Woodward to Cantwell, Mar. 12, 1864, Joseph Woodward Letterbooks, RG 28, OHA, NMHM.

172. Woodward to Surgeon M. McGill, Oct. 23, 1866, ibid.

173. Tetanus was one of those diseases that stimulated debate and then research. Indeed, many elite physicians including S. Weir, Mitchell, Da Costa, and Keen conducted experiments on tetanus (caused from infection, transmitted by animal feces, or contracted during surgery in temporary field hospitals set up near barns—it caused painful muscle spasms, patients could not swallow or breathe, and back, abdominal, and limb muscles become rigid, extremely painful). Brown-Séquard spoke at length on tetanus, including postmortem appearances, symptoms, treatment, and prevention during his lecture at the Smithsonian. See "Notes of a Lecture by Dr. Brown-Séquard Delivered at the Smithsonian Institution June 14, 1864," Reports of Diseases and Individual Cases, 1841–93, file A, no. 344, entry 621, RG 94, NARA.

174. Bollet, *Civil War Medicine*, 213.

175. Woodward to Surgeon M. McGill, Oct. 23, 1866, Joseph Woodward Letterbooks, RG 28, OHA, NMHM.

176. "Specimen Histories, Douglas USA General Hospital for June 1863, submitted by William Thomson," Reports of Diseases and Individual Cases, 1841–93, file A, no. 103, entry 621, RG 94, NARA.

177. Ibid.

178. Ibid.

179. Ibid. Emphasis in original.

180. Bollet, *Civil War Medicine*, 144.

181. "Hygeia Hospital Fortress Monroe, R. B. Bontecou's Report," Reports of Diseases and Individual Cases, 1841–93, file A, no. 59, entry 621, RG 94, NARA.

182. Resections often led to more cases of infection and took much longer than amputation.

183. "Hygeia Hospital Fortress Monroe, R. B. Bontecou's Report."

184. Ibid.

185. The fatality rate for wounds treated conservatively was 17.9 percent, for amputation it was 25 percent, and for excision, 27.5 percent. *Medical and Surgical History*, 3:879.

186. "Special Cases in Ward D Fifth Street Hospital," Submitted by Surgeons Dunglison and Hunt, June 30, 1862, Reports of Diseases and Individual Cases, 1841–93, file A, no. A-1, entry 621, RG 94, NARA.

187. Ibid.

188. Woodward and Otis, *Circular No. 6*, 3. See also Otis, *A Report on Amputations of the Hip Joint in Military Surgery*; *A Report on Excisions of the Head of the Femur for Gunshot Injury*.

189. Keen, "Surgical Reminiscences of the Civil War," 432–33.

190. Bollet, *Civil War Medicine*, 153.

191. John Carpenter to Brinton, May 7, 1863, Incoming Correspondence, RG 13, OHA, NMHM.

192. John Morgan to Brinton, Mar. 19, 1863, ibid.

193. W. F. Norris, Douglas General Hospital, to Brinton, Oct. 19, 1865, ibid.

194. A. A. Hudson, U.S. Volunteers, Carver US General Hospital, "Specimen Histories, June 21, 1865," Medical Records, 1814–1919, D file, box 28, entry 623, RG 94, NARA.

195. James H. Armsby to Brinton, Oct. 22, 1865, Incoming Correspondence, RG 13, OHA, NMHM.

196. Ibid.

197. Ibid.

198. Billings, "Medical Museums," 135.

199. Joseph Barnes to Thomas Longmore, Jan. 29, 1864, Medical Records, 1814–1919, D file, box 14, no. 23, entry 623, RG 94, NARA.

200. Fredrickson, *The Inner Civil War*, 201.

CHAPTER 6

1. Woodward, "The Army Medical Museum," 233.

2. Bynum, *Science and the Practice of Medicine*, 74–75.

3. Ibid., 75.

4. Circular No. 5, issued Jan. 4, 1867, Circulars and Circular Letters of the Surgeon General's Office, entry 63, RG 112, NARA. This is an interesting point because one of the tenets of contagionist theory was that medical attendants often contracted the disease—Woodward was not a contagionist (and was later criticized for it), but it shows the uncertainty about previously accepted doctrines during this period.

5. Pelling, *Cholera, Fever and English Medicine*. See also Rosenberg, *The Cholera Years*, 193–94.

6. Though his theories were at variance with Snow's. See Rosenberg, *The Cholera Years*, 194.

7. Quoted in Baldwin, *Contagion and the State*, 143.

8. For the very best study on theories related to cholera in the nineteenth century, see Pelling, *Cholera, Fever and English Medicine*.

9. Ibid.

10. Rosenberg, *The Cholera Years*, 150, 199. There is an important class or racial dimension to this disease. It was always associated with "lower" class and crowded tenements, and even within the military it was associated with intemperance, poor personal habits, and disobeying sanitary regulations. These views are still prevalent in some of the case reports.

11. Ibid., 194–95. In a sampling of 128 physicians, Rosenberg cites 55 as being "thoroughly contagionist," 21 were considered "contingent contagionist," 52 were anticontagionists, and 45 accepted some of the conclusions of Snow and Pettenkofer.

12. See Johansen et al., *Cholera, Chloroform and the Science of Medicine*, 392.

13. Pelling, *Cholera, Fever and English Medicine*, 236.

14. Physicians often pointed out how their findings may have differed from or enhanced the findings of European physicians—it is actually part of the American identity that developed through the war.

15. Hamlin, *Cholera: The Biography*, 165.

16. For example, from the 1860s to the 1890s Britain, France, Germany, and Russia sent out various teams to study cholera in Egypt, among other locales. By the 1880s German and French researchers were searching for a "germ," while the British were further developing ideas about sanitation and epidemiology. We now know that cholera is transmitted through the ingestion of water contaminated with the cholera bacteria or by soiled bedding and clothing. Cholera patients suffered very liquid diarrhea, which often made its way into waterways, groundwater, or drinking water supplies. It has generally not been associated with direct human-to-human contact; however, a 2002 study at Tufts University recently demonstrated the potential for human-to-human transmission; see Merrell et al., "Host-Induced Epidemic Spread of the Cholera Bacterium." The bacteria of cholera has long been studied in the laboratory as an evolving disease form.

17. For one of the best discussions of the decline of infectious disease mortality and the techniques and educational ideas of public health authorities after 1870, see Tomes, "The Private Side of Public Health"; Tomes, *The Gospel of Germs*. (However, she does not mention the war.)

18. Woodward, *Circular No. 1*, vi.

19. See, for example, Woodward, *Circular No. 5*, sec. B, "Extracts from Official Reports."

20. See, for example, editorial, *Richmond Medical and Surgical Journal* (Jan. 1867): 88–91.

21. Downs, *Sick from Freedom*, 114–16.

22. General Orders issued after the war put the enforcement of quarantine and health laws of the state in the hands of appointed military officers, state officers, and private physicians who subsequently worked together on matters of quarantine and tracing the disease. See "Bvt. Brig. General J. J. Milhau, Surgeon U. S. A. to Medical Director 3rd Military District Atlanta, Ga., Report Relative to Quarantine," Reports on Diseases and Individual Cases, 1841–93, Papers Relating to Cholera, Smallpox and Yellow Fever Epidemics, 1849–1893, entry 620, RG 94, NARA. See also Library of the Surgeon General's Office: Data Relevant to the Library in the Annual Reports of the Surgeon-General's Office, box 3, MS C 185, NLM.

23. See Maxwell, *Lincoln's Fifth Wheel*.

24. Ibid., 288. Individual physicians were fine to move between a hospital position and work for the Sanitary Commission, but some higher-ups, notably Barnes, were often jealous and felt scientific inquiry should be the exclusive domain of the medical department.

25. Rosenberg, *The Cholera Years*, 193.

26. He wrote a scathing report about the sanitary conditions in New York. For more on Harris as a sanitary reformer, see ibid., 187–91.

27. Woodward to Elisha Harris, Jan. 14, 1867, Joseph Woodward Letterbooks, OHA, RG 28, NMHM.

28. Ibid.

29. Elisha Harris incorporated the surgeon general's findings into his *Conclusions concerning Cholera*, and the Surgeon General's Office similarly incorporated his findings into Circulars No. 1 and 5. Exchanging these early findings, and having the medical department as a resource, was important for civilian physicians. Much of the material was unpublished, and Woodward emphasized that the information in the unpublished case reports "fully equals in value, and certainly exceeds in quantity, that which has thus been printed." See, for example, Woodward, "The Medical Staff of the United States Army," 15.

30. See Bvt. Brig. General J. J. Milhau, "Relative to Quarantine." He discusses the medical director of the army becoming president of the Board of Health. General Order No. 43, Medical Department of Louisiana, May 15, 1866, appointed medical officers to quarantine duty. Military quarantines existed also in the Carolinas, Florida, Texas, and Indiana, and the military was found effective in maintaining quarantines. The military did this to protect both the states and the military forces.

31. General Order No. 3, Headquarters, Second Military District, Charleston, S.C., Mar. 24, 1864, established quarantine for all vessels, which carried on into 1866. Ibid.

32. Joseph Barnes, Surgeon General, to Hon. E. M. Stanton, Secretary of War, in Annual Report of the Secretary of War for 1865. Quoted in Bollet, *Civil War Medicine*, 286.

33. Circular letter, Dec. 5, 1866, Joseph Woodward Letterbooks, RG 28, OHA, NMHM.

34. Woodward, *Circular No. 1*.

35. The reports that were submitted to Barnes refer to his directive, which was issued to trace epidemics in 1866 and 1867. J. K. Barnes, Circular No. 3, "Cholera," Apr. 20, 1867, Circulars and Circular Letters, entry 63, RG 112, NARA.

36. Harris, *Conclusions concerning Cholera*, 1874, 11.

37. Woodward to J. H. Franz, Jan. 14, 1867, Joseph Woodward Letterbooks, RG 28, OHA, NMHM.

38. J. H. Franz, "Report concerning Epidemic Cholera Which Prevailed among 11th U.S. Infantry during August and Sept. 1866," Feb. 21, 1867, Papers Relating to Cholera, Smallpox and Yellow Fever Epidemics, 1849–93, entry 620, RG 94, NARA.

39. Ibid.

40. Ibid.

41. Ibid.

42. R. B. Browne to Barnes, Aug. 1866, Papers Relating to Cholera, Smallpox and Yellow Fever Epidemics, 1849–93, entry 620, RG 94, NARA.

43. Jos. R. Smith, Medical Directors Office, 4th Military District, Vicksburg, Miss., Apr. 19, 1867, to Barnes, ibid.

44. Ibid.

45. Joseph Brown to Woodward, June 1, 1866, ibid.

46. Ibid.

47. Ibid.

48. Ibid.

49. T. A. McParlin, Fort Delaware, Nov. 20, 1866, Papers Relating to Cholera, Smallpox and Yellow Fever Epidemics, 1849–93, entry 620, RG 94, NARA.

50. Ibid.

51. Ibid.

52. The social and political strife between civilians and the military is not considered here; this study is concerned with the scientific study of cholera. For more on the social and racial inequalities of the medical response to cholera, see Rosenberg, *The Cholera Years*.

53. Geo. Taylor to Woodward, Jan. 9, 1867, Papers relating to Cholera, Smallpox and Yellow Fever Epidemics, 1849–93, entry 620, RG 94, NARA. Some physicians in the nineteenth century distinguished between direct contagion (touch) and infection in which people could inhale a "virus" after it was given off or exhaled from the skin or pores of an infected person. See Johansen et al., *Cholera, Chloroform and the Science of Medicine*, 177.

54. Geo. Taylor to Woodward, Jan. 9, 1867, Papers Relating to Cholera, Smallpox and Yellow Fever Epidemics, 1849–93, entry 620, RG 94, NARA.

55. George McGill died July 20, 1867, near Old Fort Lyon, Colorado Territory, from cholera.

56. Worboys, *Spreading Germs*, 126.

57. Special Report of Davids Island, New York Harbor, Feb. 25, 1867, submitted by George McGill, Assistant Surgeon, Papers Relating to Cholera, Smallpox and Yellow Fever Epidemics, 1849–93, entry 620, RG 94, NARA.

58. Ibid.

59. Ibid.

60. Report from William Sloan, Medical Director of the East, July 31, 1866, Papers Relating to Cholera, Smallpox and Yellow Fever Epidemics, 1849–93, entry 620, RG 94, NARA.

61. Ibid.

62. Ibid.

63. He did not make this link—but his measures would support emerging research about microorganisms and preventative medicine in the later nineteenth century.

64. Anticontagionists usually saw most cases of disease at the beginning of a stay at a new locale (e.g., with the most cases of disease up front and then waning). It was just the opposite for contagionists, who saw cases increase over time and as a result of more human-to-human contact.

65. Report from William Sloan, Medical Director of the East, July 31, 1866, Papers Relating to Cholera, Smallpox and Yellow Fever Epidemics, 1849–93, entry 620, RG 94, NARA.

66. Ibid.

67. Woodward, *Circular No. 1*, ix.

68. Ibid., 34. Report submitted by W. Carroll, Brevet Major and Assistant Surgeon, U.S.V.

69. Woodward, *Circular No. 5*, Extract from Official Reports, 34. Report submitted by W. Carroll, Brevet Major and Assistant Surgeon, U.S.V.

70. From a newspaper clipping entitled "The Public Health," box 1, Papers Relating to Cholera, Smallpox and Yellow Fever Epidemics, 1849–93, entry 620, RG 94, NARA.

71. See, for example, Woodward, *Circular No. 5.*

72. Ibid., xv.

73. Ibid., xvi.

74. Ibid., 60–61.

75. Ibid.

76. Worboys, *Spreading Germs*, 248. He was also searching for causative bacteria.

77. Ibid., 234. See also Pelling, *Cholera, Fever and English Medicine*, chap. 6.

78. Woodward was also asked to prepare a report on the pathological histology of yellow fever, and he detailed his results with photomicrographs prepared at the museum. See Woodward, "The Size of the Blood Corpuslce," *Medical Record*, New York (1880): 131; Woodward, "Remarks on the Pathological Histology of Yellow Fever."

79. Woodward, *Circular No. 1*, v. (See also Circular No. 3, rpt. in Circular No. 1, Appendix, 17.)

80. Ibid., v.

81. In the late 1880s, Joseph Kinyoun joined the Marine Hospital Service and subsequently set up a laboratory at the Staten Island Marine Hospital. It was an experimental laboratory with animals and up-to-date laboratory apparatus. He undertook an investigation of the water in the New York Bay to investigate the power to sustain the life of the cholera spirillum. He later identified the cholera comma bacillus in the stools of immigrants, which, as Victoria Harden has demonstrated, "was the first bacteriological diagnosis of cholera in the Western Hemisphere." See Harden, *Inventing the NIH: Federal Biomedical Research Policy*, 12–13. However, it is important to emphasize that this discovery was not made in isolation. Kinyoun was building on a tradition of government-sponsored research and investigation, which began on a large scale with the Civil War.

82. Special Report of Davids Island, New York Harbor, Feb. 25, 1867, submitted by George McGill, Assistant Surgeon, Papers Relating to Cholera, Smallpox and Yellow Fever Epidemics, 1849–93, entry 620, RG 94, NARA.

83. Ibid.

84. Ibid.

85. William Farr, *Cholera*, xv. Quoted in Worboys, *Spreading Germs*, 114.

86. He did not, however, go into detail here. For example, he did not say whether they formed in the person and then were released in the discharge and transmitted to another body—rather he says formed in the discharge. During the same period, Karl Thiersch (who worked with Pettenkofer and Liebig; together they were referred to as the "Munich Chemists") undertook experiments to prove the communicability of cholera person to person but found that "cholera evacuations are not at first capable of generating the disease." See Pelling, *Cholera, Fever and English Medicine*, 247.

87. He mixed sucrose and sulfuric acid with the bile to see if it would turn violet, which would indicate the presence of bile acids.

88. George McGill, "Special Report of Davids Island, New York Harbor Feb. 25th, 1867," Papers Relating to Cholera, Smallpox and Yellow Fever Epidemics, 1849–93, entry 620, RG 94, NARA.

89. Liebig and Thiersch often focused extensively on the blood since its altered appearance was associated with poor health or abnormal function. See Pelling, *Cholera, Fever and English Medicine*, 244. But many theories (Farr, Liebig, etc.) saw disease as resting in the

blood—or that a chemical could excite a reaction in the blood; thus, this detail in the blood was not uncommon.

90. Special Report of Davids Island, New York Harbor, Feb. 25, 1867, submitted by George McGill, Assistant Surgeon, Papers Relating to Cholera, Smallpox and Yellow Fever Epidemics, 1849–93, entry 620, RG 94, NARA.

91. Reports on Diseases and Individual Cases, 1841–93, Papers Relating to Cholera, Smallpox and Yellow Fever Epidemics, 1849–93, entry 620, RG 94, NARA. There are seven boxes in this series, boxes 1–3 and 5–7 mostly consider cholera and smallpox, while box 4 concerns reports related to yellow fever.

92. Reprinted in Woodward, *Circular No. 5*, 37.

93. Ibid.

94. Ibid.

95. Pelling, *Cholera, Fever and English Medicine*, 236. Simon noted in 1881 a popular experiment in London "performed on half a million human beings in South London, by the commercial water companies."

96. Woodward, *Circular No. 5*, 37.

97. Ibid.

98. Ibid, 38.

99. Ibid. Between 1854 and the 1880s there were experiments (and debates) about water supplies during cholera outbreaks between but not limited to Simon, Snow, Thiersch, Sanderson, Parkes, and Pettenkofer. The various objectives were multifactorial, but most were focused on communicability, the dangerousness of water supply during visits of cholera, and how to purify water safely. See Pelling, *Cholera, Fever and English Medicine*, 233–35.

100. For more on the development of experimental practices, see Marks, *The Progress of Experiment*, 30–31.

101. B. F. Craig, "Report on the Disinfectants and Their Use in Connection with Cholera from the Laboratory of the Surgeon General's Office," May 1, 1867, Papers Relating to Cholera, Smallpox and Yellow Fever Epidemics, 1849–93, entry 620, RG 94, NARA. Though Craig later published his report, the unpublished, handwritten report contains more questions and uncertainty about various ideas and findings than the published version. The report nicely illustrates the dynamism of the period as it related to the development of new theories and new investigative tools.

102. Ibid. Importantly, the Chemical Laboratory of the Surgeon General's Office, where Craig performed the experiments, was created during the Civil War. Indeed, Woodward noted that the creation of this laboratory was "one of the necessities of the Civil War." See, for example, Woodward, "The Medical Staff of the United States Army," 15.

103. Craig, "Report on the Disinfectants."

104. Ibid.

105. Quoted in Worboys, *Spreading Germs*, 34.

106. Ibid., 35.

107. In 1865, John Simon, British medical officer of health, told members of the Privy Council that further progress in understanding cholera required "improved methods of aetiological observation and scientific researches must first have created a far more intimate knowledge than is yet current as to the nature of the morbid processes which are to be

prevented, and as to the physical and chemical conditions of their development." Quoted in Pelling, *Cholera, Fever and English Medicine*, 237.

108. Worboys, *Spreading Germs*, 43–44. See also Romano, *John Burdon Sanderson and the Culture of Victorian Science*.

109. Worboys, *Spreading Germs*, 44.

110. Romano, *John Burdon Sanderson and the Culture of Victorian Science*, 58–59; Worboys, *Spreading Germs*, 42 and chap. 2.

111. Quoted in Worboys, *Spreading Germs*, 54.

112. Ibid. Interestingly, he suggests that in killing the "lower forms of animal life," putrefaction will be arrested, suggesting a biological interpretation of putrefaction. Carbolic alcohol had been used with success during the war.

113. Craig, "Report on the Disinfectants."

114. See Worboys, *Spreading Germs*, 34.

115. Craig, "Report on the Disinfectants."

116. Bartholow, *The Principles and Practice of Disinfection*, 4–5.

117. Ibid., 1. During the Civil War, Bartholow was in charge of hospitals in Baltimore, New York Harbor, Washington, Chattanooga, and Nashville. In 1864 he entered private practice in Cincinnati and became a professor in the Medical College of Ohio.

118. Craig, "Report on the Disinfectants." A brief note about language here. Words like virus, bacteria, germs, and poison had no fixed meaning in 1865—this was before the theories of Pasteur, Koch, and Lister gave shape to these words. A "germ" usually referred to a living organism, whereas a "zyme," poison or cellular breakdown, was usually associated with a chemical process. An "animalcule" was sometimes thought of as chemical, other times as living. During and after the Civil War, these terms were in flux because ideas about diseases, as separate or physiological entities, were all being debated, and traditional ideas were being challenged. The important point is that these terms had a different meaning than they do today.

119. Bartholow, *The Principles and Practice of Disinfection*, 2.

120. Ibid., 6.

121. The focus of this book is not the radical debates around the germ theory that ensued in the 1870s and 1880s, but rather the role of the Civil War in preparing American physicians for this transformation. Civil War physicians such as Bartholow, Keen, Weir, Mitchell, Goldsmith, and Ben Woodward were supporters of the "germ theory," however.

122. Bartholow, *The Principles and Practice of Disinfection*, 7.

123. Ibid.

124. Ibid.

125. These theories were passionately debated in Europe in the 1880s. See Worboys, *Spreading Germs*, 248–52.

126. Woodworth, *The Cholera Epidemic of 1873*, 19.

127. However, Pelling has demonstrated that these two theories "eventually emerged as being complementary." See Pelling, "Contagion, Germ Theory, Specificity," 327.

128. Rosenberg, *The Cholera Years*, 210.

129. In 1867 Woodward reported that the hygienic measures adopted during the 1867 epidemic as compared to the 1866 epidemic greatly reduced the severity of the epidemic. The proportion of deaths to the total number of cases was 1 death to 2.19 cases in 1867, whereas in 1866 it was 1 to 2.22. As Woodward observed, the disease was no less virulent in 1867, but

rather the hygienic precautions and the additional measures taken had been successful. See Woodward, *Circular No. 1*, vi.

130. Most of the letters were positive and complimentary of the military's work and management of the disease. Indeed, the Moscow Surgery Society thanked the Surgeon General's Office in particular for the cholera circular and "respectfully begs the Washington Surgeon General's Office to continue sending any of their medical publications and offers to forward all those that the Moscow society will publish." Letter to Barnes, Oct. 26, 1868, Incoming Correspondence, RG 13, OHA, NMHM.

131. Ibid. See also Rosenberg, *The Cholera Years*.

132. Woodworth, *The Cholera Epidemic of 1873*.

133. Woodworth had served in the Union army and, among his many responsibilities, cared for soldiers during Sherman's march through Georgia.

134. The Marine Hospital Service developed from a "one room bacteriological laboratory" established in Aug. 1887 at the Marine Hospital on Staten Island, New York. A 1902 act provided for both the reconfiguration of the laboratory and the renaming of the laboratory to the Marine Hospital Service. See Harden, *Inventing the NIH*, 9–18, 34–36.

135. Harris, *Conclusions concerning Cholera*, 1.

136. Ibid.

137. Bartholow, *The Principles and Practice of Disinfection*, 37.

138. Harris, *Conclusions concerning Cholera*, 2–4.

139. Joseph Lister to A. C. Girard, copied to Surgeon General Crane, Nov. 28, 1877, Special Scientific and Historical Reports, box 5, entry 629, RG 94, NARA. Girard went to England in July 1877 to study Lister's methods and wrote a report for Crane.

140. Ibid. For more on the evolution of cholera, see Hamlin, *Cholera: The Biography*.

141. Woodworth, *The Cholera Epidemic of 1873*, 5. The tensions that characterized acceptance of bacteriological theories are considered in one of my upcoming projects, which examines various Civil War physicians in the thirty years after the war.

142. Ibid., 97.

143. Hamlin, *Cholera: The Biography*, 8.

144. Ibid., 134.

145. For more on the history of cholera, see Hamlin, *Cholera: The Biography*; Baldwin, *Contagion and the State*.

CHAPTER 7

1. Editorial, *Richmond Medical and Surgical Journal* (Jan. 1867): 88–91, 88.

2. Silas Weir Mitchell, as quoted in Warner, "Physiology," in Numbers, *The Education of American Physicians*, 58.

3. Editorial, *Richmond Medical and Surgical Journal* (Jan. 1867): 88.

4. Ibid.

5. Quoted in Blustein, *Preserve Your Love for Science*, 75.

6. Rothstein, *American Medical Schools and the Practice of Medicine*, 42.

7. See Gillett, *The Army Medical Department*.

8. See especially Library of the Surgeon General's Office: Data Relevant to the Library in the Annual Reports of the Surgeon-General's Office, box 3, MS C 185, NLM; Alpheus

Benning Crosby, "Construction of a Pavilion Hospital during the Civil War, ca. 1876," MS C 254, NLM.

9. Joseph Barnes was awarded the authority to have all "slush funds" of discontinued wartime hospitals transferred to Otis and Billings for the development of the museum and library. Henry, *The Armed Forces Institute of Pathology*, 52.

10. See, for example, Cassedy, *John Shaw Billings*.

11. Henry, *The Armed Forces Institute of Pathology*, 52. Billings created these guides with his assistant, Robert Fletcher.

12. Billings, "Letter of transmittal, Specimen fasciculus," quoted in Rogers, *Selected Papers of John Shaw Billings*, 19.

13. Woodward, "The Medical Staff and the United States Army," 19. See also Miles, *A History of the National Library of Medicine*, 176–77.

14. Woodward, "The Medical Staff and the United States Army," 19.

15. John Shaw Billings, Report 1875, Library of the Surgeon General's Office: Data Relevant to the Library in the Annual Reports of the Surgeon-General's Office, box 3, MS C 185, NLM. Woodward and Otis released surgical photographs and photographs of specimens; Billings published extensively on public health and hospitals. In 1878 Otis and Woodward published an article, "Notes on the Contributions to the Army Medical Museum by Civil Practitioners," *Boston Medical and Surgical Journal 98* (1878): 163. The idea was to emphasize that the museum was a national resource, not just for military medicine.

16. Clipping from the *Richmond and Louisville Medical Journal* 11 (Feb. 1871), U.S., Army Surgeon General's Office: Correspondence Acknowledging Receipt of Circular nos. 1–7, box 1, MS C 7, NLM.

17. Woodward, "The Medical Staff of the United States Army," 21.

18. Blight, *Race and Reunion*.

19. See Downs, *Sick from Freedom*. Providing for veterans proved more successful than providing for freedmen. As Downs demonstrates, the federal government did not allot enough funds to hire proper personnel and to maintain efficient hospitals. There was a fear that freedpeople would become dependent on the government for support (the bureau was only a temporary institution). Moreover, there was the larger objective of sustaining an effective labor system, and the explicit goal was to have states assume responsibility for the healthcare of the newly freed people.

20. Figg and Farrell-Beck, "Amputation in the Civil War," 465.

21. Quoted in ibid., 472.

22. Holmes, "Widows and the Civil War Pension System," 172. Figg and Farrell-Beck, "Amputation in the Civil War," 462. The "General Law Pension System" was in place from 1862 to 1890, and was replaced with the Dependent Pension Act of 1890.

23. Holmes, "Widows and the Civil War Pension System," 172. See also Goler and Rhode, "From Individual Trauma to National Policy."

24. Holmes, "Widows and the Civil War Pension System," 172.

25. Figg and Farrell-Beck, "Amputation in the Civil War," 462.

26. Ibid., 460.

27. Grant, "The Lost Boys," 249–50.

28. Until just before his death on August 17, 1884, Woodward ran the Record and Pension Office, while the Division of Surgical Records was run by Otis (until his death on February

23, 1881); both of these divisions operated through the museum and library. See Goler and Rhode, "From Individual Trauma to National Policy," 13–14.

29. W. W. Keen, "An Autobiographical Sketch by W. W. Keen," Reminiscences for His Children; 1912 with additions 1915, p. 44, APS.

30. Da Costa to Keen, Feb. 8, 1865, W. W. Keen Correspondence, CPP. Letter in which he thanks Keen for the heart stethoscope and larynscope.

31. The patient had one pupil that was contracted to the size of a pinpoint. He was diagnosed with having a division of the sympathetic nerve. The case history is recorded in Mitchell, Morehouse, and Keen, *Gunshot Wounds and Other Injuries of Nerves*, 39. After his visit with Bernard, Keen went on a tour of Virchow's laboratory, which he enjoyed very much. W. W. Keen, "An Autobiographical Sketch by W. W. Keen," Reminiscences for His Children; 1912 with additions 1915, p. 224, APS.

32. With Drs. Mitchell, Wood, Lewis, Harlan, and Oliver, Keen saw the patient and conferred on the diagnosis. At that time, the doctors decided against the removal of the brain tumor. (According to Keen, the first modern removal of a brain tumor was done in London by Dr. Godlee in 1884, and Weir Mitchell had performed one in 1885, but it was a very new and little understood procedure.) A few weeks later, however, Keen recalled, the patient returned and at that time Keen "operated on him and when I removed the trephine button from his skull . . . there lay the tumor, just where I diagnosed it to be. . . . I passed my little finger around its margin and peeled it out as easily as one scoops a hardboiled egg out of its shell with a spoon!" He remembered that there was no hemorrhage and not a lot of blood. Though Keen worried that he bungled the aftercare, he monitored the patient, and twenty-five years later the patient, Theodore Daveler, was still alive. W. W. Keen, "An Autobiographical Sketch by W. W. Keen," Reminiscences for His Children; 1912 with additions 1915, p. 43, APS.

33. W. W. Keen Correspondence, boxes 1–3, ser. 1–2, CPP. In October 1866 Keen purchased the "lease, seven pupils at ten dollars each, a dozen dissecting tables, and half a dozen cadavers" from Dr. R. S. Sutton, so that Keen could take over teaching anatomy and operative surgery at the Philadelphia School of Anatomy. Given his lack of anatomical knowledge just five years earlier, this suggests again the important role of the Civil War in Keen's development and also in the transfer of wartime knowledge and methods to the next generation of American physicians. See W. W. Keen, "An Autobiographical Sketch by W. W. Keen," Reminiscences for His Children; 1912 with additions 1915, p. 30–40, APS.

34. John H. Brinton Manuscript Collection, box 1, RG 124, OHA, NMHM.

35. On Nov. 12, 1891, Brinton sent letters to physicians in America requesting submissions. John Hill Brinton Papers, 1853–1896, CPP.

36. John H. Brinton, "Address to the Graduating Class of Jefferson Medical College, April 27, 1892," John H. Brinton Manuscript Collection, box 1, RG 124, OHA, NMHM.

37. Letter from Brinton to the Board of Charities of Philadelphia, 1891, John Hill Brinton Papers, 1853–1896, CPP.

38. Brinton, *Personal Memoirs*, 181.

39. Mitchell, "The Medical Department in the Civil War: Address before the Physicians Club Chicago, Ills. 1902/March/25," Silas Weir Mitchell Papers, box 17, ser. 7, p. 3, CPP.

40. Ibid.

41. Ibid., 17.

42. Ibid.

43. Williams, "S. Weir Mitchell," in *Silas Weir Mitchell: Memorial Addresses and Resolutions*, 87–88.

44. Kelly and Burrages, *American Medical Biography*, "Joseph Janvier Woodward," clipping, Joseph Woodward Papers, RG 363, OHA, NMHM.

45. Review of J. J. Woodward's "Outlines of the Chief Camp Diseases of the United States Armies as Observed during the Present War," *American Journal of the Medical Sciences* 95 (1864): 159–71.

46. Ibid., 160.

47. Ibid.

48. Woodward was given honorary memberships to numerous associations, was asked to speak at medical conferences, and constantly received letters asking for advice. It is not an exaggeration to say that there are more than a thousand letters in the NMHM incoming correspondence (OHA RG 13) or Joseph Woodward Letterbooks (OHA RG 28) from physicians asking for his advice or to report interesting findings.

49. Reiser, *Medicine and the Reign of Technology*, 87.

50. Ibid., 88.

51. Wilson, *Minnesota Academy of Medicine*, 4. No large epidemics of typhus were diagnosed during the war. It was in fact very rare, though there were a few cases. See Bollet, *Civil War Medicine*, 276.

52. Ibid.

53. Ibid., 21.

54. Medical Officers Who Have Made Contributions of Worth to the Science of Medicine, Armed Forces Medical Library Document Section, MS B 281, NLM.

55. Quoted from editorial, *Boston Medical and Surgical Journal* (Feb. 1871), clipping, Library of the Surgeon General's Office: Data Relevant to the Library in the Annual Reports of the Surgeon-General's Office, MS C 185, NLM.

56. Ibid. See also *Army Medical Bulletin* (1942): 60.

57. Issac Minis Hays Papers, APS.

58. Ibid.

59. Ibid.

60. Resolutions from Billings to Hays, June 28, 1883, Issac Minis Hays Papers, APS.

61. Billings, "On Medical Museums," 4.

62. Ibid., 4.

63. Editorial, *American Practitioner*, 1871, clipping, Library of the Surgeon General's Office: Data Relevant to the Library in the Annual Reports of the Surgeon-General's Office, box 3, MS C 185, NLM.

64. Joseph Woodward, "The Medical Staff and the United States Army," 10.

65. Letters to John Shaw Billings, Nov. 28, 1888, and Mar. 7, 1888, Incoming Correspondence, RG 13, OHA, NMHM.

66. Library of the Surgeon General's Office: Data Relevant to the Library in the Annual Reports of the Surgeon-General's Office, box 3, MS C 185, NLM.

67. Henry, *The Armed Forces Institute of Pathology*, 93.

68. *The Official Correspondence between Surgeon General William Hammond, U.S.A. and the Adjutant General of the Army Relative to the Founding of the Army Medical Museum and the Inauguration of the Medical and Surgical History of the War*, 6.

69. Brieger, "The Therapeutic Conflicts and the American Medical Profession in the 1860s."

70. See Blustein, *Preserve Your Love for Science*; Duncan, "The Strange Case of Surgeon General Hammond."

71. Adams, "Confederate Medicine," 151.

72. Ibid., 152.

73. Smallpox was one of the most feared infections during the war because its manifestation was painful, grotesque, and often fatal. It occurred throughout the war, but a major pandemic struck in 1863, causing widespread disease in both armies.

74. Central Office Correspondence, Letters and Endorsements Sent, 1818–1946, entry 2, RG 112; Office of the Surgeon General, Letters Received, 1818–1870, entry 12, RG 112; Issuances and Forms: Excerpts of War Dept. Special Orders Relating to Medical Personnel, entry 57, RG 112, NARA. There are numerous letters. As one example, on Jan. 7, 1862, Dr. Blaney wrote to Dr. Finley: "I have the honor in obedience to telegraphic order received yesterday to forward the same mail herewith 20 crusts of vaccine virus. I also enclose duplicate account of virus purchased by me in accordance with your order to date. Please forward draft in payment of the same to Charles E. Allen Medical Student care of Prof. D. Brainard Chicago, Ills."

75. Jones, "Researches upon 'Spurious Vaccination,'" Medical Dept., Letters Sent, Medical Director's Office, Richmond, Va., chap. VI, vol. 416, RG 109, NARA.

76. Physicians made multiple inoculations by making scratches on a calf's belly and applying material from a vaccination pustule. Seven to ten days later they were able to take the pustular material from these lesions and use it for vaccinations on humans or to inoculate other calves to produce more material. This method became common in the 1880s, but only Italy was using this method prior to 1865. See Jones, *Circular No. 2.*

77. I have presented various parts of this research in three public lectures: "Science, Identity and Southern Medicine: Spurious Vaccination during the American Civil War, 1861–1865," Reynolds Lecture, Lister Hill Library, University of Alabama, Birmingham, Oct. 19, 2011; "The South's Vaccination Crisis: Smallpox and the American Civil War," Center for Biomedical Ethics and Humanities, University of Virginia School of Medicine, Nov. 10, 2011; "Medical Experimentation in Andersonville Prison," annual meeting of the Society of Civil War Historians, Lexington, Ky., June 14–16, 2012.

78. Stowe, *Doctoring the South*. Stowe suggests that the war did not "alter the ordinary M.D.s expectation of what constituted a desirable practice." This underscores the impact of the war. As one example, when Joseph Jones issued his circular requesting information about spurious vaccination in 1865, more than 600 essays and case reports were submitted by former Confederate medical officers. The complexities that physicians saw or experienced during the war could not be taken away and, where practicable, were incorporated into everyday medicine in the postwar period. However, the response to Jones's circular suggests there was an interest among southern physicians in producing knowledge and developing the basic sciences. Jones's research project went on for more than twenty years and became one of the cornerstones of his public health initiative in Louisiana. For another example, see Flannery, *Civil War Pharmacy*, 234–36.

79. Simon Baruch, for example, began his medical training in the Civil War South but moved to New York after the war, where he pioneered hydrotherapy, the use of public baths as a hygiene measure, investigations into balneology, and experimental treatments into appendicitis and malaria. For more on Simon Baruch, see Ward, *Simon Baruch: Rebel in the Ranks*.

80. This is the subject of my forthcoming monograph, "Science and the Practice of Medicine in the Civil War South."

81. Emphasis added. Woodward, "The Medical Staff and the United States Army," 20. See also Henry, *The Armed Forces Institute of Pathology*.

82. Breeden, *Joseph Jones, M.D.*, 172.

83. Quoted in Stowe, *Doctoring the South*, 270–71.

84. Editorial, *Richmond and Louisville Medical Journal* 5 (June 1868): 506.

85. Starr, *The Social Transformation of American Medicine*, 114.

86. By the end of the fiscal year 1865, just over 12,000 doctors had been in service in the United States Army Medical Department. See Key, "U.S. Army Medical Department and Civil War Medicine," 185.

87. John H. Brinton, "Address to the Members of the Graduating Class of the Army Medical Museum: Closing Exercises of the Session 1895–96, Army Medical School," 599–605, John H. Brinton Manuscript Collection, box 1, RG 124, OHA, NMHM.

88. Brinton, *Personal Memoirs*, 351.

Bibliography

PRIMARY SOURCES

Manuscripts and Manuscript Collections

American Philosophical Society, Philadelphia, Pa.
  Thomas Hewson Bache Diary, 1862
  Isaac Minis Hays Papers
  W. W. Keen, "An Autobiographical Sketch by W. W. Keen," Reminiscences for His
    Children; 1912 with additions 1915.
  John LeConte Papers
Library of Congress, Manuscript Division, Washington, D.C.
  James Jenkins Gillette Papers (1857–84)
  Alonzo C. Pickard Papers (1856–87)
  U.S. Sanitary Commission Papers
Library of the College of Physicians, Philadelphia, Pa.
  D. H. Agnew, Lecture Introductory to the One Hundred and Fifth Course of Instruc-
    tion in the Medical Department of the University of Pennsylvania, delivered
    Monday, October 10, 1870, Philadelphia
  H. M. Bellows, "Ward C Medical Case-Book," MSS 2/0076-04.
  John Hill Brinton Papers, 1853–1896, MSS 2/0269-01
  "Clinical Notes on Cases Seen at the Douglas Hospital at Washington, D.C., during
    the Late Civil War," Class Z10-70
  Henry Hartshorne Papers, 1823–1897, MSS 2/0030-01
  Herbert Marshall Howe Papers, 1844–1916, MSS 2/0241-03
  W. W. Keen Correspondence, 1860–1931, MSS 2/0076-04
  W. W. Keen Papers, 1881–1936
  Joseph Leidy Papers, 1845–1933, MSS 2/0170-01
  Silas Weir Mitchell Papers, 1850–1928, MSS 2/0241-03
  Silas Weir Mitchell, Turner's Lane Hospital: Case and Follow Up Studies, 1863–1892,
    MSS 2/0019, box 1, ser. 1–2.2
  West Philadelphia Hospital Record, 1864, 1N1-24-12
National Archives and Records Administration, Washington, D.C.
  Record Group 94: Records of the Adjutant General's Office, 1780s–1919
    Entry 544, Field Records of Hospitals-Pennsylvania, vol. 319
    Entry 559, Register of Surgical Operations, 1862–1865, 1875–82, 4 vols.
    Entry 561, Personal Papers of Medical Officers and Physicians
    Entry 620, Reports on Diseases and Individual Cases, 1841–93, Papers Relating to
      Cholera, Smallpox and Yellow Fever Epidemics, 1849–1893

Entry 621, Medical Records: Reports of Diseases and Individual Cases, 1841–93, file A and bound manuscripts

Entry 622, Medical Records, 1814–1919, Records relating to the sick and wounded, discharges, registers of death, records of transfers between hospitals, B file, 1860s-1870s

Entry 623, Medical Records, 1814–1919, D file

Entry 624, Medical Records, 1861–1889, files E and F, includes hospital records

Entry 628, John Brinton's Manuscripts, 1861–1865, 10 vols.

Entry 629, Medical Records, 1814–1919, Special Scientific and Historical Reports

Record Group 109: War Department Collection of Confederate Records

Medical Director's Office, Chapter VI, Volume 416 and 364

Record Group 112: The Records of the Office of the Surgeon General

Entry 2, Central Office Correspondence, Letters and Endorsements Sent, 1818–1946

Entry 4, Records Relating to Hospitals

Entry 12, Office of the Surgeon General, Letters Received, 1818–1870

Entry 26, Surgeon General's General Correspondence File

Entry 46, "Reports of the Surgeon General's Office," vols. 1–9

Entry 48, "Reports of Various Post Hospitals"

Entry 57, Issuances and Forms: "Excerpts of War Dept. Special Orders Relating to Medical Personnel"

Entry 63, Central Office Issuances and Forms: Circulars and Circular Letters of the Surgeon General's Office, 1861–85, 7 vols.

Entry 64, Circular No. 6: Original and Rough Proof of Circular No. 6: War Department, Reports on the Extent and Nature of the Materials Available for the Preparation of a Surgical History of the Rebellion, Surgeon General's Office, Washington, Nov. 1, 1865

National Library of Medicine, Bethesda, Md.

Alpheus Benning Crosby, "Construction of a Pavilion Hospital during the Civil War, ca. 1876," MS C 254

Alexander Henry Hoff Papers, 1821–1876, MS C 484

Merritte Weber Ireland, Biographical sketches of Jefferson Medical College Graduates who Served in the Civil War, MS B 169

Thomas Latimer Papers, 1861–1900, MS C 99

Library of the Surgeon General's Office: Data Relevant to the Library in the Annual Reports of the Surgeon-General's Office, MS C 185

Medical Officers Who Have Made Contributions of Worth to the Science of Medicine, Armed Forces Medical Library Document Section, MS B 281

Samuel Preston Moore Letter-Book, 1862–1863, MS B 413

Valentine Mott Correspondence, 1807–1864, MS C 281

George Miller Sternberg Papers, 1861–1917, MS C 100

United States Surgeon-General's Office, Medical Report of the Second Corps at the Battle of Gettysburg, 1863, MS C 129

U.S., Army Surgeon General's Office: Correspondence Acknowledging Receipt of Circular nos. 1–7, MS C 7

Otis Historical Archives, National Museum of Health and Medicine, Washington, D.C.

RG 2 Curatorial Records/Annual Reports, 1865–1906
RG 4 Autopsy Logbooks, 1865–1866, vols. 1–2, 1866–1919
RG 6 Curatorial Records: Circulars and Reports, 1863–1864
RG 8 Curatorial Records/Collection Logbooks, 1860–1910
RG 11 Curatorial Records: Endorsement Books, 1864–1882
RG 12 Curatorial Records: Expositions, 1876–1893
RG 13 Incoming Correspondence, 1862–1894
RG 15 Letterbooks of the Curators, 1863–1910
RG 16 Curatorial Letters Received, 1875–1889
RG 18 Curatorial Records: Notices of the Army Medical Museum Publications, 1865–1881
RG 21 Outgoing Correspondence
RG 23 Reports to the Curator, 1885–1892.
RG 25 Curatorial Records–Smithsonian Correspondence, 1867–1887.
RG 26 Special Correspondence, 1862–1887
RG 28 Joseph Woodward Letterbooks, 1864–1883
RG 38 Articles and Clippings, 1863–
RG 69 Museum Records: Publications, 1867–
RG 75 Contributed Photographs, 1862–1918
RG 76 International Exposition of 1876, Medical Department Photographs
RG 77 Medical Series Photographs, 1862–1865
RG 82 Surgical Photographs, 1862–1865
RG 83 Joseph Woodward's Photomicrographs, 1860s–1880s
RG 108 Joseph Barnes Collection
RG 124 John H. Brinton Manuscript Collection
RG 184 Harris General Hospital Photograph Album, 1862–1865
RG 226 George A. Otis Papers
RG 314 Squibb Journal, 1850s
RG 323 Surgeon General's Records, 1861–1970s
RG 330 William Thomson Photomicrographs, 1876
RG 363 Joseph Woodward Papers, Reynolds Library, University of Alabama, Birmingham, Historical Collections
Warren Webster, "The Army Medical Staff: An Address Delivered at the Inauguration of the Dale General Hospital, Feb. 22, 1865, Worchester, Massachusetts," pamphlet #6065.

Published Primary Works

Andrews, Edmund. "Hospital Gangrene." *Chicago Medical Examiner* 2 (1861): 515–16.
Atlee, Walter F. "Two Cases of Pyemia of Purulent Infection with Recovery in Which the Bisulphate of Soda Was Administered." *American Journal of the Medical Sciences* 49 (Jan. 1865): 82–84.
Bagger, Louis. "The Army Medical Museum in Washington." *Appleton's Journal* 9 (Mar. 1, 1873): 294–97.
Barnes, Joseph. "The Annual Report of the Surgeon General." *Medical and Surgical Reporter* 16 (1867): 75–77.

Bartholow, Roberts. *A Manual of Instructions for Enlisting and Discharging Soldiers: With Special Reference to the Medical Examination of Recruits, and the Detection of Disqualifying and Feigned Diseases*. Philadelphia: J. B. Lippincott, 1863.

———. *On the Antagonism between Medicines and between Remedies and Diseases: Being the Cartwright Lectures for the Year 1880*. New York: D. Appleton, 1881.

———. "Pathology and Treatment of Hospital Gangrene: Turpentine as a Local Application." *American Journal of the Medical Sciences* 49 (Jan. 1865): 274–76.

———. *A Practical Treatise on Materia Medica and Therapeutics*. New York: D. Appleton, 1887.

———. *The Principles and Practice of Disinfection*. Cincinnati: R. W. Carroll, 1867.

Beale, Lionel S. *The Microscope, In Its Application to Practical Medicine*. London: John Churchill, 1858.

Bernard, C. L., and C. H. Huette. *Illustrated Manual of Operative Surgery and Surgical Anatomy*. New York: Bailliere Brothers, 1861.

Billings, John S. "Biographical Memoir of Joseph Janvier Woodward." In *Biographical Memoirs*, 2:297–307. Washington, D.C.: National Academy of Sciences.

———. "Medical Museums." *Science* 12 (Sept. 21, 1888): 134–36.

———. "Medical Reminiscences of the Civil War." *Transactions of the College of Physicians of Philadelphia*, 3d ser., 27 (1905): 115–21.

———. "On Medical Museums, with Special Reference to the Army Medical Museum at Washington." *Medical News*, rpt. (Sept. 21, 1888): 3–43.

Bokum, Hermann. *Wanderings North and South*. Philadelphia, 1864.

Brinton, John H. "Address: Closing Exercises of the Session 1895–1896, Army Medical School." *Journal of the American Medical Association* 26 (1896): 599–605.

———. *Consolidated Statement of Gunshot Wounds*. Washington, D.C.: Government Printing Office, 1863.

———. *Personal Memoirs of John H. Brinton: Civil War Surgeon, 1861–1865*. Edited by John Y. Simon and John S. Haller. Carbondale: Southern Illinois University Press, 1996.

Brown, Harvey E. *The Medical Department of the United States Army from 1775–1883*. Washington, D.C.: Surgeon General's Office, 1873.

Brown-Séquard, Charles Edouard. *Course of Lectures on the Physiology and Pathology of the Central Nervous System*. Philadelphia: Collins, 1860.

Buck, Gurdon. *Contribution to Reparative Surgery: Showing Its Application for the Treatment of Deformities Produced by Destructive Disease or Injury, Congenital Defects from Arrest or Excess of Development and Cicatricial Contractions from Burns*. New York: Appleton, 1876.

Butler, Benjamin F. "Some Experiences with Yellow Fever and Its Prevention." *North American Review* 147 (1888): 525–41.

Catalogue of the Medical and Surgical Section of the United States Army Medical Museum. Washington, D.C.: Government Printing Office, 1867.

Clark, Henry G. "Inspection of Military Hospitals." *Boston Medical and Surgical Reporter* 67 (1863): 443–44.

Cullen, Thomas F. "Observations on the Influence of the Present War upon Medicine and Surgery." *Medical Society of New Jersey Transactions* 98 (1864): 21–44.

Da Costa, Jacob Mendes. *Medical Diagnosis*. Philadelphia: J. B Lippincott, 1864.

———. "On Functional Valvular Disorders of the Heart." *American Journal of the Medical Sciences* 57 (July 1869): 17–34.

———. "On Irritable Heart; A Clinical Study of a Form of Functional Cardiac Disorder and Its Consequences." *American Journal of the Medical Sciences* 61 (Jan. 1871): 17–52.

DeRicci, H. R. "Therapeutic Value of the Alkaline and Earthy Sulphites in the Treatment of Catalytic Diseases." *American Journal of the Medical Sciences* 49 (Jan. 1865): 236–39.

Ewing, James. "Experiences in the Collection of Museum Material from Army Camp Hospitals." *Bulletin of the International Associations of Medical Museums and Journal of Technical Methods* 8 (1922): 27.

Flower, William. *Diagrams of the Nerves of the Human Body: Exhibiting Their Origin, Divisions and Connections, with Their Distribution to the Various Regions of the Cutaneous Surface and to All the Muscles,* with additions by W. W. Keen. Philadelphia: Turner Hamilton Bookseller, 1872.

Gardner, Alexander. *Gardner's Photographic Sketchbook of the American Civil War, 1861–1865.* New York: Delano Greenridge Editions, 2001. Reprint of Philip and Solomons, Washington, D.C., 1866.

Gillman, Charlotte Perkins. *The Yellow Wallpaper and Other Stories.* Minneapolis: Filiquarian Publishing, 1892.

Goldsmith, Middleton. *A Report on Hospital Gangrene, Erysipelas and Pyaemia as Observed in the Departments of Ohio and the Cumberland with Cases Appended.* Louisville: Bradley and Gilbert, 1863.

Grace, William. *The Army Surgeon's Manual: For the Use of Medical Officers, Cadets, Chaplains, and Hospital Stewards.* New York: Balliere Brothers, 1864.

Greenleaf, Charles R. *A Manual for the Medical Officers of the United States Army.* Philadelphia: J. B. Lippincott, 1864.

Gross, Samuel D. *Autobiography of Samuel D. Gross, MD: With Sketches of His Contemporaries.* Philadelphia: George Barrie, 1887.

———. *A Manual of Military Surgery or Hints on the Emergencies of Field, Camp and Hospital Practice.* Philadelphia: Lippincott, 1861.

———. "Then and Now 1867: A Discourse Introductory to the Forty Third Course of Lectures in the Jefferson Medical College of Philadelphia." P.V. 148 No. 4. Philadelphia: Collins, 1867.

Guthrie, George James. *A Treatise on Gunshot Wounds: On Inflammation, Erysipelas, and Mortification, on Injuries of Nerves, 1827.* London: Burgess and Hill, Medical Booksellers, 1827.

Hamilton, Frank H. *A Practical Treatise on Military Surgery.* New York: Balliere Brothers, 1861.

———. *A Practical Treatise on Military Surgery and Hygiene.* New York: Balliere Brothers, 1865.

Hammond, William A. "Annual Report of the Surgeon-General, U.S.A." *Boston Medical and Surgical Journal* 67 (1863): 437–43.

———. "Circular to the Medical Profession." *Boston Medical and Surgical Journal* 68 (1863): 108–9.

———. "Experimental Researches Relative to the Nutritive Value and Physiological Effects of Albumen, Starch, and Gum When Single and Exclusively Used as Food." Philadelphia: T. K. and Collins, 1857.

————. *Military Medical and Surgical Essays Prepared for the United States Sanitary Commission*. Philadelphia: J. B. Lippincott, 1864.

————. "On Uremic Intoxication." *American Journal of the Medical Sciences* 41 (1861): 55–83.

————. *Physiological Memoirs*. Philadelphia: Lippincott, 1863.

————. *A Treatise on Hygiene with Special Reference to the Military Service*. Philadelphia: J. B. Lippincott, 1863.

Harris, Elisha. "Army Medical Museum." *American Medical Times* (June 25, 1864): 306–7.

————. *Conclusions concerning Cholera: Causes and Preventative Measures*. Cambridge: Riverside Press, 1874.

Hartshorne, Henry. *Essentials of the Principles and Practice of Medicine: A Handbook for Students and Practitioners*. Philadelphia: Henry C. Lea, 1869.

————. "On Heart Disease in the Army of the U.S. of America." *Summary of the Transactions of the College of Physicians of Philadelphia. American Journal of the Medical Sciences* 48 (July 1864): 89–94.

Jones, Joseph. *Circular No. 2, Vaccination: Spurious Vaccination*. Louisiana, 1884.

————. "Researches upon 'Spurious Vaccination' or the Abnormal Phenomena Accompanying and Following Vaccination in the Confederate Army during the Recent American Civil War, 1861–1865." Nashville: University Medical Press, W. H. F Printer, 1867.

Keen, W. W. *Animal Experimentation and Medical Progress*. Boston: Houghton Mifflin, 1914.

————. *Medical Research and Human Welfare*. Boston: Houghton Mifflin, 1917.

————. *A Sketch of the Early History of Practical Anatomy: The Introductory Address to the Course of Lectures on Anatomy at the Philadelphia School of Anatomy, Tuesday, October 11, 1870*. Philadelphia, 1870.

————. "Surgical Reminiscences of the Civil War." In *Addresses and Other Papers*. Philadelphia: W. B. Saunders, 1905.

————. *The Treatment of War Wounds*. Philadelphia: W. B. Saunders, 1917.

————. "Tribute to S. Weir Mitchell." In *Silas Weir Mitchell, M.D., L.L.D, F.R.S, 1829–1914: Memorial Addresses and Resolutions*, edited by Cornelius Wilson, 11–21. Philadelphia: College of Physicians, 1914.

Keen, W. W., Silas Weir Mitchell, and George Morehouse. "On Malingering, especially in Regard to Simulation of Diseases of the Nervous System." *American Journal of the Medical Sciences* 48 (Oct. 1864): 367–94.

Lamb, Daniel. *History of the U.S Army Medical Museum, 1862–1917: Compiled from the Official Records of Dr. Daniel S. Lamb Pathologist at the Museum*. Washington, D.C.: Army Medical Library, 1917.

Lea, Carey. "On the Transformation of Alkaline Sulphites in the Human System." *American Journal of the Medical Sciences* 49 (Jan. 1865): 84–87.

Letterman, Jonathan. *Medical Recollections of the Army of the Potomac*. New York. Appleton, 1866.

Lister, Joseph. "On a New Method of Treating Compound Fracture, Abscess, etc. With Observations on the Conditions of Suppuration." *Lancet* 1 (1867): 357–59.

————. "On the Antiseptic Principle in the Practice of Surgery." *British Medical Journal* 2 (1867): 246.

Lowenfels, Walter, ed. *Walt Whitman's Civil War*. New York: Da Capo Press, 1960.

Mitchell, John K. *Remote Consequences of Injuries and Nerves, and Their Treatment.* Philadelphia: Lea Brothers, 1895.

Mitchell, Silas Weir. *Clinical Lessons of Nervous Diseases.* Philadelphia: Lea Brothers, 1897.

———. *Doctor and Patient.* Philadelphia: Lippincott's, 1887.

———. *Fat and Blood: An Essay on the Treatment of Certain Forms of Neurasthenia and Hysteria.* Philadelphia, 1899.

———. "Influence of Nerve Lesions on Local Temperatures: Comparison of Clinical and Experimental Results." *Archives of Scientific and Practical Medicine* 1 (1873): 351.

———. *Injuries of Nerves and Their Consequences.* Philadelphia: J. B. Lippincott, 1872.

———. *The Medical Department in the Civil War: Address delivered before the Physicians' Club of Chicago, February 25, 1913.* Whitefish, Mont.: Kessinger Publishing, rpt. 2010.

———. "On the Production of Reflex Spasms and Paralysis in Birds by the Application of Cold to Definite Regions of the Skin." *American Journal of the Medical Sciences* (Jan. 1868): 10–16.

———. "Phantom Limbs." *Lippincott's Magazine of Popular Literature and Science* 8 (1871): 563–69.

———. "Relation of Pain to Weather: Being a Study of the Natural History of a Case of Traumatic Neuralgia." *American Journal of the Medical Sciences* 73 (1877): 305–29.

———. "Report on the Progress of Physiology and Anatomy." *North American Medico-Chirurgical* 2 (1858): 105–19.

———. "Some Personal Recollections of the Civil War." *Transactions of the College of Physicians of Philadelphia* 27 (1905): 87–94.

———. "Stumps and Spasmodic Disorders: Chorea of Stumps." *Medical and Surgical Reporter* 32 (1875): 100.

Mitchell, Silas Weir, and Robert Catlin. *The Relation of Pain to Weather: Studied during Eleven Years of a Case of Traumatic Neuralgia.* Philadelphia: Collins Printer, 1883.

Mitchell, Silas Weir, George Read Morehouse, and W. W. Keen. *Circular No. 6: Reflex Paralysis, the Result of Gunshot Wounds, Founded Chiefly upon Cases Observed in the United States General Hospital, Christian Street, Philadelphia.* Washington, D.C.: Surgeon General's Office, March 1864.

———. *Gunshot Wounds and Other Injuries of Nerves.* Philadelphia: J. B. Lippincott, 1864.

———. "On the Antagonism of Atropia and Morphia, Founded upon Observations and Experiments Made at the USA Hospital for Injuries and Diseases of the Nervous System." *American Journal of the Medical Sciences* 50 (1865): 67–76.

Morton, William T. G. "The First Use of Ether as an Anesthetic at the Battle of the Wilderness in the Civil War." *Journal of the American Medical Association* 42 (1904): 1068–73.

Nightingale, Florence. *Notes on Nursing: What It Is, and What It Is Not.* London: Harrison, 1859.

The Official Correspondence between Surgeon General William Hammond, U.S.A. and the Adjutant General of the Army Relative to the Founding of the Army Medical Museum and the Inauguration of the Medical and Surgical History of the War. New York: D. Appleton, 1883.

Olmsted, Frederick Law. *The Papers of Frederick Law Olmsted: Defending the Union.* Vol. 4: *The Civil War and the U.S. Sanitary Commission 1861–1863.* Edited by Jane Turner Censer. Baltimore: Johns Hopkins University Press, 1986.

Otis, George. "Contributions from the Army Medical Museum." *Boston Medical and Surgical Journal* 96 (1877): 361.

———. *List of Specimens in the Anatomical Section of the United States Army Medical Museum*. Washington, D.C.: Government Printing Office, 1878.

———. "Notes on Contributions to the Army Medical Museum by Civil Practitioners." *Boston Medical and Surgical Journal* 98 (1878): 163.

———. *Photographs of Surgical Cases and Specimens Taken at the Army Medical Museum, with Histories of 375 Cases*. 8 vols. Washington, D.C.: Surgeon General's Office, 1866–81.

———. *A Report of Surgical Cases Treated in the Army of the United States from 1865 to 1871*. Washington, D.C.: Government Printing Office, 1871.

———. *A Report on Amputations of the Hip Joint in Military Surgery*. Washington, D.C.: Government Printing Office, 1867.

———. *A Report on Excisions of the Head of the Femur for Gunshot Injury*. Washington, D.C.: Government Printing Office, 1869.

Peters, DeWitt C. "Gunshot Wound of the Internal Carotid and Vertebral Arteries—Fracture of the Atlas—Secondary Hemorrhage and Death." *American Journal of the Medical Sciences* 49 (1865): 373–74.

———. "Interesting Cases of Gunshot Wounds." *American Medical Times* 8 (1864): 3–4.

Pryer, W. C. "Hospital Gangrene in the DeCamp General Hospital." *American Medical Times* 8 (1864): 4–6.

Smart, Charles. "The Army Medical Museum and the Library of the Surgeon General's Office." *Journal of the American Medical Association* 24 (1895): 577–80.

Surgical Memoirs of the War of the Rebellion Collected and Published by the United States Sanitary Commission. Edited by Frank Hastings Hamilton. New York: Hurd and Houghton, 1871.

The Toner Lectures: Instituted to Encourage the Discovery of New Truths for the Advancement of Medicine. Washington, D.C.: Smithsonian Institution, 1873.

United States Sanitary Commission. *The Sanitary Commission of the United States Army: A Succinct Narrative of Its Works and Purposes*. New York: United States Sanitary Commission, 1864.

United States Surgeon General's Office. *Catalogue of the United States Army Medical Museum*. 3 vols. Washington, D.C.: Government Printing Office, 1866–67.

———. *The Medical and Surgical History of the War of the Rebellion (1861–1865)*. 6 vols. Washington, D.C.: Government Printing Office, 1870–88.

———. *Photographs of Surgical Cases and Specimens Taken at the Army Medical Museum*. 7 vols. Washington, D.C.: Government Printing Office, 1866–72.

United States War Department. *The War of the Rebellion: A Compilation of the Official Records of the Union and Confederate Armies*. 128 vols. Washington, D.C.: Government Printing Office, 1880–1901.

Virchow, Rudolph. *Cellular Pathology, as Based upon Physiological and Pathological Histology*. Translated by Frank Chance, with a new introduction by Lelland J. Rather. New York: Dover Publications, 1971.

von Tagen, C. H. *Biliary Calculi: Perineorrhaphy; Hospital Gangrene and Its Kindred Diseases; with their Treatments*. New York and Philadelphia: Boericke & Tafel, 1881.

Welch, William H. "S. Weir Mitchell: Physician and Man of Science." In *Silas Weir Mitchell, M.D., L.L.D, F.R.S, 1829–1914: Memorial Addresses and Resolutions*, edited by Cornelius Wilson, 97–127. Philadelphia: College of Physicians, 1914.

West, Nathaniel. *History of U.S.A General Hospital, at West Philadelphia, Pa. From Oct. 8, 1862 to October 8, 1863*. Philadelphia: Hospital Press, 1863.

Whitman, Walt. *The Sacrificial Years: A Chronicle of Walt Whitman's Experiences in the Civil War*. Edited by John Harmon McElroy. Boston: David R. Godine, 1999.

——. *Specimen Days and Collect*. Glasgow: Wilson and McCormick, 1883.

——. *The Wound Dresser: A Series of Letters Written from the Hospitals in Washington during the War of the Rebellion*. New York: Small, Maynard, 1898.

Williams, Talcott. "S. Weir Mitchell." In *Silas Weir Mitchell, M.D., L.L.D, F.R.S, 1829–1914: Memorial Addresses and Resolutions*, edited by Cornelius Wilson, 73–94. Philadelphia: College of Physicians, 1914.

Wilson, Cornelius, ed. *Silas Weir Mitchell, M.D., L.L.D, F.R.S, 1829–1914: Memorial Addresses and Resolutions*. Philadelphia: College of Physicians, 1914.

Woodward, Joseph J. "Abstract of Lecture on Photomicrography Applied to Class Demonstrations: Delivered before the Biology and Microscopic Section of the Academy of Natural Science of Philadelphia, May 30, 1869." *Monthly Microscopic Journal* 2 (1869): 165.

——. "The Army Medical Museum at Washington." *Lippincott's Magazine of Popular Literature and Science* 7 (Mar. 1871): 233–42. Washington, D.C.: J. B. Lippincott and Office of the Librarian of Congress.

——. "Brief Rejoinder to Some Recent Articles by Dr. Roberts Bartholow." *Cincinnati Medical News* 10 (Nov. 1877): 119.

——. *Catalogue of the Medical Section of the United States Army Medical Museum*. Washington, D.C.: Government Printing Office, 1867.

——. *Circular No. 1: Report on Epidemic Cholera and Yellow Fever in the Army of the United States during the year 1867*. Washington, D.C.: Government Printing Office, 1868.

——. *Circular No. 5: Report on Epidemic Cholera in the Army of the United States during the Year 1866*. Washington, D.C.: Government Printing Office, 1867.

——. "Hospital Gangrene (Letter to Prof. Detmold)." *American Medical Times* (1863): 179.

——. *The Hospital Steward's Manual*. Philadelphia: J. B. Lippincott, 1862.

——. "The Medical Staff and the United States Army, and Its Scientific Work: An Address Delivered to the International Medical Congress at Philadelphia." Wednesday Evening, Sept. 6, 1876.

——. "Memorandum on Pleurosigma Angulatum and Pleurosigma Forosum." Washington, D.C.: Surgeon General's Office, 1871.

——. "On Photomicrography with the Highest Powers and Practiced in the Army Medical Museum." *American Journal of the Medical Sciences* 42 (1866): 189.

——. "On the Permanent Preservation of Histological Preparations as Practiced at the Army Medical Museum, Washington, D.C." *American Journal of the Medical Sciences* 57 (Jan. 1869): 277–81.

——. "On the Use of Aniline in Histological Researches; with a Method of Investigating the Histology of the Human Intestine, and Remarks on Some of the Points to Be Observed in the Study of the Diseased Intestine in Camp Fevers and Diarrhoeas." *American Journal of the Medical Sciences* 49 (Jan. 1865): 106–13.

———. "On the Use of Monochromatic Sunlight as an Aid to High Power Definition." *American Naturalist* (1872): 472.

———. *Outlines of the Chief Camp Diseases of the United States Armies as Observed during the Present War*. Philadelphia: J. B. Lippincott, 1863.

———. "Remarks on the Pathological Histology of Yellow Fever, Prepared at the Request of the National Board of Health: Supplement No. 4." *National Bulletin of Health* (Washington, 1880).

———. "Report on the Causes and Pathology of Septicemia." *Transactions of the American Medical Association* 17 (1866): 171.

———. "Report on the Sickness and Mortality in the U.S. Army for the Year Ending June 30, 1862." *American Medical Times* (1863): 166.

———. Review of *Cellular Pathology* by Rudolph Virchow. *American Journal of the Medical Sciences* 41 (1861): 465.

Woodward, Joseph J., and George A. Otis. *Circular No. 6: Reports on the Extent and Nature of the Materials Available for the Preparation of a Medical and Surgical History of the Rebellion*. Philadelphia: J. B. Lippincott, 1865.

Woodworth, John. *Cholera Epidemic of 1873, the Introduction of Epidemic Cholera through the Agency of the Mercantile Marine: Suggestions of Measures of Prevention*. Washington, D.C.: Government Printing Office, 1875.

Journals

American Journal of the Medical Sciences, 1861–75
American Medical Association Transactions, 1861–70
American Medical Times, 1861–70
Boston Medical and Surgical Journal, 1861–70
Medical and Surgical Reporter, 1861–66
New York Medical Record, 1880

Periodicals and Newspapers

New York Times, 1861–66
Harper's Weekly, 1861–65
Lippincott's Magazine of Popular Literature and Science, 1871–85

SECONDARY WORKS

Ackerknecht, Erwin. "Anti-contagionism between 1821–1867." *Bulletin of the History of Medicine* 22 (1948): 562–93.

———. *Medicine and the Paris Hospital, 1794–1848*. Baltimore: Johns Hopkins University Press, 1967.

———. *A Short History of Medicine*. Baltimore: Johns Hopkins University Press, 1982.

Adams, George. "Confederate Medicine." *Journal of Southern History* 6 (1940): 151–66.

———. *Doctors in Blue: The Medical History of the Union Army in the Civil War*. New York: Henry Schuman, 1952.

Alberti, Samuel J. M. M. *Morbid Curiosities: Medical Museums in Nineteenth-Century Britain*. Oxford: Oxford University Press, 2011.

Allen, Phyllis. "Etiological Theory in America Prior to the Civil War." *Journal of the History of Medicine and Allied Sciences* 2 (1947): 514–39.

Alotta, Robert I. *Civil War Justice: Union Army Executions under Lincoln*. Shippensburg: White Mane Publishing, 1989.

Aminoff, Michael J. *Brown-Séquard: An Improbable Genius Who Transformed Medicine*. New York: Oxford University Press, 2011.

Austin, Anne. *The Woolsey Sisters of New York: A Family's Involvement in the Civil War and a New Profession*. Philadelphia: American Philosophical Society, 1971.

Bell, Andrew McIlwaine. *Mosquito Soldiers: Malaria, Yellow Fever, and the Course of the American Civil War*. Baton Rouge: Louisiana State University Press, 2010.

Berman, Gary E. "Civil War Embalming: A Short History." *Journal of Civil War Medicine* 1 (July–Aug. 1997): 3–4.

Blake, John. "Anatomy." In *The Education of American Physicians: Historical Essays*, edited by Ronald Numbers, 29–47. Berkeley and Los Angeles: University of California Press, 1980.

Blight, David W. *Race and Reunion: The Civil War in American Memory*. Cambridge, Mass.: Belknap Press of Harvard University Press, 2001.

Blumenthal, Henry. *Americans and French Culture, 1800–1900: Interchanges in Art, Science, Literature and Society*. Baton Rouge: Louisiana State University Press, 1975.

Blustein, Bonnie Ellen. *Preserve Your Love for Science: Life of William A. Hammond, American Neurologist*. New York: Cambridge University Press, 1991.

———. "To Increase the Efficiency of the Medical Department: A New Approach to Civil War Medicine." *Civil War History* 33 (1987): 22–39.

Bollet, Alfred. *Civil War Medicine: Challenges and Triumphs*. Tucson: Galen Press, 2002.

Bonner, Thomas N. *Becoming a Physician: Medical Education in Britain, France, Germany and the United States, 1750–1945*. New York: Oxford University Press, 1995.

———. "The German Model of Training Physicians in the United States, 1870–1914: How Closely Was It Followed?" *Bulletin of the History of Medicine* 64 (1990): 18–34.

Booth, Christopher C. "Clinical Research." In *Companion Encyclopedia of the History of Medicine*, edited by W. F. Bynum and Roy Porter, 1:205–29. London: Routledge, 1993.

Bracegirdle, Brian. "The Microscopial Tradition." In *Companion Encyclopedia of the History of Medicine*, edited by W. F. Bynum and Roy Porter, 1:102–19. London: Routledge, 1993.

Breeden, James O. *Joseph Jones, M.D.: Scientist of the Old South*. Lexington: University Press of Kentucky, 1975.

Brieger, Gert. "Sanitary Reform in New York City: Stephen Smith and the Passage of the Metropolitan Health Bill." *Bulletin of the History of Medicine* 40 (1966): 407–29.

———. "The Therapeutic Conflicts and the American Medical Profession in the 1860s." *Bulletin of the History of Medicine* 41 (1967): 215–22.

Brock, Thomas D. *Robert Koch: A Life in Medicine and Bacteriology*. Washington, D.C.: American Society for Microbiology, 1999

Brooks, Stewart. *Civil War Medicine*. Springfield: Charles C. Thomas, 1966.

Bruce, Robert. *The Launching of American Science, 1846–1876*. New York: Alfred A. Knopf, 1987.

Burke, Joanna. *Dismembering the Male: Men's Bodies, Britain and the Great War*. Chicago: University of Chicago Press, 1996.

Burney, Ian A. *Bodies of Evidence: Medicine and the Politics of the English Inquest, 1830–1926*. Baltimore: Johns Hopkins University Press, 2000.

Burns, Stanley B. *Early Medical Photography in America (1839–1883)*. New York: Burns Archive, 1983.

———. *Shooting Soldiers: Civil War Medical Photography by R. B. Bontecou*. New York: Burns Archive, 2011.

Bynum, W. F. *Science and the Practice of Medicine in the Nineteenth Century*. New York: Cambridge University Press, 1991.

Canale, D. J. "'The Firm' Mitchell, Morehouse and Keen and Civil War Neurology." In *Years of Change and Suffering: Modern Perspectives on Civil War Medicine*, edited by James M. Schmidt and Guy R. Hasegawa, 127–42. Roseville, Minn.: Edinborough Press, 2009.

Capa, Cornell, ed. *The International Center of Photography Encyclopedia of Photography*. New York: Crown Publishers, Pound Press, 1984.

Carter, Codell K. *The Rise of Causal Concepts of Disease: Case Histories*. Aldershot: Ashgate, 2003.

Cartwright, Lisa. *Screening the Body: Tracing Medicine's Visual Culture*. Minneapolis: University of Minnesota Press, 1997.

Cassedy, James H. *American Medicine and Statistical Thinking, 1800–1860*. Cambridge, Mass.: Harvard University Press, 1984.

———. *John Shaw Billings: Science and Medicine in the Gilded Age*. Bethesda, Md.: National Library of Medicine, 2009.

———. *Medicine in America: A Short History*. Baltimore: Johns Hopkins University Press, 1991.

Catton, Bruce. *The Civil War*. Boston: Houghton Mifflin, 1960.

Chapman, Charleton B. *Order Out of Chaos: John Shaw Billings and America's Coming of Age*. Boston: Boston Medical Library, 1994.

Clinton, Catherine, and Nina Silber, eds. *Battle Scars: Gender and Sexuality in the American Civil War*. New York: Oxford University Press, 2006.

Coco, Gregory A. *Killed in Action: Eyewitness Accounts of the Last Moments of 100 Union Soldiers Who Died at Gettysburg*. Gettysburg: Thomas Publications, 1992.

Coleman, William. "The Cognitive Basis of the Discipline: Claude Bernard on Physiology." *Isis* 76 (March 1985): 49–70.

———. "Koch's Comma Bacillus: The First Year." *Bulletin of the History of Medicine* 61 (1987): 315–42.

Coleman, William, and Frederick Holmes, ed. *The Investigative Enterprise: Experimental Physiology in Nineteenth-Century Medicine*. Berkeley and Los Angeles: University of California Press, 1992.

Conway, Herbert, and Richard B. Stark. *Plastic Surgery at the New York Hospital One Hundred Years Ago*. New York: Paul Hoeber, 1953.

Cooter, Roger. "Medicine and the Goodness of War." *Canadian Bulletin of Medical History* 12 (1990): 637–47.

Cooter, Roger, Mark Harrison, and Steve Sturdy, eds. *Medicine and Modern Warfare*. Atlanta: Rodopi, 1999.

———. *War, Medicine and Modernity*. Gloucestershire: Sutton, 1999.

Cope, Zachary. "The Medical Balance-Sheet of War." In *Some Famous General Practitioners and Other Medical Historical Essays*, edited by Zachary Cope, 169–83. London: Pitman Medical Publishing, 1961.

Cunningham, Andrew. "Transforming the Plague: The Laboratory and the Identity of Infectious Disease." In *The Laboratory Revolution in Medicine*, edited by Andrew Cunningham and Perry Williams, 209–45. Cambridge: Cambridge University Press, 1992.

Cunningham, Andrew, and Perry Williams. *The Laboratory Revolution in Medicine*. Cambridge: Cambridge University Press, 1992.

Cunningham, H. H. *Doctors in Gray: The Confederate Medical Service*. Baton Rouge: Louisiana State University Press, 1958.

Daston, Lorraine, and Peter Galison. *Objectivity*. New York: Zone Books, 2010.

Davis, Audrey B. *Medicine and Its Technology: An Introduction to the History of Medical Instrumentation*. Westport, Conn.: Greenwood Press, 1981.

Davis, William. *The Embattled Confederacy*. Vol. 3 of *The Image of War: 1861–1865*. New York: Doubleday, 1982.

———. *The Guns of '62*. Vol. 2 of *The Image of War: 1861–1865*. New York: Doubleday, 1982.

———. *Shadow of the Storm*. Vol. 1 of *The Image of War: 1861–1865*. New York: Doubleday, 1981.

Dean, Eric T., Jr. *Shook over Hell: Post-Traumatic Stress, Vietnam, and the Civil War*. Cambridge, Mass.: Harvard University Press, 1997.

———. "'We will all be lost and Destroyed': Post-Traumatic Stress Disorder of the Civil War." *Civil War History* 37 (1991): 138–53.

Denney, Robert E. *Civil War Medicine: Care and Comfort of the Wounded*. New York: Sterling Publishers, 1994.

Devine, Shauna. "Producing Knowledge: Civil War Bodies and the Development of Medical Science in the Nineteenth Century." Ph.D. diss., University of Western Ontario, 2010.

Downs, Jim. *Sick from Freedom: African-American Illness and Suffering during the Civil War and Reconstruction*. New York: Oxford University Press, 2012.

Duffin, Jacalyn. *Lovers and Livers: Disease Concepts in History*. Toronto: University of Toronto Press, 2005.

———. "Vitalism and Organicism in the Philosophy of R. T. H. Laennec." *Bulletin of the History of Medicine* 62 (1988): 525–45.

Duffy, John. *From Humors to Medical Science: A History of American Medicine*. Urbana: University of Illinois Press, 1993.

———. *The Healers: A History of American Medicine*. Urbana: University of Illinois Press, 1979.

———. *The Sanitarians: A History of American Public Health*. Urbana: University of Illinois Press, 1990.

Duncan, Louis. *The Medical Department of the United States Army in the Civil War*. Gaithersburg, Md.: Butternut, 1985.

———. "The Strange Case of Surgeon General Hammond." *Military Surgeon* 64 (1929): 98–110, 252–62.

Dupree, Hunter A. *Science in the Federal Government: A History of Policies and Activities.* Baltimore: Johns Hopkins University Press, 1986.

Dupuy, T. N., and R. E. Dupuy. *Encyclopedia of Military History.* New York: Harper and Row, 1970.

Ellis, Richard H., ed. *The Case Books of Dr. John Snow.* London: Wellcome Institute for the History of Medicine, 1994.

Epler, Percy H. *The Life of Clara Barton.* New York: Macmillan, 1926.

Epstein, Julia. *Altered Conditions: Disease, Medicine and Storytelling.* New York: Routledge, 1995.

Faust, Drew Gilpin. "Altars of Sacrifice: Confederate Women and the Narratives of War." *Journal of American History* 76 (1990): 1200–1228.

———. *This Republic of Suffering: Death and the American Civil War.* New York: Knopf, 2008.

Fett, Sharla M. *Working Cures: Healing, Health, and Power on Southern Slave Plantations.* Chapel Hill: University of North Carolina Press, 2002.

Figg, Laurann, and Jane Farrell-Beck. "Amputation in the Civil War: Physical and Social Dimensions." *Journal of the History of Medicine and Allied Sciences* 48 (1993): 454–75.

Fissell, Mary. "The Disappearance of the Patient's Narrative and the Invention of Hospital Medicine." In *British Medicine in an Age of Reform*, edited by Roger French and Andrew Wear, 92–109. New York: Routledge, 1991.

Flannery, Michael A. "Another House Divided: Union Medical Service and Sectarians during the American Civil War." *Journal of the History of Medicine* 54 (Oct. 1999): 489–90.

———. *Civil War Pharmacy: A History of Drugs, Drug Supply and Provision, and Therapeutics for the Union and Confederacy.* New York: Pharmaceutical Products Press, 2004.

Foucault, Michel. *The Birth of the Clinic: An Archaeology of Medical Perception.* Trans. A. M. Sheridan Smith. New York: Pantheon, 1973.

Fox, Daniel M., and Christopher Lawrence. *Photographing Medicine: Images and Power in Britain and America since 1840.* New York: Greenwood Press, 1988.

Fox, William F. *Regimental Losses in the American Civil War.* Albany: Albany Publishing Company, 1889.

Frassanito, William A. *Gettysburg: A Journey in Time.* Gettysburg: Thomas Publications, 1975.

Fredrickson, George M. *The Inner Civil War: Northern Intellectuals and the Crisis of the Union.* New York: Harper and Row, 1965.

Freemon, Frank. "The First Neurological Research Center: Turner's Lane Hospital during the American Civil War." *Journal of the History of the Neurosciences* 2 (1993): 135–42.

———. *Gangrene and Glory: Medical Care during the American Civil War.* Urbana: University of Illinois Press, 2001.

———. "The Health of the American Slave Examined by Means of Union Army Medical Statistics." *Journal of the National Medical Association* 77 (1985): 49–52.

———. "Lincoln Finds a Surgeon General: William A. Hammond and the Transformation of the Union Army Medical Bureau." *Civil War History* 33 (1987): 5–21.

Fye, Bruce W. *The Development of American Physiology: Scientific Medicine in the Nineteenth Century.* Baltimore: Johns Hopkins University Press, 1987.

——. "S. Weir Mitchell, Philadelphia's Lost Physiologist." *Bulletin of the History of Medicine* 57 (1983): 188–202.

Garrison, Fielding. *Notes on the History of Military Medicine*. Washington, D.C.: Government Printing Office, 1922.

Gelfand, Toby. *Professionalizing Modern Medicine: Paris Surgeons and Medicine Science and Institutions in the 18th Century*. Westport, Conn: Greenwood Press, 1980.

Geison, Gerald L. *The Private Science of Louis Pasteur*. Princeton: Princeton University Press, 1995.

Giesberg, Judith. *Civil War Sisterhood: The U.S. Sanitary Commission and Women's Politics in Transition*. Boston: Northeastern University Press, 2000.

Gillett, Mary C. *The Army Medical Department, 1818–1865*. Washington, D.C.: United States Army Center of Military History, 1987.

Glatthaar, Joseph T. "The Costliness of Discrimination: Medical Care for Black Troops in the Civil War." In *Inside the Confederate Nation: Essays in Honor of Emory M. Thomas*, edited by Lesley J. Gordon and John C. Inscoe, 251–71. Baton Rouge: Louisiana State University Press, 2005.

Goler, Robert, and Michael Rhode. "From Individual Trauma to National Policy: Tracking the Uses of Civil War Veteran Medical Records." In *Disabled Veterans in History*, edited by David Gerber, 163–84. Ann Arbor: University of Michigan Press, 2000.

Goodman, Jordan, Anthony McElligott, and Lara Marks, eds. *Useful Bodies: Humans in the Service of Medical Science in the Twentieth Century*. Baltimore: Johns Hopkins University Press, 2003.

Grant, Susan Mary. "The Lost Boys: Citizen Soldiers, Disabled Veterans and Confederate Nationalism in the Age of People's War." *Journal of the Civil War Era* 2 (2012): 233–54.

Green, Carol C. *Chimborazo: The Confederacy's Largest Hospital*. Knoxville: University of Tennessee Press, 2004.

Grob, Gerald. *The Deadly Truth: A History of Infectious Disease in America*. Cambridge, Mass.: Harvard University Press, 2002.

Hacker, D. J. "A Census Based Account of the Civil War Dead." *Civil War History* 57 (2011): 307–48.

Haller, John. *American Medicine in Transition, 1840–1910*. Urbana: University of Illinois Press, 1981.

——. *Farmcoats to Ford: A History of the Military Ambulance, 1790–1925*. Carbondale: Southern Illinois University Press, 1992.

Hamlin, Christopher. *Cholera: The Biography*. London: Oxford University Press, 2009.

Hannaway, Caroline, and Ann La Berge. *Constructing Paris Medicine*. B.V. Amsterdam, Wellcome Series in the History of Medicine. Atlanta: Rodopi, 1998.

Harden, Victoria. *Inventing the NIH: Federal Biomedical Research Policy, 1887–1937*. Baltimore: Johns Hopkins University Press, 1986.

Harrison, Mark. "The Medicalization of War—The Militarization of Medicine." *Social History of Medicine* 9 (1996): 267–76.

Hasegawa, Guy R. "The Civil War's Medical Cadets: Medical Students Serving in the Union." *Journal of the American College of Surgeons* 193 (2001): 1–12.

Henry, Robert. *The Armed Forces Institute of Pathology: Its First Century, 1862–1962*. Washington, D.C.: Government Printing Office, 1964.

Herschbach, Lisa Marie. "Fragmentation and Reunion: Medicine, Memory and Body in the American Civil War." Ph.D. diss., Harvard University, 1997.

Hessler, James A. *Sickles at Gettysburg: The Controversial Civil War General Who Committed Murder, Abandoned Little Round Top and Declared Himself the Hero of Gettysburg*. New York: Savas Beatie, 2009.

Hilde, Libra. *Worth a Dozen Men: Women and Nursing in the Civil War South*. Charlottesville: University of Virginia Press, 2012.

Holmes, Amy E. "'Such is the price we pay': American Widows and the Civil War Pension System." In *Toward a Social History of the American Civil War*, edited by Maris A. Vinovskis, 171–96. New York: Cambridge University Press, 1990.

Humphrey, David C. "Dissection and Discrimination: The Social Origins of Cadavers in America, 1760–1915." *Bulletin of the New York Academy of Medicine* 49 (1973): 819–25.

Humphreys, Margaret. *Intensely Human: The Health of the Black Soldier in the American Civil War*. Baltimore: Johns Hopkins University Press, 2008.

Iacovetta, Franca, and Wendy Mitchinson, eds. *On the Case: Explorations in Social History*. Toronto: University of Toronto Press, 1998.

Johansen, Peter Vinten, Howard Brody, Nigel Paneth, Steven Rachman, and Michael Rip. *Cholera, Chloroform and the Science of Medicine: A Life of John Snow*. New York: Oxford University Press, 2003.

Johns, Frank S., and Ann Page. "Chimborazo Hospital and J. B. McCaw, Surgeon in Chief," *Virginia Monthly Magazine of History and Biography* 62, no. 2 (1954): 190–200.

Jones, Gordon. "Sanitation in the Civil War." *Civil War Times Illustrated* 5 (Nov. 1966): 12–18.

Jones, Russell. "American Doctors and the Parisian Medical World, 1830–1840." *Bulletin of the History of Medicine* 47 (1973): 40–65.

———. "American Doctors in Paris, 1820–61: A Statistical Profile." *Journal of the History of Medicine and Allied Science* 25 (1970): 143–57.

Kaufman, Martin. *American Medical Education: The Formative Years, 1765–1910*. Westport, Conn.: Greenwood Press, 1976.

Kelly, Catherine. *War and the Militarization of British Army Medicine, 1793–1830*. London: Pickering and Chatto, 2011.

Kett, Joseph. *The Formation of the American Medical Profession: The Role of Institutions, 1780–1860*. New York: Greenwood, 1980.

Key, Jack D. "U.S. Army Medical Department and Civil War Medicine." *Military Medicine* 133 (1968): 181–91.

King, Lester. *Transformations in American Medicine: From Benjamin Rush to William Osler*. Baltimore: Johns Hopkins University Press, 1991.

Kramer, Howard. "The Effect of the War on the Public Health Movement." *Mississippi Valley Historical Review* 35 (1948): 449–62.

Kuz, Julian E., and Bradley P. Bengston. *Orthopaedic Injuries and Treatment during the Civil War*. Kennesaw: Kennesaw Mountain Press, 1996.

La Berge, Ann. "Dichotomy or Integration? Medical Microscopy and the Paris Clinical Tradition." In *Constructing Paris Medicine*, edited by Caroline Hannaway and Ann La Berge, 275–312. B.V. Amsterdam, Wellcome Series in the History of Medicine. Atlanta: Rodopi, 1998.

La Berge, Ann, and Caroline Hannaway. "Paris Medicine: Perspectives Past and Present." In *Constructing Paris Medicine*, edited by Caroline Hannaway and Ann La Berge, 1–70. B.V. Amsterdam, Wellcome Series in the History of Medicine. Atlanta: Rodopi, 1998.

Laderman, Gary. *The Sacred Remains: American Attitudes toward Death, 1799–1883*. New Haven: Yale University Press, 1996.

Latour, Bruno. *The Pasteurization of France*. Cambridge, Mass.: Harvard University Press, 1988.

———. *Science in Action: How to Follow Scientists and Engineers through Society*. Cambridge, Mass.: Harvard University Press, 1987.

Latour, Bruno, and Steve Woolgar. *Laboratory Life: The Social Construction of Scientific Facts*. Princeton: Princeton University Press, 1986.

Lawson, Melinda. *Patriot Fires: Forging a New American Nationalism in the Civil War North*. Lawrence: University Press of Kansas, 2002.

Leavitt, Judith Walzer. "Public Health and Preventative Medicine." In *The Education of American Physicians: Historical Essays*, edited by Ronald Numbers, 250–72. Berkeley and Los Angeles: University of California Press, 1979.

Lederer, Susan. *Subjected to Science: Human Experimentation in America before the Second World War*. Baltimore: Johns Hopkins University Press, 1995.

Lein-Schroeder, Glenna R. *Confederate Hospitals on the Move: Samuel H. Stout and the Army of the Tennessee*. Columbia: University of South Carolina Press, 1994.

Lenman, Robin, ed. *The Oxford Companion to the Photograph*. Oxford: Oxford University Press, 2005.

Lenoir, Timothy. "Laboratories, Medicine and Public Life in Germany, 1830–1849: Ideological Roots of the Institutional Revolution." In *The Laboratory Revolution in Medicine*, edited by Andrew Cunningham and Perry Williams, 14–72. Cambridge: Cambridge University Press, 1992.

Lesch, John E. *Science and Medicine in France: The Emergence of Experimental Physiology, 1790–1855*. Cambridge, Mass.: Harvard University Press, 1984.

Linderman, Gerald F. *Embattled Courage: The Experience of Combat in the American Civil War*. New York: Free Press, 1987.

Litvin, Martin. *The Young Mary 1817–1861: Early Years of Mother Bickerdyke, America's Florence Nightingale, and Patron Saint of Kansas*. Galesburg, Ill.: Log City Books, 1977.

Long, Lisa A. *Rehabilitating Bodies: Health, History, and the American Civil War*. Philadelphia: University of Pennsylvania Press, 2004.

Loudon, Irvine S. L. "Childbirth." In *Companion Encyclopedia of the History of Medicine*, edited by W. F. Bynum and Roy Porter, 2:1050–71. London: Routledge, 1993.

———. *Death in Childbirth: An International Study of Maternal Care and Maternal Mortality 1800–1950*. Oxford: Clarendon Press, 1992.

Ludmerer, Kenneth. *Learning to Heal: The Development of American Medical Education*. New York: Basic Books, 1985.

MacDonald, Helen. *Human Remains: Dissection and Its Histories*. New Haven: Yale University Press, 2005.

Marks, Harry. *The Progress of Experiment: Science and Therapeutic Reform in the United States, 1900–1990*. Cambridge: Cambridge University Press, 1997.

Mattingly, Cheryl, and Linda C. Garro, eds. *Narrative and the Cultural Construction of Illness and Healing*. Berkeley and Los Angeles: University of California Press, 2001.

Maulitz, Russell C. "American Doctors and Parisian Medical World, 1830–1840." *Bulletin of the History of Medicine* 47 (1973): 40–65.

———. *Morbid Appearances: The Anatomy of Pathology in the Early Nineteenth Century*. New York: Cambridge University Press, 1987.

———. "The Pathological Tradition." In *Companion Encyclopedia of the History of Medicine*, edited by W. F. Bynum and Roy Porter, 1:169–91. London: Routledge, 1993.

Maxwell, William Quentin. *Lincoln's Fifth Wheel: The Political History of the United States Sanitary Commission*. New York: Longmans, 1956.

McCleary, Erin. "Science in a Bottle: The Medical Museum in North America, 1860–1940." Ph.D. diss., University of Pennsylvania, 2001.

McPherson, James. *Battle Cry of Freedom: The Civil War Era*. New York: Oxford University Press, 1988.

———. *For Cause and Comrades: Why Men Fought in the Civil War*. New York: Oxford University Press, 1997.

Merrell, D. S., S. M. Butler, F. Qadri, N. A. Dolganov, A. Alam, M. B. Cohen, S. B. Calderwood, G. K. Schoolnik, and A. Camilli. "Host-Induced Epidemic Spread of the Cholera Bacterium." *Nature* 417, no. 6889 (2002): 642–45.

Miles, Wyndam B. *A History of the National Library of Medicine*. Bethesda, Md.: National Library of Medicine, 1982.

Morantz-Sanchez, Regina. *Sympathy and Science: Women Physicians in American Medicine*. Chapel Hill: University of North Carolina Press, 2000.

Neff, John. *Honoring the Civil War Dead: Commemoration and the Problem of Reconstruction*. Lawrence: University of Kansas Press, 2005.

Neushul, Peter. "Fighting Research: Army Participation in the Clinical Testing and Mass Production of Penicillin during the Second World War." *In War, Medicine and Modernity*, edited by Roger Cooter, Mark Harrison, and Steve Sturdy, 203–24. Gloucestershire: Sutton, 1999.

Nudelman, Franny. *John Brown's Body: Slavery, Violence, and the Culture of War*. Chapel Hill: University of North Carolina Press, 2004.

Numbers, Ronald, ed. *The Education of American Physicians: Historical Essays*. Berkeley and Los Angeles: University of California Press, 1979.

Osler, William. *An Alabama Student and Other Biographical Essays*. New York: Oxford University Press, 1909.

Parsons, Gail Pat. "Puerperal Fever, Anticontagionists, and Miasmatic Infection, 1840–1860: Toward a New History of Puerperal Fever in Antebellum America." *Journal of the History of Medicine and Allied Sciences* 52 (1997): 424–52.

Pelling, Margaret. *Cholera, Fever and English Medicine, 1825–1865*. Oxford: Oxford University Press, 1978.

———. "Contagion, Germ Theory, Specificity." In *Companion Encyclopedia of the History of Medicine*, edited by W. F. Bynum and Roy Porter, 1:309–34. London: Routledge, 1993.

Pernick, Martin S. *A Calculus of Suffering: Pain Professionalism and Anesthesia in Nineteenth-Century America*. New York: Columbia University Press, 1985.

Pickstone, John V. *Ways of Knowing: A New History of Science, Technology and Medicine.* Chicago: University of Chicago Press, 2000.

Rable, George C. *Fredericksburg! Fredericksburg!* Chapel Hill: University of North Carolina Press, 2002.

———. *God's Almost Chosen People: A Religious History of the American Civil War.* Chapel Hill: University of North Carolina Press, 2010.

Rapkiewicz, Amy, Alan Hawk, Adrienne Noe, and David Berman. "Surgical Pathology in the Era of the Civil War: The Remarkable Life and Accomplishments of Joseph Janvier Woodward." *Archives Pathology Laboratory Medicine* 129 (Oct. 2005): 1313–15.

Reiser, Stanley Joel. "Creating Form Out of Mass: The Development of the Medical Record." In *Transformations and Tradition in the Sciences*, edited by Everett Mendelson, 303–16. Cambridge: Cambridge University Press, 1984.

———. *Medicine and the Reign of Technology.* Cambridge: Cambridge University Press, 1978.

Rhode, Michael G. "'The extent of these materials is simply enormous': The Creation and Publication of the Medical and Surgical History of the War of the Rebellion from 1862–1888." Annual Meeting of the American Association for the History of Medicine, May 2, 2004, 1–11.

Rhode, Michael G., and J. T. H. Connor. "Curating America's Premier Medical Museum: The Legacy of John Shaw Billings to the Professional and Public Understanding of Medicine." *Anglo-American Medical Relations: Historical Insights* (June 19–21, 2003): 1–17.

———. "A Repository for Bottled Monsters and Medical Curiosities: The Evolution of the Army Medical Museum." In *Defining Memory: Local Museums and the Construction of History in America's Changing Communities*, edited by A. K. Levin, 177–96. Lanham, Md.: Alta Mira Press, 2007.

Richardson, Ruth. *Death, Dissection, and the Destitute.* Chicago: University of Chicago Press, 1987.

Rogers, Frank B. *Selected Papers of John Shaw Billings: Compiled with a Life of Billings by Frank. B. Rogers.* Baltimore: Medical Library Association, 1965.

Romano, Terrie M. *John Burdon Sanderson and the Culture of Victorian Science.* Baltimore: Johns Hopkins University Press, 2002.

Rosen, George. *A History of Public Health.* Expanded Edition. Baltimore: Johns Hopkins University Press, 1993.

———. *The Specialization of Medicine with Particular Reference to Ophthalmology.* New York: Froben, 1944.

Rosenberg, Charles. *The Care of Strangers: The Rise of America's Hospital System.* Baltimore: Johns Hopkins University Press, 1992.

———. *The Cholera Years: The United States in 1832, 1849, and 1866.* Chicago: University of Chicago Press, 1962.

———. *Explaining Epidemics and Other Studies in the History of Medicine.* Cambridge: Cambridge University Press, 1992.

———. *No Other Gods: On Science and American Social Thought.* Baltimore: Johns Hopkins University Press, 1976.

———. "Social Class and Medical Care in Nineteenth-Century America: The Rise and Fall of the Dispensary." *Journal of the History of Medicine and Allied Sciences* 29 (1974): 32–54.

——. "The Therapeutic Revolution: Medicine, Meaning, and Social Change in 19th Century America." In *Explaining Epidemics and Other Essays in the History of Medicine*. Cambridge: Cambridge University Press, 1992.

Rothstein, William G. *American Medical Schools and the Practice of Medicine: A History*. New York: Oxford University Press, 1987.

——. *American Physicians in the Nineteenth Century: From Sects to Science*. Baltimore: Johns Hopkins University Press, 1972.

Rutkow, Ira. *Bleeding Blue and Gray: Civil War Surgery and the Evolution of American Medicine*. New York: Random House, 2005.

Sappol, Michael. "The Odd Case of Charles Knowlton: Anatomical Performance, Medical Narrative, and Identity in Antebellum America." *Bulletin of the History of Medicine* 83 (2009): 460–98.

——. *A Traffic of Dead Bodies: Anatomy and Embodied Social Identity in Nineteenth-Century America*. Princeton: Princeton University Press, 2002.

Savitt, Todd. "Use of Blacks for Medical Experimentation and Demonstration in the Old South." *Journal of Southern History* 48 (1982): 331–48.

Schantz, Mark S. *Awaiting the Heavenly Country: The Civil War and America's Culture of Death*. Ithaca: Cornell University Press, 2008.

Schmidt, James M., and Guy R. Hasegawa, eds. *Years of Change and Suffering: Modern Perspectives on Civil War Medicine*. Roseville, Minn.: Edinborough Press, 2009.

Schultz, Jane E., ed. *This Birth Place of Souls: The Civil War Nursing Diary of Harriet Eaton*. London: Oxford University Press, 2011.

——. *Women at the Front: Hospital Workers in Civil War America*. Chapel Hill: University of North Carolina Press, 2004.

Schultz, Suzanne M. *Body Snatching: The Robbing of Graves for the Education of Physicians in Early Nineteenth Century America*. North Carolina: McFarland, 1992.

Shryock, Richard. *American Medical Research*. New York: The Commonwealth Fund, 1947.

——. *The Development of Modern Medicine: An Interpretation of the Social and Scientific Factors Involved*. New York: Knopf, 1947.

——. "A Medical Perspective on the Civil War." *American Quarterly* 14 (1962): 161–73.

——. *Medicine and Society in America, 1660–1860*. New York: New York University Press, 1960.

Smith, Dale C. "Austin Flint and Ausculation in America." *Journal of the History of Medicine and Allied Sciences* 33 (1978): 129–49.

——. "Gerhard's Distinction between Typhoid and Typhus and Its Reception in America, 1833–1860." *Bulletin of the History of Medicine* 54 (1980): 368–85.

——. "Military Medical History: The American Civil War." *Magazine of History* 19 (September 2005): 17–19.

——. "The Rise and Fall of Typhomalarial Fever: I. Origins." *Journal of the History of Medicine and Allied Sciences* 37 (April 1982): 182–220.

Smith, George Winston. *Medicines for the Union Army: The United States Army Laboratories during the American Civil War*. New York: Pharmaceutical Products Press, 2001.

Starr, Paul. *The Social Transformation of American Medicine*. New York: Basic Books, 1982.

Steiner, Paul. *Disease in the Civil War: Natural Biological Warfare in 1861–1865*. Springfield: Charles Thomas, 1968.

Stevens, Rosemary. *American Medicine and the Public Interest: A History of Specialization.* Berkeley and Los Angeles: University of California Press, 1971.

———. "Sweet Charity": State Aid to Hospitals in Pennsylvania, 1870–1910. *Bulletin of the History of Medicine* 58 (1984): 287–314.

Stone, James L. "W. W. Keen: America's Pioneer Neurological Surgeon." *Neurosurgery* 17 (1985): 997–1010.

Stowe, Steven M. *Doctoring the South: Southern Physicians and Everyday Medicine in the Mid-Nineteenth Century.* Chapel Hill: University of North Carolina Press, 2004.

Tomes, Nancy. *The Gospel of Germs: Men, Women and the Microbe in American Life.* Cambridge, Mass.: Harvard University Press, 1988.

———. "The Private Side of Public Health: Sanitary Science, Domestic Hygeine and the Germ Theory, 1870–1900." *Bulletin of the History of Medicine* 64 (1900): 509–39.

Waller, John. *The Discovery of the Germ: Twenty Years That Transformed the Way We Think about Disease.* New York: Columbia University Press, 2002.

Ward, Patricia S. *Simon Baruch: Rebel in the Ranks of Medicine, 1840–1921.* Madison: University of Wisconsin Press, 1990.

Warner, Deborah Jean. "The Campaign for Medical Microscopy in Antebellum America." *Bulletin of the History of Medicine* 69 (1995): 358–83.

Warner, John Harley. *Against the Spirit of the System: The French Impulse in American Medicine.* Baltimore: Johns Hopkins University Press, 1998.

———. "Ideals of Science and Their Discontents in Late Nineteenth Century American Medicine." *Isis* 82 (1991): 454–78.

———. "Physiology." In *The Education of American Physicians: Historical Essays,* edited by Ronald Numbers, 48–71. Berkeley and Los Angeles: University of California Press, 1980.

———. "The Rise and Fall of Professional Mystery: Epistemology, Authority and the Emergence of Laboratory Medicine in Nineteenth Century American Medicine." In *The Laboratory Revolution in Medicine,* edited by Andrew Cunningham and Perry Williams, 110–41. Cambridge: Cambridge University Press, 1992.

———. "The Selective Transport of Medical Knowledge: Antebellum American Physicians and Parisian Medical Therapeutics." *Bulletin of the History of Medicine* 59 (1985): 213–31.

———. *The Therapeutic Perspective: Medical Practice, Knowledge and Identity in America, 1820–1855.* Cambridge, Mass.: Harvard University Press, 1986.

Warner, John Harley, and Guenter Risse. "Reconstructing Clinical Activities: Patient Records in Medical History." *Society for the Social History of Medicine* 5 (1992): 183–205.

Warner, John Harley, and Lawrence Rizzolo. "Anatomical Instruction and Training for Professionalism from the 19th to the 21st Centuries." *Clinical Anatomy* 19 (2006): 403–14.

Washington, Harriet A. *Medical Apartheid: The Dark History of Medical Experimentation on Black Americans from Colonial Times to the Present.* New York: Harlem Moon, 2006.

Watson, Harry. *Liberty and Power: The Politics of Jacksonian America.* New York: Hill and Wang, 1990.

Weisz, George. *Divide and Conquer: A Comparative History of Medical Specialization.* New York: Oxford University Press, 2006.

———. *The Medical Mandarins: The French Academy of Medicine in the Nineteenth and Early Twentieth Centuries.* New York: Oxford University Press, 1995.

Wilson, Leonard G. *Minnesota Academy of Medicine, 1887–2012.* Minneapolis, Minn.: privately printed, 2012.

Wintermute, Bobby A. *Public Health and the U.S. Military: A History of the Army Medical Department, 1818–1917.* New York: Routledge, 2011.

Wooley, Charles. *The Irritable Heart of Soldiers and the Origins of Anglo-American Cardiology: The U.S. Civil War (1861) to World War I (1918).* Aldershot: Ashgate, 2002.

Worboys, Michael. *Spreading Germs: Disease Theories and Medical Practice in Britain, 1865–1900.* Cambridge: Cambridge University Press, 2000.

Index

Abscesses, 60, 63–64, 66–67, 86, 112, 128, 203, 205, 213

Absorption, 107, 303 (n. 55). *See also* Disease

Adams Express Company, 36, 195, 287 (n. 116)

Agnew, C. R., 220

Alcohol, 35, 49, 82, 123, 128, 239, 240, 332 (n. 112)

Allen, H., 68

American Association for the Relief of Misery on the Battlefield, 220

American Journal of the Medical Sciences, 66, 75, 259, 285 (n. 84)

American Medical Association, 4–5, 136, 138, 140, 171, 257, 262, 267, 268, 310 (n. 38). *See also* Specialists/specialization

American Microscopial Society, 82–83

American Public Health Association, 221, 290 (n. 193)

Amputations, 23, 28, 33, 39–40, 46–47, 60–62, 66, 94, 97, 101, 116, 142, 155–56, 165, 190, 192, 196–97, 202–3, 207, 209–10, 253–55, 268, 275, 286 (n. 105), 314 (n. 134), 326 (n. 185); primary vs. secondary, and resections, 203–8, 326 (n. 182)

Anatomy, knowledge and, 3, 4, 6–11, 15, 17, 18, 22, 24, 31, 34, 36, 37, 40, 51, 53–55, 59, 62, 74, 77, 80, 81, 91, 138, 145, 159, 173–74, 177, 180, 182, 183, 194–95, 256–58, 261, 268, 271, 291 (n. 2), 293 (n. 31), 312 (n. 92), 317 (n. 1), 335 (n. 33). *See also* Dissections; Postmortems

Anatomy acts, 3, 7–8, 173, 183, 258, 271

Anesthesia, 165, 316 (n. 185); chloroform, 117, 165, 201–2, 316 (n. 184); ether, 98, 117, 123, 165, 168, 205, 316 (n. 185)

Aniline dyes, 77, 79, 87–89. *See also* Histology, pathological

Animalcules, 80, 93, 108, 111, 112, 131. *See also* Disease

Anti-contagion, 100, 130, 217, 218, 238, 327 (n. 10), 329 (n. 64). *See also* Disease

Antietam, Battle of, 2, 156, 175, 177–78, 195–96, 211, 319 (n. 32), 321 (n. 78), 322 (n. 106), 324 (n. 144)

Antiseptics, 7, 70, 103, 109, 111, 114, 116, 119, 121, 122, 131, 239, 240, 243, 244, 246, 247, 262, 302 (n. 47)

Apprenticeship. *See* Medical education: apprenticeship and

Armory Square Hospital, 20, 175

Armsby, James, 39, 194, 323 (n. 129)

Army Medical Department, 8–9, 13–17, 21–30, 72, 104, 159, 174, 177–78, 185, 188–93, 198, 212–13, 220, 230, 240, 244–46, 251, 263, 280 (n. 46), 285 (n. 88), 328 (nn. 28, 29); unprepared for war, 13–15, 281 (n. 7)

Army Medical Museum, 1, 9, 13, 16, 21, 27–29, 33, 34, 36, 92, 141, 179, 185; circular no. 2 and, 2, 9–10, 13, 21–22, 27–30, 33, 45, 49, 52, 54, 62, 66, 73, 158, 166, 177, 189–90, 193–94, 200, 269, 286 (n. 105), 292 (n. 8); class and, 320 (n. 43); collecting specimens and, 10–12, 19–22, 27–50, 52, 54, 64, 66, 73–92, 133, 139, 141, 166, 177, 180–214, 250, 252, 256, 262–69, 272, 292 (n. 17); corpses on battlefield and, 35; Europe and, 37, 50–51, 54, 71, 75, 77, 78, 83, 89, 91, 92, 113, 131, 137, 179, 187, 188, 209, 249, 251, 260, 263, 270; hierarchy of knowledge and, 41–44, 58, 81, 91, 133; identity and, 38–45, 50, 51, 54, 132, 210, 211, 214, 249, 261, 262, 263, 271, 272; in postwar period, 242, 253, 255, 262–64, 269, 282 (n. 24), 283 (n. 56), 290 (n. 193), 324 (n. 146); preservation of specimens and, 35, 36, 49, 59; public and, 174, 179, 180, 181, 182, 184; scientific medicine and, 37–41, 49–52, 59, 76–78, 81, 84, 88–89, 179; and South, 10, 266, 267. *See also* Experiment, medical; Medical science and practice; Specialists/specialization; Woodward, Joseph J.

Army Medical School, 16, 184, 213, 265, 287 (n. 124), 320 (n. 59), 321 (n. 64), 322 (nn. 87, 90, 98), 324 (n. 146), 338 (n. 87)

Army of the Potomac, 18, 31, 33, 48, 55, 161, 261, 288 (n. 157)

Army of the Tennessee, 55, 292 (n. 15)

Arterial ligations, 65, 256

Artificial limb program, 254, 271

Asepsis, 7, 209

Atlee, Walter, 118

Auscultation, 19, 159

Autoinoculation, 303 (n. 54)

Autopsies. *See* Dissections; Postmortems

Bacteria, 69, 94–95, 106, 109, 110, 231, 293 (nn. 34, 43), 298 (n. 129), 300 (n. 6), 303 (nn. 54, 55), 305 (n. 99), 327 (n. 16), 332 (n. 118)

Bacteriology, 153, 212, 228, 231, 232, 243–44, 248, 260, 265, 303 (n. 55), 330 (n. 81); Robert Koch's work on, 70–71, 89, 212, 219, 231, 247, 248, 260, 294 (n. 53); Joseph Lister's work on, 70–72, 105–6, 241, 243, 246, 247, 261, 270, 294 (n. 53), 302 (n. 47), 306 (n. 112); Louis Pasteur's work on, 212, 239, 241–42. *See also* Disease

Baldwin, W. O., 268

Barnes, Joseph K., 36, 51, 78, 113, 118, 213, 220–25, 230, 237, 242, 259, 264–65, 287 (n. 120), 328 (n. 24), 334 (n. 9)

Bartholow, Roberts, 18, 24, 28, 74, 118, 126–28, 151–52, 190, 242–43, 246, 284 (n. 75), 332 (n. 117)

Bartlett, A. J., 197

Bartlett, Elisha, 5

Baruch, Simon, 266–67, 337 (n. 79)

Beale, Lionel, 78, 83, 86, 296 (n. 93)

Bernard, Claude, 137, 153, 256, 335 (n. 31); experimental physiology and, 153

Bichat, Xavier, 54, 141, 271

Billings, John Shaw, 18, 20, 31, 37, 38, 45–50, 156, 182, 185, 212, 252, 262–64, 271, 289 (n. 166); design of Johns Hopkins, 48, 49, 262, 290 (n. 193); National Library of Medicine, 250–52, 262, 264, 282 (n. 24), 334 (nn. 9, 15). *See also* Army Medical Museum; Surgeon General's Office, and medical literature

Blood, 11, 46, 58, 63–69, 73, 75, 81, 86, 93, 95, 97, 105–12, 116, 127, 137, 143, 155, 160, 175, 181, 201, 205, 207, 234, 235, 239, 270, 293 (n. 45), 298 (n. 120), 302 (n. 33), 303 (nn. 51, 54), 304 (n. 70), 330 (n. 89), 335 (n. 32)

Bodies: body-snatchers and, 53, 173; burial, 176, 177, 179, 197, 318 (n. 19); contests and, 188–97. *See also* Army Medical Museum

Bolton, Richard, 9

Bontecou, R. B., 68–69, 91–92, 96, 99, 115, 121, 183, 193, 194, 204, 207, 208, 213

Brain, 36, 46, 47, 58, 65, 69, 132, 141, 142, 191, 199, 202, 257, 293 (n. 43), 311 (n. 61), 312 (n. 92), 335 (n. 32)

Brainerd, Daniel, 5

Brinton, John, 24, 27–28, 33–41, 48, 51, 111–13, 122–23, 131–35, 139, 180–200, 256, 257, 258, 272; contests over bodies and, 180–200

British Journal of Photography, 81

Bromide of potassa, 122, 126–28, 307 (nn. 133, 136)

Bromine, 11, 98, 114, 119–31, 153, 165, 242, 250, 268, 275, 305 (n. 99), 306 (n. 111), 307 (nn. 123, 133, 136, 138)

Brown, Harvey E., 21

Brown, J. B., 211

Brown, John, 17

Brown, Joseph, 224–25

Browne, R. B., 224

Brown-Séquard, Charles Edouard, 153, 313 (n. 111), 325 (n. 173)

Buck, Gurdon, 41, 165–70, 316 (n. 189), 317 (nn. 200, 202, 205)
Budd, William, 217
Bull Run, Battle of, 45, 143

Calhoun, J. T., 13, 191, 196, 201, 228
Calomel, 265
Campbell Hospital, 20, 116, 192
Cancer research, 17, 34, 42, 90–91, 199, 259, 264, 299 (n. 158)
Cantwell, J. T., 201–2
Carbolic acid, 105, 181, 201, 240–41, 261, 302 (n. 47), 332 (n. 112)
Cardiac diseases, as medical specialty, 158–64. *See also* Da Costa, Jacob; Heart diseases
Carpenter, John S., 210
Carroll, William, 229–30
Carver Hospital, 20
Case histories, 1, 11–12, 28, 29, 30, 31, 32, 33, 37, 43, 44, 50, 55–59, 60–62, 74, 78, 86, 97, 99, 101, 117, 118, 123, 133, 140, 150, 157–59, 160, 165, 167, 169, 170, 171, 181, 192, 196, 198, 200, 203, 209, 211, 216, 218, 220–22, 229, 230, 233, 250, 253, 270, 272, 286 (n. 101), 287 (n. 127), 300 (nn. 4, 14), 317 (n. 200), 324 (n. 142), 328 (n. 78). *See also* Knowledge production
Cells, 42, 47, 65, 66, 75, 77, 80, 85, 86, 93, 97, 100, 108, 111–13, 126, 129, 131, 227, 234–35, 260, 295 (n. 77–79), 303 (n. 61), 304 (n. 67)
Cell theory, 75–76. *See also* Virchow, Rudolph
Chancellorsville, Battle of, 47, 191, 196
Chattanooga, general hospital in, 74
Chemical investigations, 2, 67, 75, 98, 100, 114, 217, 219, 227, 239, 241, 242, 243, 269, 291 (n. 201), 301 (n. 26), 303 (n. 62); in medical practice, 107, 109–16, 118–19, 122, 126–31, 137, 177, 219, 227, 228, 233, 237, 239, 242–44, 265, 269, 306 (n. 112), 332 (nn. 107, 118); tests of urine, 66, 74, 127, 137, 233, 237, 270
Cholera, 11, 44, 70, 215–16, 253–54, 268,

271, 327 (nn. 10, 11); cattle plague and, 240–42; Congress and, 245–48; etiology, 216–19; germ theories and, 223–24, 226, 227–29, 232; international research and, 218–19, 222, 245–48, 327 (n. 16); investigations and, 216, 219, 222, 232–44, 328 (n. 29), 330 (nn. 81, 86), 331 (n. 29); management of, 222–30, 236, 239–48, 332 (n. 129); microscopy and, 219, 234–36; northern and southern physicians and, 216, 219, 220; prevention of, 232, 236, 237; spread of, 219, 220, 221, 224–25; transmission of knowledge and, 220–30, 244–48, 333 (n. 130); water purification and, 235, 236, 237, 238–48, 331 (n. 99)
Christian Street Hospital, 139, 141, 142, 147
Cincinnati Academy of Medicine, 126, 142
Civil War, U.S.: Europe and, 8, 11, 15, 19, 24, 28, 37, 51, 54, 70, 71, 75, 77, 78, 82, 83, 89, 91, 92, 113, 131, 137, 140, 143, 144, 169, 171, 179, 209, 216, 218, 219, 222, 237, 245, 246, 247, 249, 251, 254, 257, 260, 262, 263, 270; medical literature and, 7; medical professionalization and, 7, 8, 11, 16, 17, 19, 21, 28, 30, 38, 41, 50, 51, 53, 54, 71, 73, 89, 131, 133, 134, 135, 137, 140, 144, 171, 172, 174, 179, 180, 182, 184–87, 200, 209–12, 214, 216, 249, 255–58, 262, 263, 265, 267, 271, 278 (n. 26); other American wars compared with, 1; size and scope of, 1, 174–75, 212, 215
Clark, Alonzo, 5
Clark, Henry, 28
Cliffburne hospital, 18, 45
Clinical trials, 117, 118, 122, 123, 125, 126, 129, 131, 152, 153, 164, 242, 271, 294 (n. 55), 301 (n. 16), 307 (n. 138)
Cogswell, Mason, 196
Cogwell, George B., 195
Confederate Medical Department, 9
Contagion, 100–106, 108, 124, 125, 129, 130–31, 217–18, 223, 226–27, 230, 232, 245, 269, 326 (n. 4), 329 (n. 53). *See also* Disease
Contributions to Reparative Surgery, 167
Corpse, 35, 176, 177, 178, 179, 216

causes of, 95–95; disease theories, 100–107; investigations of, 96, 97, 111, 114–19, 120–24, 126, 128–31; management of, 115, 119, 120–24, 165, 238, 243, 268, 271, 274, 300 (n. 3), 301 (n. 17), 307 (n. 138)

Examining boards, medical, 16, 17,

Executions in Civil War, 186, 321 (n. 73)

Experiment, medical, 2, 4, 5, 9, 11, 15, 23, 38, 40, 75, 79, 80–82, 86, 88–90, 93, 96, 98, 108, 110–20, 122–23, 126–29, 131, 134, 137–38, 142, 144, 147, 151–55, 160, 166, 169, 171, 174, 202, 216, 219, 224, 233, 235–38, 241–43, 246, 249, 252, 256–57, 263, 265–66, 269, 270, 272, 278 (n. 22), 285 (n. 90), 299 (n. 149), 300 (n. 15), 301 (n. 16), 303 (n. 62), 304 (n. 62), 307 (nn. 135, 136), 309 (n. 16), 311 (nn. 54, 60), 325 (n. 173), 330 (nn. 81, 86), 331 (nn. 95, 102). *See also* Medical education

Faber, Hermann, 88

Fairfax Seminary Hospital, 190

Farr, William, 301 (n. 26), 330 (n. 89)

Faxon, W. L., 42

Fellows of the College of Physicians of Philadelphia, 259

Field hospitals, 55–59

Filbert Street Hospital, 139, 141, 158

Finley, Clement, 13, 14, 23, 281 (n. 7)

Finley Hospital, 20

Flint, Austin, Sr., 5, 24, 184

Fomites, 104, 223. *See also* Disease

Fort Monroe (Va.) Post Hospital, 74, 193

Fort Republic, Battle of, 46

Fort Sumter, 13

Foucault, Michel, 188

Franco-Prussian War, 106, 209

Franz, J. H., 222–23

Frederick, general hospital in, 40–41, 102–3, 125, 130, 141, 170

Fredericksburg, Battle of, 61, 116, 146, 175, 178, 190, 307 (n. 138)

Freedmen's Bureau, 220, 253

French, George, 261

Frey, Heinrich, 82

Gangrene, 1, 10, 18, 23, 32, 63, 71, 74, 93, 94, 95, 165, 192, 201, 202, 238, 242, 243, 256, 268, 271, 273, 275, 300 (n. 6), 301 (n. 17), 303 (nn. 61, 62), 304 (n. 67); theories of disease causation, 100–107; causes of, 94–95; management, 102–3, 106, 107, 114–24, 128–30, 204 (n. 77); study of, 63, 94–103, 107, 108, 111–14, 119, 121–30, 303 (nn. 61, 62), 304 (n. 67). *See also* Disease

Gardner, Alexander, 178, 319 (n. 32)

General hospitals, 2, 26, 36, 56, 59, 60, 72–73, 75, 94, 118, 122, 136, 139, 154, 176, 213, 222, 250, 292 (n. 68)

General Law Pension System, 253. *See also* Pension program

Gerhard, William, 6, 54

Gerlach, Joseph von, 82–83

German medicine, influence on American medicine, 6, 7, 50, 51, 70, 76, 125, 144, 199, 219, 231, 239, 249, 269, 278 (n. 26), 279 (n. 27), 296 (n. 82), 327 (n. 16)

Germ theory, 12, 70, 71, 93, 106, 217, 227, 238, 240, 241, 243, 246, 268. *See also* Antiseptics; Disinfectants; Public health

Gettysburg, Battle of, 44, 47, 57, 64, 117, 175, 178, 191, 195, 197, 200, 201

Gilbert, R. H., 193

Girard, A. C., 246–47

Goldsmith, Middleton, 24, 74, 97–98, 101–7, 119–28, 131, 294 (n. 64), 302 (n. 41), 303 (n. 55)

Greenleaf, Charles R., 28

Gross, Samuel D., 5, 23–24, 28, 44–45, 133, 165, 184, 190, 192, 257, 267, 283 (n. 59), 284 (n. 68)

Gross, S. W., 193

Gunshot Wounds and Other Injuries of Nerves, 257

Hamilton, Frank, 94, 220

Hammond, William, 9–10, 14–18, 21–23, 26–28, 30–31, 33–34, 36, 38, 41, 43, 47, 54, 61, 64, 72, 94, 97, 102, 106, 109–10, 113, 115–16, 122, 131, 136, 138, 158, 167, 177, 185, 189, 193–95, 199, 203–5, 207, 258, 265, 269,

215, 217, 230, 244, 256, 258–59; transmission of, 29, 30, 39, 41, 49–52, 88, 96, 97, 98, 114, 123–24, 131, 154, 193, 244. *See also* Army Medical Museum; Case histories

Koch, Robert, 70–71, 89, 212, 219, 231, 247–48, 260, 271, 294 (nn. 53, 55), 313 (n. 120), 332 (n. 118)

Kolliker, Rudolph Albert von, 296 (n. 98)

Laboratory, 7, 10, 15, 33, 36, 41, 48–49, 70–72, 75–76, 82, 85, 98, 113–14, 125, 131, 136, 137, 153, 216, 231–33, 235, 237, 240, 242, 244, 247, 252, 262, 265–66, 268–69, 290 (n. 193), 291 (n. 201), 294 (nn. 58, 65), 304 (n. 62), 327 (n. 16), 330 (n. 81), 331 (n. 102), 335 (n. 31)

Lawson, Thomas, 13

Lea, M. Carey, 118

LeConte, John, 59, 135, 282 (n. 32), 309 (nn. 12, 16)

Lee, Robert E., 178, 191, 272

Leidy, Joseph, 24, 45, 60, 62–63, 188, 289 (n. 161)

Letterman, Jonathan, 18, 43, 47–48, 55, 190, 280 (n. 157)

Liddel, John, 191–92

Liebig, Justus von, 239, 294 (n. 53), 301 (n. 26), 305 (n. 97), 330 (nn. 86, 89)

Lincoln Hospital, 20, 181, 295 (n. 81)

Lippincott's Magazine, 180, 214, 257

Lister, Joseph, 70–71, 105–6, 241, 243, 246–47, 261, 270, 294 (n. 53), 302 (n. 47), 306 (n. 111), 332 (n. 118), 333 (n. 139)

Louis, Pierre, 62

Lying-in hospitals and puerperal fever. *See* Puerperal fever

Mack, A. J., 264

Maddox, R. L., 80–81, 84, 297 (nn. 102, 103)

Madison, Mills, 135

Malaria, 28, 70, 74, 261, 268–69, 337 (n. 79)

Malvern Hill, Battle of, 59, 178, 322 (n. 106)

March, Alden, 195

Marine Hospital Service, 221, 245, 255, 290 (n. 193), 330 (n. 81), 333 (n. 134)

Markoe, Thomas, 193–94

McBride, Alex, 119

McClellan, E., 231, 245

McDougall, Charles M., 27, 193–94, 317 (n. 200)

McDowell, Ephraim, 5

McGill, George, 24, 68, 202, 226–29, 233–35, 329 (n. 55)

McKelway, A. J., 159

McParlin, Thomas, 48, 225, 235–37

Measles, 13, 74

Medical and Surgical History of the War of the Rebellion, 11, 28, 30, 86, 95, 111, 123, 250, 259

Medical and Surgical Reporter, 51

Medical cadets, 14–15, 20, 26–27, 282 (n. 26)

Medical College of Ohio, 45

Medical education: apprenticeship and, 2, 24, 261, 278 (n. 26); competing sects of, 3, 4, 6; controversy over cadavers and, 3, 8, 53–54, 173–77; lowered standards, 3, 4, 6, 278 (n. 26); medical profession and, 1–2, 4–5, 11, 16–17, 22, 25, 37–38, 42, 50, 54, 73, 79, 80, 83, 125, 137, 172, 249–52, 261; medical schools, proliferation of, 3; microscope and, 6, 9, 33, 71–75, 80, 82–90, 131, 179, 180, 248, 256, 260, 269, 289 (n. 160), 294 (n. 160), 299 (n. 160); wartime development of, 2, 4, 23, 25–28, 37, 49, 50, 54, 58–59, 73, 80, 137, 166, 172, 179, 187, 188, 198–99, 209, 250–52, 258, 260

Medical entrance exams, 14, 16, 17, 18, 19, 26, 45, 282 (nn. 26, 30, 34)

Medical Gazette, 51

Medical museums, 37, 49, 182, 187. *See also* Army Medical Museum

Medical News and Library, 28

Medical photography. *See* Photography; Photomicrography

Medical profession, identity of, 38, 41, 51, 54, 132, 169, 176, 210, 211, 214, 249, 257, 263, 271, 272, 327 (n. 14). *See also* Medical education

Medical science and practice, 4, 5, 6, 11, 24,

New York Harbor, 221, 223, 225, 226, 230, 237

Nitric acid, 46, 87, 98, 102–3, 110, 114, 125, 165, 228, 275, 303 (n. 62)

Norris, William F., 180, 214, 257

Nurses, 14, 15, 20, 102, 103, 117, 122, 130, 229, 324 (n. 158)

Nussbaum, Johann, 105

Olmsted, Fredrick Law, 14

Ontological conceptions of disease, 97, 106, 130, 303 (n. 53)

Osler, William, 83, 262, 271, 278 (n. 26)

Osteomyelitis, 32, 202

Otis, George, 28, 37, 51, 78, 84, 180, 187, 188, 209, 252, 259, 260, 264, 291 (n. 204), 321 (n. 82), 334 (nn. 15, 28)

Ovariotomy, 261

Pain: in diagnosis, 45, 46, 55, 57–60, 69, 117, 122, 143–50, 154, 156–57, 160, 163, 165, 202, 205, 304 (n. 77), 316 (n. 185); as stimulus to research, 148–60, 163, 202, 325 (n. 173)

Parasitic diseases, 99

Paris Clinical School, 4–5, 20, 49, 53, 76, 179, 277 (n. 140). *See also* Army Medical Museum

Pasteur, Louis, 70–71, 113, 212, 239, 241–43, 271, 294 (n. 53), 302 (n. 49), 332 (n. 118)

Pathological anatomy, 4, 6, 9–10, 21, 36–37, 41–42, 54, 58, 62, 76–78, 86, 91, 96, 185, 192, 256–58, 269, 299 (n. 160). *See also* Army Medical Museum

Pathological societies, 51, 187; of London, 187; of New York, 187; of Philadelphia, 187; of San Francisco, 187; Smithsonian Institution and, 187

Pension program, 253–55, 317 (n. 194), 324 (n. 148), 334 (n. 22)

Pepper, William, 5, 300 (n. 3)

Percussion, 19, 137, 159–62

Pericarditis, 161

Permanganate of potassa, 114, 115, 238, 241, 318 (n. 22)

Peters, DeWitt, 25, 115, 191

Pettenkofer, Max von, 217–18, 227, 230, 234–35, 237–38, 240, 248, 330 (n. 86), 331 (n. 99)

Photography, 1, 39, 80, 81, 82, 83, 90, 91, 167, 169, 171, 174, 177, 178, 187, 188, 194, 197, 253, 260

Photomicrography, 79, 80, 82, 85–90, 92, 93, 250, 259, 297 (n. 98). *See also* Army Medical Museum; Woodward, Joseph J.

Physicians, quality of in 1861, 22–27

Physiological conceptions of disease, 97, 106, 332 (n. 118); versus ontological conceptions, 106. *See also* Disease

Physiology, 3, 6, 7, 9, 11, 15, 17, 31, 36, 37, 48, 62, 66, 75, 84, 106, 114, 118–19, 125, 126, 137, 138, 145, 151, 152, 159, 182, 249, 252, 256, 257, 263, 269, 290 (n. 193), 299 (n. 160), 310 (n. 39), 313 (n. 111), 315 (nn. 151, 168)

Plastic operations, 41, 165–67, 308 (n. 4), 316 (n. 193)

Pneumonia, 13, 28, 42, 44, 61, 70, 265, 293 (n. 27), 300 (n. 6)

Porcher, Peyre Francis, 9

Postmortems, 4, 27, 44–46, 48, 53, 55, 56–62, 66, 69, 70, 85, 86, 93, 104, 117, 162, 181, 192, 191, 196, 199, 200, 201, 206, 213, 227, 233, 261, 287 (n. 127), 292 (n. 8), 295 (n. 81)

Posttraumatic stress disorder, 157, 314 (n. 137)

Poultices, 57, 69, 201

Prosthetic, 254, 271

Public health, 7, 45, 70, 131, 215, 218, 220, 221, 230, 231, 243, 245, 247, 253, 269, 290 (n. 193), 334 (n. 15), 337 (n. 78); prevention and, 2, 11, 28, 70, 77, 84, 102, 111, 113, 116, 119, 122, 124–31, 151, 164–65, 202, 207, 215, 218, 221–28, 231, 232, 236–46, 250, 265, 270, 302 (nn. 41, 47), 324 (n. 158), 325 (n. 173). *See also* Cholera; Erysipelas; Gangrene

Puerperal fever, 104–6, 130, 302 (nn. 41, 49), 303 (n. 55)

Pus, 39, 57, 60–67, 75, 86, 97, 101, 108–12, 117, 156, 205–7, 213, 234, 243, 302 (n. 33),

303 (nn. 54, 60), 304 (nn. 62, 67, 68);
globules, 108, 111, 112, 234, 235; ichorous,
57, 97, 111, 302 (n. 33); laudable, 111, 302
(n. 33)
Putrefaction, 95, 97, 112, 131, 239–44, 332
(n. 112)
Pyemia, 1, 32, 66–67, 94–95, 107, 111, 118, 131,
196, 202–3, 207–8, 293 (n. 45), 300 (n. 4)

Quarantines, 104; cholera and, 217–33,
244–48, 327 (n. 22), 328 (nn. 30, 31)
Quartermaster's Department, 35, 176, 233
Quick, Lavington, 18, 286 (n. 112), 322 (n. 93)
Quinine, 28, 46, 58, 60, 120, 122, 148, 149, 208

Reconstructive surgery. *See* Plastic
operations
Reed, Walter, 89, 252, 265
Reflex paralysis, 140, 142, 145–48
Remak, Robert, 144, 311 (n. 67)
Research, medical. *See* Medical science and
practice—research
Richmond Medical Journal, 119
Rokitansky, Carl von, 96
Royal College of Surgeons (London), 187
Royal Commission on the Cattle Plague,
240

Satterlee General Hospital, 59, 60, 62, 64,
288 (n. 132), 292 (n. 25), 307 (n. 138)
Schafhert, Frederick, 188
Schell, H., 65
Sects, medical: botanic medicine, 4, 6,
277 (n. 11); exclusion of, from medical
department, 8; homeopathy, 4, 6, 8,
9, 54, 277 (n. 11), 292 (n. 10), 320 (n. 58);
Thomsonianism, 4, 6, 277 (n. 11)
Semmelweis, Ignaz, 104, 130, 302 (nn. 41,
49), 303 (n. 55), 305 (n. 90)
Sepsis, 108–9, 112, 269, 302 (n. 41)
Sherman, T. W., 39
Sickles, Daniel, 197–98
Sim, T., 197
Simon, John, 219, 236, 331 (nn. 95, 99, 107)
Simpson, Sir James Young, 165

Sloan, William, 228
Smallpox, 124, 218, 253, 261, 268, 269, 331
(n. 91), 337 (nn. 73, 77); vaccination, 124,
261, 265–66, 337 (nn. 76, 77, 78)
Smith, D. P., 190, 191
Smith, Edward H., 38, 287 (n. 132)
Smith, Jos. R., 224, 284 (n. 75), 287 (n. 120)
Smithsonian Institution, 15, 50, 90, 187,
263, 290 (n. 201), 309 (n. 16), 313 (n. 111), 321
(n. 82), 325 (n. 173)
Snow, John, 217–18, 230, 235, 237, 326 (n. 6),
327 (n. 11), 331 (n. 99)
Specialists/specialization, 5, 9, 10, 133, 134,
136–72, 271, 308 (n. 1); American Medical
Association and, 136, 137, 171–72, 268, 271;
medical practice and, 132, 133–72; rela-
tionship to GPs, 132, 133, 171–72, 268, 271;
wartime organization of, 134–39, 146, 154,
158–73. *See also* Electricity, as medical
treatment; Medical technology
Specialty hospitals, 15, 24, 132, 135, 136,
139, 171, 172, 270. *See also* Turner's Lane
Hospital
Spinal commotion. *See* Reflex paralysis
Stanton, Edwin, 14, 31, 282 (n. 26)
Stanton, general hospital in, 191
Sternberg, George Miller, 89, 265
Stethoscope, 4, 335 (n. 30)
Stewards, hospital, 26, 266, 284 (n. 76)
Stewart, Jacob, 260–61
Stillé, Alfred, 41, 262
Stillé, C. J., 220
Stone, Alexander, 261
Stone, H., 196
Stone, W., 39
Stout, Samuel, 9
Surgeon General's Library, 16, 89, 112, 172,
185, 252, 255, 264–65; John Shaw Billings
and, 184, 250, 252, 263–64; Congress and,
250–51; national and international col-
laboration and, 251, 252, 263–65; Joseph
Woodward and, 251
Surgeon General's Office, and medical
literature, 51, 250–51
Surgery, 3, 7, 17, 19, 21–23, 27–28, 32–36, 38,

40, 45, 51, 65, 70, 96, 164, 166–67, 169, 185, 187, 198, 202–4, 209, 213, 243, 247, 249, 256–58, 261, 267, 299 (n. 160), 302 (n. 47), 316 (n. 192), 317 (nn. 202, 205), 325 (n. 173), 325 (n. 33); ligation, 65, 256; trephining, 46, 141, 180, 213, 289 (n. 175). *See also* Amputations; Plastic operations

Suturing, 39, 46, 47, 166, 168, 169, 201

Taylor, George, 226, 329 (n. 53)
Taylor, M. K., 42, 288 (n. 151)
Tetanus, 1, 62, 142, 196, 202, 269, 293 (n. 32), 325 (n. 173)
Thomson, William, 61, 200, 262, 293 (n. 28), 299 (n. 151), 325 (n. 164)
Tissues, 2, 11, 30, 66, 68, 71, 75, 79, 80, 82, 83, 85–89, 95–99, 107–8, 110, 111–12, 118, 138, 145, 150, 168, 203, 205–7, 234, 239, 270, 295 (n. 77), 296 (n. 93), 298 (nn. 131, 136), 304 (nn. 68, 69)
Todd, L. S., 43
Toner, J. M., 90
Toner Lectures, 90, 299 (nn. 153, 158)
Town, F. L., 189, 287 (n. 112), 322 (n. 93)
Trephining. *See* Surgery
Turner's Lane Hospital, 132, 134, 138–43, 150–54, 157–59, 163–64, 256–57. *See also* Specialists/specialization
Turpentine, 87, 114, 118, 233
Typhoid fever, 6, 13, 71, 120, 315 (n. 152)
Typhus, 6, 74, 261, 268

Union Medical Department, structure of, 22–29. *See also* Army Medical Department
Union soldiers, 1, 9, 13, 19, 24, 27, 37, 43, 47, 84, 95, 104, 115, 118, 148, 165, 172, 174, 175–83, 185, 186, 188, 192, 197, 198, 200, 207, 213, 230, 236, 253, 258, 259, 266, 315 (n. 152), 319 (n. 41), 324 (nn. 148, 158); as research subjects, 29, 33, 41, 53, 71, 79, 83, 87, 90, 94, 115, 118, 139, 150–58, 159–64, 170, 173, 185, 212, 297 (n. 98), 301 (n. 16). *See also* Medical science and practice—research

United States Dispensary, 115
United States Sanitary Commission, 14–15, 135, 165, 220, 267, 281 (nn. 7, 15, 17), 324 (n. 158), 328 (n. 24)
University of Pennsylvania, 27, 33, 44, 62, 155, 157, 188, 252, 289 (n. 167), 291 (n. 204), 300 (n. 3)

Vaccination, 124, 261, 265–66, 337 (nn. 76, 77, 78). *See also* Smallpox
Veterans, government support of, 253, 254, 334 (n. 19). *See also* Pension program
"Vibrio," 108, 131, 219, 235, 247–48
Virchow, Rudolph, 75–79, 84, 86, 87, 97, 100, 107, 234, 241, 256, 259, 260, 271, 294 (n. 53), 295 (nn. 77, 79)

Wagner, C., 32, 38, 39, 47
Wapping Heights, Battle of, 196
War, impact of on medicine, generally considered, 5, 278 (n. 16)
Weeks, G. R., 123
Weir, R., 17, 41, 125, 130, 141
Welch, William, 15
Welch, William H., 14, 262, 268, 271
West Philadelphia Hospital, 45, 102, 103, 284 (n. 64), 307 (n. 138)
Whitman, Walt: on death, 172, 175, 178; on hospitals, 20, 21, 286 (n. 104)
Williams, Talcott, 259
Williamsburg, Battle of, 46, 159, 207
Wilson, Henry, 280 (n. 46). *See also* Wilson Bill
Wilson Bill (Bill no. 188), 14, 25, 280 (n. 46)
Wood, H., 68–69
Wood, James R., 193
Woodman, A. M., 8
Woodward, Benjamin, 23, 24, 111, 113, 120, 121, 284 (n. 67), 294 (n. 64), 304 (nn. 64, 68)
Woodward, Joseph J., 17, 18, 24, 27, 28, 33, 34, 76, 99, 332 (n. 48); and Army Medical Museum, 31, 33, 35, 37, 41–43, 48–50, 54, 133, 180, 181, 192, 198, 199, 201–2, 252, 252, 259, 260, 264, 267, 271, 331 (n. 102), 332 (n. 129), 334 (nn. 15, 28); and cholera,

215, 216, 220–25, 230–39, 241–42, 244, 328
(n. 29); and gangrene, 96, 108–9, 118, 130,
303 (n. 61); and microscopy, 64, 73–76,
77–94, 108–9, 291 (n. 93), 296 (n. 98),
297 (n. 104), 298 (n. 142), 301 (n. 26), 309
(n. 16), 330 (n. 78). *See also Army* Medical Museum; Pathological anatomy;
Photomicrography
Woodworth, John, 55–56, 245, 333 (n. 133)

Wyman, Morrill, 6

Yellow fever, 70, 90, 222, 265, 268, 302
(n. 43), 330 (n. 78), 331 (n. 91)

Zentmeyer, M., 71, 72, 80, 81, 297 (n. 104).
See also Microscope
Zymotic theory, 99, 229, 239, 301 (n. 26). *See
also* Disease